WITHDRAWN
WRIGHT STATE UNIVERSITY LIBRARIES

DEC 2 7 1994

Evaluating Family Mental Health
History, Epidemiology, and Treatment Issues

CRITICAL ISSUES IN PSYCHIATRY
An Educational Series for Residents and Clinicians

Series Editor: Sherwyn M. Woods, M.D., Ph.D.
University of Southern California School of Medicine
Los Angeles, California

Recent volumes in the series:

CASE STUDIES IN INSOMNIA
    Edited by Peter J. Hauri, Ph.D.

CHILD AND ADULT DEVELOPMENT: A Psychoanalytic Introduction for Clinicians
    Calvin A. Colarusso, M.D.

CLINICAL DISORDERS OF MEMORY
    Aman U. Khan, M.D.

CONTEMPORARY PERSPECTIVES ON PSYCHOTHERAPY WITH LESBIANS AND GAY MEN
    Edited by Terry S. Stein, M.D., and Carol J. Cohen, M.D.

DECIPHERING MOTIVATION IN PSYCHOTHERAPY
    David M. Allen, M.D.

DRUG AND ALCOHOL ABUSE: A Clinical Guide to Diagnosis and Treatment, Third Edition
    Marc A. Schuckit, M.D.

ETHNIC PSYCHIATRY
    Edited by Charles B. Wilkinson, M.D.

EVALUATING FAMILY MENTAL HEALTH: History, Epidemiology, and Treatment Issues
    John J. Schwab, M.D., Judith J. Stephenson, S.M., and John F. Ice, M.D.

EVALUATION OF THE PSYCHIATRIC PATIENT: A Primer
    Seymour L. Halleck, M.D.

THE FREEDOM OF THE SELF: The Bio-Existential Treatment of Character Problems
    Eugene M. Abroms, M.D.

HANDBOOK OF BEHAVIOR THERAPY IN THE PSYCHIATRIC SETTING
    Edited by Alan S. Bellack, Ph.D., and Michel Hersen, Ph.D.

NEUROPSYCHIATRIC FEATURES OF MENTAL DISORDERS
    James W. Jefferson, M.D., and John R. Marshall, M.D.

RESEARCH IN PSYCHIATRY: Issues, Strategies, and Methods
    Edited by L.K. George Hsu, M.D., and Michel Hersen, Ph.D.

SEXUAL LIFE: A Clinician's Guide
    Stephen B. Levine, M.D.

STATES OF MIND: Configurational Analysis of Individual Psychology, Second Edition
    Mardi J. Horowitz, M.D.

A Continuation Order Plan is available for this series. A continuation order will bring delivery of each new volume immediately upon publication. Volumes are billed only upon actual shipment. For further information please contact the publisher.

Evaluating Family Mental Health
History, Epidemiology, and Treatment Issues

John J. Schwab, M.D.
Judith J. Stephenson, S.M.
John F. Ice, M.D.

University of Louisville
Louisville, Kentucky

PLENUM PRESS • NEW YORK AND LONDON

Library of Congress Cataloging-in-Publication Data

```
Schwab, John J.
    Evaluating family mental health : history, epidemiology, and
  treatment issues / John J. Schwab, Judith J. Stephenson, John F.
  Ice.
       p.    cm. -- (Critical issues in psychiatry)
    Includes bibliographical references and index.
    ISBN 0-306-44436-4
    1. Family--Mental health. 2. Family--Mental health--Kentucky-
  -Louisville--Longitudinal studies. 3. Family--Mental health-
  -Research. 4. Family--History.  I. Stephenson, Judith J. II. Ice,
  John F. III. Title. IV. Series.
    [DNLM: 1. Family. 2. Mental Health. 3. Mental Disorders.
  4. Interpersonal Relations.   WM 105 S398e 1993]
  RC455.4.F3S385 1993
  616.89'156--dc20
  DNLM/DLC
  for Library of Congress                                   93-28471
                                                                CIP
```

ISBN 0-306-44436-4

© 1993 Plenum Press, New York
A Division of Plenum Publishing Corporation
233 Spring Street, New York, N.Y. 10013

All rights reserved

No part of this book may be reproduced, stored in a retrieval system, or transmitted in any form or by any means, electronic, mechanical, photocopying, microfilming, recording, or otherwise, without written permission from the Publisher

Printed in the United States of America

Foreword

At the time of this writing, there is much uncertainty about the form of this country's future healthcare system and the role of psychiatry and other mental health disciplines in that system. Current experience with various managed healthcare programs is not encouraging. Most often patients with severe psychiatric disturbances receive, at best, some form of crisis intervention or brief treatment. Marital and family approaches to treatment receive even less support.

This discouraging socioeconomic context makes the work of John Schwab and his colleagues even more important than it would be in more favorable times. Their message is clear: The family is crucial to an understanding of psychiatric disorders and must often be the major focus in the treatment of these disorders.

This book is unique in its direct reflection of the senior author's long-term professional interests—the family, epidemiology, and history. A careful reading provides family therapists and researchers with wonderful opportunities to examine the ways in which history, socioeconomic and political contexts, and epidemiology can be used to increase understanding of the family.

This history of the family is unusually thorough; in particular, I found fascinating the information about early Egyptian families (3000 B.C.) and their accordance of high status of women.

The pilot study of a small group chosen as a representative sample of families in Louisville, Kentucky, provides important leads to be explored in a larger study. Over 50 percent of the families were considered symptomatic, and although the risk factors (low socioeconomic status, single parenthood, and high levels of stress) for family symptomatic status are not surprising, it is intriguing that in many families different members are symptomatic at different times. This finding lends credence to the family system construct that some families may "require" a patient, even if the person occupying the patient role varies over time.

The third feature of this work is the analysis of child guidance clinic records from a 65-year period. The findings support the existence of increasing levels of particular individual and marital–family disorders, as well as much that has recently been of widespread concern about the current state of the American family.

At a time when bookstores are filled with pop psychology and self-help manuals, this scholarly work will be most welcome to those professionals who embrace complex models of human behavior, probability approaches to causality, and an appreciation of how much we have yet to learn.

Jerry M. Lewis, M.D.
Timberlawn Psychiatric Research Foundation
Dallas, Texas

Preface

Anxiety about the well-being of the family mounted steadily during the 1980s and now extends to include concerns about the character of our society and its moral fabric. But there is confusion about what is wrong and what needs to be rectified. The worries about the family and fears of its possible disintegration are matched by both veiled and loud denunciations of its having failed, with consequences being drug abuse, defective education, violence, poor-quality manufactured goods, and an indulged and cynical (if not narcissistic) generation of young persons.

But the family does not need blame; it needs help. After the manuscript of this book was prepared, our data showing that increasing percentages of families receiving psychiatric care had multiple problems were supported by the winter 1992 report from Family Service America in the *Family Album,* with its headline, "American Families in Trouble": "The majority of families seeking help from family service agencies . . . are suffering from multiple problems and require several kinds of services" (p. 1). The report on 16,000 families that have used family service agencies states that "the average number of serious problems families faced was three. Since 1970, problems that have increased among clients include drug/alcohol abuse, abuse-violence, single-parenting, work-related problems, and physical health problems" (p. 1). The most frequent problems also included marital and parenting concerns. In commenting on the report, Dan Fax, the executive director of the Family and Children's Agency of Metropolitan Louisville, stated that "we have definitely seen an increasing trend toward families who are facing more than one problem" (p. 1).

Thus, the widespread concerns about the family are confirmed by reports of families' multiple problems and indicators that the high divorce-remarriage-redivorce rates have had destabilizing, if not deleterious, effects on a generation of young persons. Inasmuch as many of the multiple problems faced by American families are paralleled by a host of national problems—especially the deficit, unemployment, epidemic violence, and pervasive distrust of leaders and institutions—our studies of family mental health are aimed at two objectives. One is to gain a historical as well as scientific perspective on the status and well-being of the contemporary family. Some historians have found associations between the rise and fall of great civilizations and the health and instability of the family as a social unit. Therefore, we think that an in-depth historical view of the family and the social scene is timely as we approach the end of both a century and a millenium. The other objective is to attempt to clarify the interactions and influences of three levels of biosocial organization upon each other: the wider society and the community, the family, and the individual. Many works on the family present it as an almost singular entity or institution, without a past and existing in isolation, uninfluenced by other institutions and the social climate.

We view the family in Aristotelian terms as the basic social unit; its two traditional functions are to produce children who will become autonomous members of society and to stabilize the parents' emotional and sexual lives. In our opinion, the family can best be understood as a system that operates according to the principles of general living systems theory, as elaborated by James Grier Miller (1978). We hope that our research efforts will simplify some of the confusion about the well-being and fate of the family and enhance appreciation of the reciprocal effects of the society, the family, and the individual. To do so, we have focused on the family and mental disorder; accumulating evidence points both to a possible increase in mental illness and to the intergenerational continuity of mental health and illness.

In Chapter 1, we look at "the crisis": the American family in the 1980s, when the key words related to it were *divorce, stepfamilies, domestic partners, homeless families* (almost a contradiction in terms), and *single-parent families*. In a decade that is now seen as characterized by an orgy of American self-indulgence, not Emersonian "self-reliance," the family was blamed for society's ills; the traditional, institutionally based family was considered out of fashion, if not derided as obsolete, by many of our nation's leaders and others of the elite. As the 1990s began, some of the concerns changed to cries of alarm as the working poor and poverty became common household realities and an economic recession failed to recede before President Bush's pronouncements of its being over, just as the waves did not heed Canute's commands to become calm a thousand years ago.

PREFACE

To place the concerns about the family in perspective, in Chapter 2 we look at the long history of the family, from its origins in the recesses of prehistory to its battered, torn nuclear existence in the United States as the twentieth century draws to a close. Our historical research shows that the Egyptians prized families and family sentiments at least 1,500 years before Moses, and that family stability waxed and waned in accord with the vitality of the society and its leadership. We then trace the three roots of the modern Western family (its classical legacy, its Judeo-Christian heritage, and its Anglo-Saxon traditions) that culminated in the emergence of the nuclear family in England during the eleventh and twelfth centuries—not during the Industrial Revolution in the eighteenth century, as had been postulated. Also, new research has provided substantial evidence of there being strong sentiments of love in Western nuclear family relationships for hundreds of years.

In Chapter 3, we see that concern about the well-being of the family as an institution in Western society surfaced in the 1880s and was manifest by 1900. We look at scholars' views of the family in every decade of the twentieth century and relate the many changes taking place in family life to the social history of the particular decade or era. A dominant group of scholars argued that the family was merely adapting to the challenges and opportunities of life in the twentieth century; in contrast, others expressed concern about the increasing appearance of family pathologies and indicators of family disorganization. From an erudite historical perspective, Carle Zimmerman (1947) saw that the vitality of the state and the well-being of the family marched in step. As early as the mid-1930s, Zimmerman anticipated that the increasing family instability would reach crisis proportions in the last decades of this century.

Chapter 4 is devoted to a summary of research on the family. We offer a review of the beginnings of research, such as Le Play's studies of family types and budgets in the 1850s, and also of such topics in this century as marital adjustment. We review studies of stress and the family and of family functioning and competence. Then we look at the changing view of the family and mental disorder, especially studies of the family and schizophrenia and of the manifold aspects of depression and the family.

In Chapter 5, we turn to a succinct description of our other approaches to the study of the family. We supply a short description of the research setting (Louisville and Jefferson County, Kentucky) that includes its history, and then we describe the methods used in our three studies. The first was a straightforward 3-year review of almost 1,000 articles and books on the family, mainly in Western society. The second was our epidemiological study of a random sample of families from the greater Louisville community over a 15-month period. The third was a historical-chart review of records from our child guidance clinic (dating between 1923 and 1988) that was designed to ascertain changes in children's and their families' presenting problems over time. We hoped that the historical-clinical record study would complement our historical and research reviews, as well as the results of the epidemiological study.

We present some of the major results of our studies of the Louisville families, including their sociodemographic characteristics, symptom status, and risk factors (especially living in a single-parent family, low socioeconomic status, and stressors). In addition, we looked at members' perceptions of their family environments and associations between such variables as cohesion and symptom status. We found more symptomatology in the random sample of families in the community than we anticipated, and some of the families were both multisymptomatic and polysymptomatic (in that two or more members had symptoms and there were at least two different syndromes and/or substance abuse problems). Our follow-up evaluations of 34 of the original 43 families that continued in the study to its completion provided Time 1 and Time 3 comparisons that included changes in the family and in symptomatology. Discriminant function analyses and logistic regressions of Time 1 family environment subscale scores predicted family symptom status at about an 80% degree of accuracy 15 months later (when the Time 3 interviews were conducted).

In Chapter 6, we present data on both the young and the adult children who participated in the study. A large percentage (about 30%) of the 34 children under age 16 were found to be symptomatic, and in some families, there was a "ping-ponging" of symptomatology among the children from Time 1 to Time 3. In 1983, when we first went into the families' homes, our interviewers were surprised to find an apparently large number of adult children, some of whom had come back to live with their parents after once being launched, but had been defeated by the recession and/or divorce. Since the early 1980s, there has been a definite trend for adult children to "come back home" that has been studied by demographers and other social scientists and noted by the media. We classified the adult children into three groups (those still preparing for adulthood, those in the stage of extended youth, and returnees), ascertained some of their characteristics and problems, and evaluated the extensive symptomatology they presented.

Chapter 7 contains a description of the general approach to and the major findings from our historical clinic study—analyses of selected random samples of children's records from our child guidance clinic, 1923–1988. We found that there had been changes in the children's presenting problems (in particular, aggressive disorders had become much more prominent in the later years of the study), as well as in their family structures and parents' problems. The number of single-parent families has grown steadily, and there has been a definite increase in marital conflicts, in more recent decades. Many of the findings from previous decades support the observations discussed in our review of the literature in Chapter 3; the most ominous finding, however, is that the percentage of families with multiple problems has been increasing rapidly.

We devote Chapter 8 to the clinical implications of our historical, epidemiological, and clinical research. We hope that the findings provide a backdrop against which clinicians can assess their everyday work with patients and their families. We thought about the findings in terms of our clinical experiences during the past four decades and attempted to enhance the clinical significance of the research results by adding some of our observations and suggestions. The epidemiological study was supported largely by National Institute of Mental Health Grant No. MH36140, 1983–1985.

In Chapter 9, we present a summary of what we consider to be some of the major results of our work—in the library, office, research facilities, clinics, and respondents' homes—since the early 1980s. Also, we describe what we have learned about conducting an epidemiological study of families in their homes, point out our deficiencies and limitations, and make suggestions about future studies. We are aware that the summary is not comprehensive and, as would be expected, that some of the conclusions are tinged by bias. In many ways, we regard this chapter as the prologue for a companion volume that we hope to publish in 1994. It will contain more information about family interactions, our epidemiological study of the families in the community, and ratings of the videotapes of the family interviews, as well as our general living systems family functioning model. The companion volume also will include the results of the Time 4 1-year follow-up report on the families that participated in the original study. In addition, we will present the first data on the 16 families that participated in the clinical-neighborhood study and compare the results of that case-control approach with those of our epidemiological study.

It has taken us more than two years to prepare the manuscript for the current volume. Although we had anticipated that it would be completed in about one "long" year, we beg the publisher's indulgence. The book is multiauthored, but there has been a division of labor. Dr. Schwab did most of the work on the first four chapters. Our research assistants, Diane Eiland and Paul Winkler, made significant contributions to Chapter 5, and their assistance with the authorship deserves special recognition. Ms. Stephenson carried out practically all of the data analyses and did much of the preliminary writing for Chapters 6 and 7. The late Dr. Ice reviewed all of the data on the children and their families, including the children's detailed reports and the videotapes of all the families. In addition to assuming primary responsibility for the discussion of the children, he oversaw much of the child psychiatry residents' superb work on the chart reviews for the historical clinic study. To Chapter 8, he added observations gleaned from his many years of experience as a senior child psychiatrist and professor in Louisville, Kentucky.

The last two chapters were written by Dr. Schwab, but both Ms. Stephenson and Dr. Ice enriched them with their critiques and additions. As senior author, Dr. Schwab bears responsibility for the entire manuscript, including the opinions and biases in it. Whether it is possible to be objective or dispassionate about the family and the social and political history of one's own era, especially an era as tumultuous as that in the United States since the mid-1960s, is debatable. Indeed, whether it is desirable is at least arguable.

We have received a great deal of help from friends, colleagues, students, and other family researchers in many parts of the United States. Helen Gray, one of the persons to whom the book is dedicated, deserves special mention. She gave unsparingly of her clinical wisdom accumulated in several decades of work in child psychiatry. In our department, Roger A. Bell, who was the project director for the epidemiological study, gave us considerable assistance and, generously, much of his time. We thank Allan Tasman, professor and chairman of the University of Louisville Department of Psychiatry and Behavioral Sciences, for supporting our efforts during the past year. Our child psychiatry residents—Lisa Graziano, Kris Houser, and Katherine Raymer—devoted substantial time and effort to the reviews of the hundreds of charts for the historical-clinic study. Florence Prentice, who will be one of the coauthors of the companion volume, helped with the final preparation of the manuscript.

As every epidemiologist knows, much of the hard work (which too often is not recognized) was carried out by our interviewers, headed by Mickey Vaughn. We thank them and their part-time associates and assistants for working long hours to make sure that the project succeeded.

In these troubled times for the family, we dedicate this work to the 43 families in Louisville, Kentucky, who gave generously of their time to the research studies we are reporting. An average family gave about 20 to 30 hours to the research. Their willingness to extend themselves in the hope that their efforts would eventually help others is a testimony to

PREFACE

altruism that can lessen the anguish of those who despair of the human condition. Also, we recognize the help and patience of the members of our families, who tolerated our long hours away from home and our often seemingly self-absorbed interest in this work. Their only compensation has been our gratitude and the knowledge that their altruism and desire to help others are inspiring.

We owe an immense debt to the secretaries, other personnel, and colleagues in our department who went beyond the duties and responsibilities of their various positions to assist us with the library work, the literature reviews, and many of the tasks involved in managing large amounts of data. Although Ms. Eiland was responsible for the preparation of the manuscript, she was ably assisted by Heddy Rubin, Patty Smith, and Sherri Chandler. In addition, Ms. Rubin worked closely with Dr. Schwab to help him with innumerable secretarial and other tasks, many of which were bound to be tedious, demanding, and, at times, boring. Louise Chiles proofread the manuscript; we thank her for her attention to detail and for her suggestions regarding redundancies and errors. Susi Walsh, unit business manager for the Department of Psychiatry and Behavioral Sciences, helped us greatly. In the 1980s, Jenny Khaliel, Libby Kokott, and Deborah Wilson were research assistants in the department who worked with Dr. Schwab and spent many hours toiling to help with the literature review and the data analyses.

Shortly after this manuscript was sent to the publisher, John Ice tragically passed away. His death is a loss to us and to our future research efforts. We had already begun the statistical and clinical evaluations of our general living systems model of family functioning that constitutes the centerpiece of the companion volume that we hope to complete in 1994. But more important, his death is a loss to the Greater Louisville community. He was the senior child psychiatrist in the state, a distinguished teacher, and an outstanding clinician whose efforts had benefited children and their families for 40 years.

Contents

1. The Crisis 1

   Introduction: Concerns 1
   Divorce 3
   Children of Divorce 6
   Structural Changes in the Family 9
      Stepfamilies 10
      Grandparenting 12
   Changes in Roles 13
   Effects of Poverty on the Family 14
   Economic Factors and Antifamilism 20
      Antifamilism and the American Character 21
   Concluding Remarks 26

2. History of the Family 31

   Ancient Times and Myths 31
      The Beginnings of the Modern Family 31
      The Egyptian Family 34
   Early Social Scientists' Views of the Family 37
   Economic Influences on the Origin of the Family 42
   The Family and the Incest Taboo 43
   Current Views of the Origin of the Family 44
   The Biological and Sociocultural Bases of the Family 46
   The Three Roots of the Modern Family 46
      The Classical Root 46

The Judeo-Christian Root	51
The Anglo-Saxon Root	53
The Nuclear Family	56
The Emotional Basis for Marriage and Family	60
The Reformation and the Industrial Revolution	63
The Early American Family	65
The Black Family	70
Concluding Remarks	82

3. A Century of Concern ... 85

Background: The Late Nineteenth Century	85
The Turn of the Century and the Early 1900s	90
The Roaring Twenties: Social Change, Changing Family Functions, and Companionate Marriage	96
The Great Depression	105
Individualism versus Familism	108
World War II	112
The Postwar Family and the 1950s	114
The Searing Sixties	132
The 1970s and the Looming Crisis	142
Concluding Remarks	155

4. Family Research ... 157

The Pioneer Researchers	157
Social Research	157
Anthropological Studies	162
Psychoanalytic Contributions	163
Family Studies	167
Systems Theory	169
Developments During the 1950s and 1960s	171
The Transactional Approach: Spiegel and Associates	173
Bowen's Family Systems Theory	174
Conceptual Frameworks in Family Sociology	178
Minuchin's *Families of the Slums*	181
Recent Family Sociological Research	183
Family Studies of Schizophrenia	187
Family Studies of Depression	194
Theories of Depressive Illness	194

Effects of Depression on the Family 195
Our Pilot Longitudinal Family Study 197
Research Perspectives on Depression and the Family 198
  Assortative Mating 198
  Marital Interactions and Depression 200
  Stressful Life Events, Social Support, Chronic Depression,
    and Depression in the Family 206
The Family Life Cycle 208
Marital and Family Satisfaction in Dual-Career
  African-American Families 210
Family Functioning 212
  The McMaster Model of Family Functioning 212
  The Olson Circumplex Model 213
  The Beavers System Model 216
  Reiss's Problem-Solving Model 217
  The Moos and Moos Family Environment Scale 219
  Lewis: Family Competence 219
  Belsky's Pennsylvania State University Infant
    and Family Development Project 223
Concluding Remarks 225

5. Our Family Studies 227

Background and Methods 227
  Background 227
  Methods for the Epidemiological Study 230
Sociodemographic Characteristics, Symptom Status,
  and Family Risk Factors 234
  Sociodemographic Characteristics 234
  Family Symptom Status 240
  Family Risk Factors and Symptom Status 243
  Family Life Cycle Stage, Stress, Symptoms,
    and Family Vignettes 247
Perception of the Family Environment 250
  FES Profiles of Families with and without
    Symptomatic Children 255
  FES Profiles of Symptomatic and Asymptomatic
    Families 255
  Predicting Family Symptomatic Status from
    the FES Subscale Scores 257
  Areas of Family Responsibility 259
  Marital Satisfaction 261

Changes in Symptomatology Over Time	265
Introduction	265
Sociodemographic Characteristics of the Dropout and Completing Families	266
Dropout Families' Time 1 Symptom Status	268
Completing Families at Time 1	269
Completing Families at Time 3	274
Changes in Symptom Status Over Time	276

6. The Younger and Adult Children ... 285

Younger Children	285
Sociodemographic Characteristics	285
Developmental Histories	286
Social Histories	286
Parents' Expectations and Values	287
Parental Discipline	288
Time Spent With Children	289
What Parents Did With Children	290
Symptomatic Status	290
Summary	298
Older Adolescents and Adult Children	299
Sociodemographic Characteristics	301
Feelings About Current Marital Status	304
Time 1 Symptomatic Status	305
Adult Children in the Home and the Family Environment Scale	310
Some Possible Individual and Family Reactions to Adult Children	312

7. The Historical-Clinic Chart Study ... 315

Background and History of the Clinic	315
Study Sample	316
Study Protocol	316
Results	317
Sociodemographic Characteristics	317
Children's Presenting Problems	318
Families' Problems	322
Conclusions	324

8. Clinical Implications ... 331

The Extent of Symptomatic Distress in Families ... 331
Change and Variability in Symptomatology in the Family ... 332
Identification of Family Members at Risk ... 333
Family Histories and the Intergenerational
 Continuity of Symptomatology ... 333
Comorbidity ... 334
Treatment-Resistant Families ... 334
Family Risk Factors ... 335
Family Stress ... 336
Family Environment ... 338
   Cohesion ... 338
   Expressiveness and Communication ... 339
Depression in the Family and Social Supports ... 339
The Use of Research Measures in Clinical Practice ... 340
Videotapes of the Families ... 342
Home Visits ... 342
The Problems of Poverty ... 343
Children ... 344
   Subclinical Cases ... 344
   Intergenerational Boundaries ... 345
   Adult Children ... 346
   Trends in Children's and Families' Problems ... 347
Individualism Versus Familism ... 350
Supportive Family Therapy ... 351

9. Summary and Conclusions ... 353

Introduction: Concerns and Questions ... 353
Our Studies ... 358
   The History of the Family ... 358
   The Pilot Epidemiological Study ... 363
   The Historical-Clinic Chart Study ... 386
Conclusions ... 388

References ... 393

Index ... 411

CHAPTER 1

The Crisis

> The family is a hot issue. Judging by the proliferation of magazine cover stories, television features, talk show discussions, academic research, and public policy discourse being devoted to the state of the American family . . . what civil rights and Vietnam were to the Sixties and women's rights and the environment were to the Seventies, family issues have become to the Eighties.
> —Pogrebin (1983, p. 2)

INTRODUCTION: CONCERNS

Accumulating reports from varied sources indicate that there is widespread concern about the status and well-being of the American family. Recently, 1,550 psychologists cited the family as the number one problem in our society (American Psychological Association, 1991). Moreover, the general public is somewhat pessimistic about what has been happening to the family and about its future. In a 1989 Gallup poll, 49% of 757 adult respondents reported that the family was worse off than it was 10 years ago; in contrast, only 39% reported that it was better off (Smith, 1990, p. 18). In response to questions about the family 10 years in the future, 42% reported that it would be better and 42% that it would be worse. Tragically, a new study of adolescent suicide revealed that 6% of those surveyed had attempted suicide (Jennings, 1990, p. 1); family problems were named as the reason for attempting suicide by 47%, whereas only 20% named depression. The emphasis on "family values" during the 1992 Republican National Convention indicated, as Pogrebin asserted, that family issues were the hot topic in the 1980s, and that they were heating up in the 1990s with the continuing recession, controversies about gay rights, and the many reports of stepfamilies' problems, sexual abuse, and incest.

Concerns about marriage and the family are prominent topics in novels, magazines, newspapers, and radio and television programs, as well as in the scientific literature. In a special issue on "The 21st Century Family," *Newsweek* (which created a regular family section in 1985) reported that

> as Americans head into the 21st century, *the family itself has become one of the biggest stories of our generation.* At once venerated and vulnerable, this most basic of society's institutions is *facing unprecedented change.* . . . The very nature of the family is in transition with the explosive increase in stepfamily households and the growth of other non-traditional families. . . . Technological, demographic and economic trends are shaping everything from our attitudes about child care and financial planning to how we build our houses and have our babies. (Smith, 1990, pp. 8–9; italics added)

Concerns about the family also spring from everyday clinical experience and the statistics on disruption of the family. Much of our daily work is devoted to patients' worries about their marriages, other personal relationships, and their families. Recently, a talented musician in her mid-30s who was changing careers sought therapy for her increasing phobias and symptoms of depression. She was studying in order to be admitted to medical school, but worries about her husband's fidelity and her 9-year-old son's regressed behavior—fighting at school and occasional bed-wetting—had reduced her ability to study efficiently. Her major reason for trying to get into medical school was insecurity; her marriage was unstable, and as she put it, "all of our friends have been getting divorced. I need a profession." She wanted to be emotionally as well as vocationally prepared for life after divorce.

Another representative case is that of a 29-year-old high school teacher whose obsessive-compulsive symptoms had increased in severity since he had become engaged a few months earlier to a social worker with whom he had been living for 3 years. He attributed his increased symptoms and recent loss of libido to worries about the commitment he was making and the responsibilities he would be assuming.

Even more poignantly, a 10-year-old girl was brought for treatment because she was moody, refusing to eat, staying in her room as much as possible, and crying at school. She told that her father had "forgotten" her birthday and had sent her only one little Christmas gift. When asked about her family, she replied that she had two mothers, two fathers, three stepbrothers, and nine grandparents, but she could name only six of these—she called the others only "mom" or "pop." Many patients ask about how to deal with their young children's anxieties about the possibility that their parents will divorce. Talk about divorce is common among schoolchildren, even those as young as 7 or 8 years old, and the problems of being a child of divorce often are so great that support groups for these children have been started in some elementary schools in New York.

The ominous facts that have made headlines in recent years are that (a) the divorce rate has doubled since 1965; (b) one half of all new first marriages end in divorce; (c) six of ten second marriages will probably fail; (d) one third of all children born in the 1980s will live in a stepfamily before age 18; (e) one of every four children is being raised by a single parent; (f) more than 20% of children today were born out of wedlock; and (g) at least one of every five children lives in poverty, with the percentage as high as 40% to 50% among African-Americans and Hispanics (Smith, 1990). Such data indicate that the "typical American family" is changing, if not disappearing.

Of those indicators that the family is an institution in jeopardy, the most telling is that the divorce rate has more than quintupled during this century, from 0.7 per 1,000 in 1900 to a peak of 5.2 per 1,000 in 1980; in 1989, it was 4.8 per 1,000. In contrast, the marriage rate has fluctuated less than 50% although it has been influenced by varying economic circumstances, other social processes, and wars. The low was 8.4 per 1,000 in 1958, and the high was 12.2 per 1,000 in 1945; in 1980, the rate was 10.6 per 1,000 (*Information Please Almanac*, 1990, p. 807). In asking "What Happened to the Family?" Footlick (1990) stated flatly, "The American family does not exist. Rather, we are creating many American families, of diverse styles and shapes. . . . We are living through a period of historic change in American family life" (p. 15). This change includes a strong antifamilistic trend. For example, many young persons hesitate to marry. In 1989, the median ages at first marriage, 26.2 years for males and 23.8 for females, were the highest since they were first tabulated in 1890. Significantly, the percentage of the population under age 40 that had never married rose for men from 39.6% in 1960 to 50.8% in 1989 and for women from 28.1% to 40.6% (*World Almanac*, 1990, p. 551). Thus many persons regard marriage as being less appealing than in the past.

DIVORCE

In "The Road to Polygamy," his review of Phillips' (1990) monumental volume, *Putting Asunder: A History of Divorce in Western Society*, Stone (1989) pointed out that "divorce is merely a legal condition; marital breakdown is a social fact" (p. 12). He suggested that the extent of marital breakdown may be much greater than indicated by the divorce rate, and that the rising divorce rate in the late nineteenth and twentieth centuries needs to be viewed in relation to the death rates. Until the 1960s, the marriages ended by divorce tended to be equivalent to those ended by spousal death, but since then they have been much greater. Stone insisted that

> the scale of marital breakdown in the West since 1960 has no historical precedent that I know of, and seems unique. There has been nothing like it for the past 2,000 years, and probably much longer. In retrospect, the 1960s look more and more like a watershed in the culture of the West, of which liberal divorce laws are only a minor symptom. (p. 14)

He quoted Watkins, Menken, and Bongaarts's (1987) research, which showed that in 1800 American women could expect to be married for 27 years and, in accord with the lengthened life span, in 1960 for 42 years; in 1980, though, they could expect to be married for only 35 years (Stone, 1989, p. 14).

The divorce rates, as to be expected, increased sharply for a few years immediately after both world wars. Although they declined a few years later, each time they leveled off at higher than the prewar rate. Stone stated, "The two world wars of the twentieth century have therefore had long-term as well as short-term social and psychological consequences. They seem permanently to have raised divorce rates to quite new levels" (p. 14). He concluded that divorce in the 1980s often was viewed as freedom from "an agonizing relationship" (p. 14); however, "it also often ends up as a financial bonanza for men, a financial and personal catastrophe for women, and a psychological disaster for the children" (p. 15).

Divorce is becoming part of the American way of life. In her article in *Fortune*, entitled "The CEO's Second Wife," Julie Connelly (1989) stated that

> in the corporate world, as in much of the rest of society, it took the roaring Eighties to make divorce fully respectable. As the decade began, Americans inaugurated their first divorced President, a man who somehow managed to convince a nation that he was the embodiment of old-fashioned family values. If the CEO of the United States could shed and rewed, why not the CEO of a Fortune 500 company? (p. 53)

For years, a stable marriage had been almost a *sine qua non* for an executive on his way to the top. But, according to Connelly, "gutsy change is finally rattling the windows of the nation's most conservative secular institution, the corporation. Chief executives set the tone for acceptable behavior in their companies, and though the majority are still on their first marriages, a growing minority have discovered serial monogamy" (p. 53).

The joys of divorce and remarriage were extolled in Connelly's article by Helen Singer Kaplan, a psychiatrist and the second wife of the chairman of *Toys "R" Us*, who insisted: "The change has been radical. . . . There's no longer a prejudice against divorce and remarriage—almost the reverse. In some cases the man with the old, nice, matronly first wife is looked down on. He's seen as not keeping up appearances. Why can't he do better for himself?" (p. 53). But Boston psychologist Harry Lovenson, in the same article, stated, "The culture of self-indulgence has just crept up to the CEO level" (p. 53).

Many of the second wives, according to Connelly (1989), are "trophy" wives who are considerably younger than their husbands, well educated, and often successful in business. They are thin, well groomed, and resemble "the social X-rays" described in Tom Wolfe's *Bonfire of the Vanities*. They spend freely, strive to build their husbands' reputations, and increase the prominence of both partners by attending benefits for charitable causes and working on committees. One such marriage that captured the headlines (and was parodied in the "Doonesbury" comic strip in 1991) was that of 41-year-old Georgette Mosbacher to 62-year-old former Houston oil man and ex-secretary of commerce Robert Mosbacher.

The divorcing husband tends to see the first wife as critical and negative and as a person who "didn't keep up" (Connelly, 1989, p. 55). Generally, she is the big loser; her share of the couple's assets range from zero to 25% (in a marriage that lasted 5 years) to 45% (in a marriage of 15 or more years). In addition to financial losses, the ex-wife loses status, relationships, and social acquaintances. Connelly quoted a young second wife's pessimistic statement: "If I had a daughter, I'd tell her never to be a first wife" (p. 56).

The young second wife gains by marrying "someone who has become a Very Important Man" (p. 57). According to Connelly, the second marriages appear to be doing well; the new second wife often has learned from her earlier marriage. Helen Singer Kaplan stated that she believed a second marriage could compensate for the pain of the first. Often the new wife sees her role primarily as that of a companion, if not a "playmate," whose task is to interest her powerful new husband and solidify their relationship. The CEO's second marriage differs dramatically from his first by "one word: children. There usually aren't any" (p. 61). A second wife was quoted as saying forthrightly: "I don't see room for children in our life. *I just don't know how you can combine a marriage and kids*" (p. 6l; italics added).

The antifamilistic sentiments expressed by many of the people Connelly interviewed signify the antifamilism revealed by the statistics on marriage and the family in the 1980s. Antifamilism on the part of the nation's leaders has an adverse effect on marital and family stability throughout our society, but such social influences are seldom unidirectional. What is happening at the top of the society in a democracy both influences and is influenced by what is happening at other levels. One of our major theses in this book is that the individual, the family, and the wider society are three interacting, mutually influential levels of human activity. Thus, the family cannot be studied in isolation. To enlarge our perspective on this thesis, we can note that King George III's serious manic-depressive illness, from which he suffered intermittently for many years, aroused sympathy for him and interest in mental illness; it is considered to be responsible for increased mental hospital admissions in London in the early 1800s (Burrows, 1828). How the divorces of President Reagan and some CEOs of Fortune 500 corporations and their second wives' endorsements of divorce influence divorce rates is an unanswerable question at this time, but it merits consideration.

Is divorce the modern social epidemic? It appears so. Many adults see marriage as a "fragile institution—not something one can count on" (Footlick, 1990, p. 16). The view of divorce as a social epidemic was advanced by Dicks (1967) in his comments on the increased divorce rate in England and Wales after World War II. He emphasized that the rapid rate of social change and the stresses of modern life produced an "emotional overdependence" in marriage, and he raised the possibility that the strains of everyday life were being manifested as relational problems rather than more traditionally as psychosomatic or mental illnesses (pp. 1–27).

In *Extraordinary Popular Delusions and the Madness of Crowds*, Mackay (1932) described such epidemics as the medieval dance crazes, the witch mania in western Europe in the seventeenth century, and the tulip mania that swept over Holland and Great Britain in the late 1600s. In his foreword to Mackay's book, Bernard Baruch commented on those "great human mass movements" and the necessity to recognize them in their early stages in order to "avoid the more harmful of their full effects" (p. xiv).

CHILDREN OF DIVORCE

The most serious consequence of divorce is the effect it can have on the couple's children. The number of children of divorce under age 18 roughly tripled from 299,000 (6.3 per 1,000 children under age 18) in 1950 to almost 1.1 million (17.3 per 1,000 children) in 1985 (*World Almanac*, 1990, p. 840). Therefore, the changes taking place in the family have repercussions that influence the nature of our society in the future.

Accumulating evidence reveals that children of divorce are a high-risk group for mental and physical disorders. A two-year follow-up study by Guidubaldi and Perry (1985) of a national sample of children of divorce showed that they had poorer academic and health ratings than children of intact families. Jellinek and Slovik (1981) reported that "approximately 15% to 25% of all children whose parents divorce will have at least moderate dysfunction and will be disproportionately represented in child psychiatry clinic populations" (p. 559). Boys are more vulnerable to the trauma of parental divorce than girls. When divorce is associated with financial and social losses to the family (as it frequently is), those losses increase the negative effects on the children.

Jellinek and Slovik (1981) described the problems encountered by children of divorce. For infants or toddlers, divorce can have an adverse effect when the mother's ability to function is compromised. The preschooler is vulnerable because his or her frame of reference includes the whole family, and the young child cannot understand the complexities of divorce. School-age children often feel guilty about or responsible for the divorce. Problems of prepubertal children of divorce are depression, psychosomatic disorders, and aggressive behavior. The effects of divorce on adolescents are difficult to evaluate because teenagers are in the process of separating from the family, but insufficient monitoring can lead to a somewhat hasty sexual and social development. The protraction of adolescence for many young persons, especially those in the middle class, can be attributed in part to their parents' divorce-remarriage rate. Footlick quoted Bumpass's statement that parenting children "stretches into their 20s and beyond. . . . Divorce has left a devastated generation in its wake, and for many youngsters, the pain is compounded by poverty and neglect" (Footlick, 1990, p. 16).

Special risk factors for children of divorce are (a) a personal or family history of mental disorders; (b) a poor quality of family life before the divorce; (c) parental conflict after the divorce; and (d) parental emotional instability. Of the risk factors, parental conflict before the divorce and continued strife afterward are the most destructive to the child of divorce (Jellinek & Slovik, 1981, p. 559). Unfortunately, about 30% of parents continue to quarrel even 2 years after divorce.

The effect of divorce on young children, however, is a controversial topic. Although substantial data indicate that divorce affects children adversely, some point out that living with a divorced parent who is happily remarried is better than continuing to live with unhappy, quarreling parents. Richman and his colleagues (1982) found that continuing marital discord is a major risk factor for children; children living in disharmonious homes were two to five times more likely to have emotional distress than those living in harmonious homes.

Clinically, we have seen the long-term, disturbing effects of divorce on children. Young adults in their 20s and early 30s express fears about their ability to relate meaningfully to persons they want to marry and are tentative about making commitments, although they state emphatically that they want to marry and have families. They trace anxieties about marriage to their parents' marital conflicts and divorces and plaintively describe fears that they will be doomed to repeat the parental pattern.

Only systematic longitudinal studies over at least 15- to 20-year periods can supply information that clarifies the consequences of the extent of marital breakdown in the United States today. Although Judith Wallerstein's (1989) 10- to 15-year follow-up study of 60 divorced couples and their 131 children is limited because there was no control group, some of the results are startling. At the 10-year follow-up, Wallerstein found that about 41% of the children were "entering adulthood as worried, underachieving, self-deprecating and sometimes angry young men and women" (p. 21). One common problem was the child's delayed emotional response to the divorce. Another was that of the "overburdened child," whose emotional well-being was sacrificed to the care of a parent. Wallerstein and Blakeslee (1989) emphasized: "Since most children live with their mothers after divorce, the single most important protective factor in a child's psychological development and well-being over the years is the mother's mental health and the quality of her parenting" (p. 302).

Many of the divorced spouses had negative emotions that persisted; one half of the women and one third of the men were "intensely angry at their former spouses" even 10 years after the divorce. "Anger has become an ongoing, and sometimes dominant, presence in their children's lives as well" (Wallerstein, 1989, p. 29). Over a 10-year period, 40% of the men and a larger percentage of the women reported that their lives were unsatisfactory and had been marred by divorce (p. 42). The financial losses sustained by divorced middle-class women aggravated their problems of divorce, and in families in the lower socioeconomic brackets, divorce often was associated with poverty for the children.

Although the most worrisome aspect of divorce is the still unknown long-term effects on the children, when couples with young children were asked in a 1989 Gallup poll whether those not getting along should (a) stay together "for the sake of the children" or (b) separate rather than raise the children in a "hostile atmosphere," 70% endorsed separation, and only 24% advocated the couple's staying together. Somewhat contradictorily, however, familism was also endorsed: 68% reported that it was important for a family to make financial sacrifices so that one parent could stay home to raise the children, whereas only 27% felt it was important for both parents to work so that the family could benefit from the highest possible income (Footlick, 1990, p. 18).

We have emphasized the divorce rate for three major reasons. First, it is a statistical indicator of family breakdown and of major changes in the family members' lives. Second, divorce is a severe psychosocial stressor. The separation of the family members and the breaking of bonds and ties is followed by changes—economic and emotional—that can be felt over two to three generations. Third, mental disorder rates, especially for depression, are higher in separated and divorced persons than in the married, widowed, or never married (Schwab, Bell, Warheit, & Schwab, 1979; Weissman, 1991).

STRUCTURAL CHANGES IN THE FAMILY

The drastic changes in relationships and living arrangements that are taking place are increasing concerns about the family. The changes in the size and composition of families are indicative of the strong antifamilistic trend sweeping through our society. Households have been getting smaller and contain fewer children than ever before. In 1989, the average number of persons per household was at a record low of 2.62, and the average number of children per household was at the extreme low of 0.69 (down roughly 35% in 25 years). Moreover, the percentage of family households (married, with or without children) declined from 87% in 1960 to 71% in 1988, while nonfamily households (men and women living alone, and unmarried couples) increased from 13% in 1960 to 29% in 1988 (*World Almanac*, 1990, pp. 551, 841).

Since World War II, a number of developments have led to the multiplication of forms of marriage, families, and even, in a sense, kinship. One is the high divorce rate since the mid-1960s; another is the growing power of the women's liberation movement and the emergence of gay rights advocates and other groups. A third is the dominance of the technoculture, with increased mobility and the advances in communication made possible by television and computers. A fourth is the emergence of relatively unchecked individualism as the dominant ethos in Western society (especially in the United States), which has been accompanied by an emphasis on the self, a loss of community with its cohesion and boundaries, and the dominance of government. The most fundamental, however, may be the spreading secularism—and concomitant decline of religion—that has weakened the ground on which most institutions stand. In addition, we can only ponder the possible effects on the stability of the family and its members of such events as World War II, World War I, and the Great Depression. We need to recognize that all of these developments may be causes as well as results and that they both stimulate and reinforce each other.

In the past, social scientists classified families into four types: (a) the traditional *monogamous* family, the "ideal" type in Western society; (b) the *polygynous* family of one husband and two or more wives, accepted in some ancient societies and occasionally in modern times (e.g., in Kuwait where the Emir marries a virgin "almost every Thursday night" and divorces her the next day; Lorch, 1991, p. 32); (c) the rare *polyandrous* family of two or more men (often brothers or coworkers) and one wife; and (d) *group marriage*, which has been practiced by certain religious groups, a tribe in New Guinea, the Masai in Africa (Burgess & Locke, 1945, p. 12), and some small groups in rural Utah. This classification system, however, has become inadequate.

As a consequence of the high divorce and remarriage rates and other changes, there has been a proliferation of structural changes in the family unit. These include many forms of stepfamilies, blended and reconstituted families, "domestic partners" (cohabitation without marriage), and the large number of single-parent families. In May 1989, the San Francisco Board of Supervisors passed legislation that recognized homosexual and unmarried heterosexual couples as families (Seligman, 1990, p. 38). The number of same-sex couples living together has risen slowly during the past 20 years, as has the number of unmarried opposite-sex couples living together. Arthur Leonard maintains that the "family has become a fluid concept" (Smith, 1990, p. 38) and reported that in 1988, only about 27% of the 91 million households in the United States fit the traditional family model. The appalling lack of an institutional and social foundation, boundaries or even structure for the family was expressed in Barbara Bush's (1992) declaration, "Your family is what you think it is."

Stepfamilies

The number of stepfamilies is booming; it rose from almost 4 million in 1980 to about 5.5 million in 1990 (ABC News, 1992). In 1985, almost 7 million children lived in stepfamilies—an increase of 11.6% in 5 years (Kantrowitz & Wingert, 1990, p. 24). This percentage is probably low, inasmuch as it does not count young children who are living in "unofficial stepfamilies," e.g. with a parent(s) or other adults who are in unconventional living arrangements. Stepchildren make up about 20% of all children in married-couple families, and that percentage is projected to increase markedly; about 40% of all children born in the 1980s will live with a stepparent before age 18. During the 1990s, more children will live in stepfamilies than with both biological parents (ABC News, 1992).

Furstenberg reported that "most people have a personal connection with a stepfamily. . . . If it's not their parents, it's their child or their grandparents or their husband's parents" (Kantrowitz & Wingert, 1990, p. 24). The high divorce rate of the past 20 years (50% of marriages begun in the 1970s have ended in divorce) portends an increased number of stepfamilies in the future, and because six of ten second marriages are expected to end in divorce, everybody—parents, children, and relatives—will be sent "into a new emotional maelstrom" (p. 27).

Stepfamilies travel a rocky road as they attempt to meld persons from different families and with unshared life histories into a cohesive, functioning group. Often there are conflicting values and goals, and some members have divided loyalties and guilt about the past that complicate their relationships with each other. Children in pre- or early adolescence (ages 9 to 15), seem to have the most trouble. Visher reminds us poignantly that "every stepfamily is a family born of loss" (Kantrowitz & Wingert, 1990, p. 27).

Perhaps the most serious stepfamily problem is the apparent increase in incestuous relationships and the many reports of sexual abuse in stepfamilies. A stepfather is eight times more likely to have a sexual relationship with a stepchild than a father with his natural children (ABC News, 1992). The variety of relationships in stepfamilies (e.g., each spouse may have children from one or more previous marriages) and the lack of continuity lower restraints to sexuality, which already has been heightened by life together and by lack of supervision by parents who are working and not at home much. In view of these problems and the breakdown of traditional boundaries, questions are being raised about the definition of incest. The legal definition is narrow in some states and broad in others; nevertheless, incest almost always has a destructive effect on families and long-term deleterious effects on the children and adolescents involved.

Stepfamilies have become remarkably complex. Although the complexities involve primarily the children who may have been "merged" and, secondarily, the new husband and wife, it is also necessary to consider other, possibly far-reaching influences of nontraditional family forms.

One is that the family members do not know who their kin are. "In a recent national survey of stepchildren, Furstenburg found that nearly one-quarter did not include their stepsiblings as part of their family even though they were living with them" (Kantrowitz & Wingert, 1990, p. 34). Fundamental questions include whether stepchildren can count on their stepparents and whether stepchildren will care for aging stepparents.

Grandparenting

Grandparents doing the parenting (becoming "skip-generation" parents) became another increasingly common family form in the 1980s. About 3 million children, or 4.6% of all children, were living with grandparents in 1988, in contrast to 2.2 million or 3.2% in 1970. In about 50% of those households, the mother was living with the children and grandparents, but in 30% neither parent was present (*World Almanac*, 1990, p. 842). Generally, the parents were having problems with drugs, alcohol, and/or mental or physical illness along with financial difficulties, and the children were being neglected or abused. The grandparents stepped in to help with the children temporarily but, as the parents continued to have difficulties, the grandparents became the de facto parents.

Seligman (1990) noted Sylvie de Toledo's study of the emotional effects of skip-generation rearing. Many of the children had difficulties in school, with authority, or making friends or were either physically aggressive or isolated. According to de Toledo, the children "have a profound sense of abandonment and loss and rejection by their parents. . . . They worry consciously and unconsciously that they may once again be abandoned" (Seligman, 1990, p. 46) when an obviously aging grandparent becomes ill or dies. Many child and young adult patients who are being or were reared by their grandparents describe years of anxiety about their grandparents' age and health and about who would be their caretakers if the grandparents die.

In Louisville, Kennedy and Keeney (1987, 1988) studied 54 grandparents who were taking care of their children who were patients at the authors' clinic. The grandparents participated in newly formed group psychotherapy programs in which they received peer support, guidance about parenting decisions, and valuable information about current parenting techniques and problems. Also, they found it helpful to ventilate their feelings (usually anger) toward the children's parents and, especially, their own anxieties about what would happen to the children if they became incapacitated or died. Kennedy and Keeney outlined their therapeutic program and emphasized the need for a range of services for those "intergenerational extended" families.

CHANGES IN ROLES

Many of the concerns about changes in roles and families that became apparent in the late 1960s have continued to grow. Arlie Hochschild stated that "husbands, wives, children are not getting enough family life. Nobody is. People are hurting" (Footlick, 1990, p. 17). Surveys of marital satisfaction have shown, generally, that women are less satisfied than men. Their dissatisfaction can be traced in large part to the problems described by Hochschild (1989). Her study of two-career parents found that the employed-outside-the-home wife and mother works at least one month per year more than her husband. About 20% of the men shared the "second shift" equally, 70% did between one third and one half of the household work and chores, and 10% did less than one third. But even when the second shift was shared, the women tended to have the more responsible, difficult jobs of caring for the children and the house, while the men had such less demanding jobs as paying the bills, maintaining the yard, and handling repairs.

Hochschild reported that there has been increased sharing between husbands and wives since the 1960s, but little increase since the early 1980s. She postulated that women had stopped pushing their husbands to share in order to reduce marital tensions. Ellen Goodman (1989) stated that the "fear of divorce quieted many women's demands," but pointed out that women whose husbands did not share the work at home reported that they thought about divorce more often than those whose husbands did. Also, the women who divorced listed "'neglect of home and child' as their chief complaint" (p. A9).

The changes in roles reflect changes in the structure of the family and cultural trends, particularly greater equality for women and families' economic difficulties. The proliferation of nontraditional family forms and the financial pressures accentuated by creeping inflation make it increasingly necessary for mothers to work. Two thirds of all mothers (twice the 1955 rate) are now in the labor force; one half of all mothers of infants work outside the home.

Parents have conflicts about work and family obligations. Some middle- and upper-class mothers have adapted by "sequencing"—working to establish themselves in a job or career for a few years, then staying at home to care for their children, and then returning to work after the children have reached school age. But most working mothers do not have this option. The shrinking real incomes for those in the middle and lower socioeconomic brackets during the 1980s made it necessary for most mothers to be wage earners, and family time was further reduced by the necessity for many fathers and mothers to work at more than just one job (when it was possible to find jobs) because of the low wages, inflation, and the long recession during the Bush presidency. In discussing "the growing time deficit," Hewlett (1991) stated that "the amount of contact time between parents and children has dropped a staggering 40% over the past 25 years" (p. D4).

EFFECTS OF POVERTY ON THE FAMILY

The destructive effects of poverty on many families increased during the supposedly affluent 1980s. Of the 33 million poor Americans, the 13 million children (20% of all children) are the frontline casualties. The United States in 1990 fell to 21st in the world in infant survival rates—behind Japan, East Germany, Ireland, Australia, and Canada—and from 16th to 17th in life expectancy. Students (including 40% of nonwhites) often do not graduate because of financial pressures (Kozol, 1990, p. 49). In writing about the poor, Kozol (1990) emphasized that "the way we treat our children tells us something of the future we envision. The willingness of the nation to relegate so many of these poorly housed and poorly fed and poorly educated children to the role of outcasts in a rich society is going to come back to haunt us. . . . Low-income children, who receive the least at home, receive the least from public education" (pp. 48–49).

The antifamilism of the nation's leaders was expressed decisively by their actions in the 1980s and early 1990s. The gains made during the 1960s and 1970s by Head Start, Upward Bound, and other programs designed to aid poor families stopped in 1981 when the Reagan administration reduced funding for them. Payments to welfare families with children have dropped to 35% below the 1970 level; about a half million families lost all welfare payments; 1 million children stopped receiving food stamps; and 2 million children were excluded from the school lunch programs.

As the problems of recession increased in 1991, many debt-ridden states further reduced payments for welfare and Aid to Families with Dependent Children (AFDC). The December 1991 budgetary shortfall in California was accompanied by Governor Pete Wilson's proposal of a state referendum on a 25% cut in welfare payments. According to De Parle (1991) in "The Welfare Attack," 16 states had cut AFDC payments, and Michigan had "virtually eliminated its general assistance program" (p. A11). Supporters of welfare cuts argued that in the long run the reductions would benefit the poor because social programs are disincentives. But Senator Moynihan objected, "I would not think you're going to change the behavior of a 4-year-old child by feeding it less," and De Parle stated that "others saw only misery" (p. A11). Danziger called the anger about welfare "a reverse class anger. . . . Instead of saying, 'look at the huge amounts of money the rich made in the 1980s; can we get some of it back in taxes?', it's 'Let's squeeze a little bit of money out of the most impoverished group'" (p. A11).

The most dire effects of poverty on the family are hunger, homelessness, and disease. Economic recession and the reduction of welfare benefits at a time when one in ten persons is on an increasingly limited food stamp program have resulted in many children going to bed hungry, even to the point of malnutrition.

Although family and home are synonymous, at least in most Americans' thinking, homelessness has become a great festering plague that has spread to affect about 500,000 persons, many of whom are children (Caton, 1990, pp. 19–28). According to Caton, there is a lack of data on homeless families. She cited a Boston study by Bassuk and her colleagues that showed that the average age of homeless mothers was 27 years and that one half were separated, divorced, or widowed; each had an average of 2.4 children. Most of the homeless mothers had come from families that had been disrupted by parental separation, divorce, or death, and about one third reported that they had been abused. In Washington, D.C., the number of homeless children increased fivefold in 1986. By 1987, about one half of the persons in homeless shelters in New York City were children; their average age was 6 years (Kozol, 1990, p. 52). CBS News reported on December 16, 1991, that increasing numbers of the homeless were young people and, frighteningly, one third were families, often with children. Kozol (1988) described the deplorable, heart-rending life of homeless families in the older New York City hotels where many were lodged. In the shelters, diseases that Americans thought had been conquered—whooping cough and tuberculosis—are now common.

Poverty has deleterious effects on family members' mental and physical health. Children's deaths from measles, for example, have increased in the past 5 to 10 years. The United States now ranks 56th in the world (after Albania) in the percentage of children receiving measles vaccinations. The association between poverty and increased mental illness rates is one of the most consistent findings in psychiatric epidemiology. George Man Burrows attributed the increased admissions to public mental hospitals in England between 1800 and 1804 to the failure of the harvests of 1800 (Burrows, 1828, pp. 61–62). In 1855, Jarvis's (1971) classic study in Massachusetts found increased mental illness rates among two groups—the poor and the recent immigrants. Since World

War II, major community-wide studies—such as the Stirling County study by Leighton, Harding, Macklin, MacMillan, and Leighton (1963); Srole et al. (1962) and Srole and Fischer's (1986) midtown Manhattan study; our Florida health study (Schwab et al., 1979); and the nationwide Epidemiologic Catchment Area (ECA) studies (Freedman, 1984) of the early 1980s—have all reported a significant inverse relationship between lower socioeconomic status and mental illness. Holzer and his colleagues' (1986) incisive analyses of the more than 19,000 adult respondents interviewed for the ECA study showed that mental illness rates were disproportionately much higher in the lowest socioeconomic status quintile than even in the low, but next higher, quintile.

Such data signal individual and family distress and are signs of societal malaise, if not decadence. In 1989, the Institute of Medicine (IOM) reported that at least 7.5 million children (12% of those under age 18) had definite mental disorders and that more than 20% of poor children may suffer from such disasters (IOM, 1990). In 1985, only 2.5 million emotionally disturbed children received treatment. Poverty, homelessness and "growing up in 'crowded inner-city neighborhoods' . . . created 'persistent psychosocial adversity' for children" (p. A21).

Family poverty has resulted in an increased number of children aged 14 to 18 leaving school to work for very low wages, sometimes in dangerous jobs. Kolata (1992) reported that 4 million children were legally (and another 2 million illegally) working in factories, in businesses, or on farms. Injury rates "were $3\frac{1}{2}$ times the adult rate," a disproportionately large number were being seen in emergency rooms for injuries sustained on the job, and "several hundred each year are killed" (p. 1). At a conference on child labor at the Mount Sinai Medical Center in New York, Dr. Philip Landrigan (Kolata, 1992) blamed the increase in child labor on three factors: the increasing number of families that slipped into poverty in the 1980s, the flood of immigrants from countries where children are exploited, and reduced federal and state funding for inspecting workplaces.

Kolata (1992) concluded that "child-labor abuses are . . . pervasive in U.S. workplaces," and Jeffrey Newman of the National Child Labor Committee stated that he "is seeing a return of child labor scandals reminiscent of those that occurred at the turn of the century. . . . It's very sad and it doesn't speak well to our understanding and commitment to children" (pp. 1, 18). Such phenomena can be understood only by diagnosing them as vestigial, as evidence of social regression as well as pathology. They are painful reminders of hideous years in our past, of slavery and sweatshops, and are reflections of the shallowness and artificiality of much of modern life.

Bane and Ellwood (1989) emphasized that "the first clue to understanding children's poverty *comes from looking at family structure*" (p. 1048; italics added). Patterns of children's poverty are attributable to (a) the poverty rate in two-parent families with incomes that fluctuate with economic conditions; (b) the increase of children in single-parent homes—from about 9% of all children in 1960 to about 22% in 1987; and (c) the high poverty rate—in the 50% to 70% range since 1960—in female-headed families. About half of the increase in poverty from 1979 to 1987 was caused by the worsening poverty rates among two-parent families; another fourth was caused by the increased number of children in single-parent homes; and the rest was the result of increasing poverty rates among female-headed families (pp. 1048–1049). Real median family income declined from 1979 to 1987, and although employment had increased, wages were so low that the "unemployed poor" became the "working poor . . . many people are able to work without being able to support a family" (p. 1049).

Poverty rates in single-parent families are very high, according to Bane and Ellwood, because "65% of absent fathers contribute no child support or alimony" (p. 1051), many single mothers who are not well educated and who have to be both the providers and the nurturers of the children make low wages, and the declining welfare benefits are below the poverty level. Contrary to official pronouncements and to opinions voiced by many upper-middle-class white suburbanites, Bane and Ellwood found little evidence that expanded welfare benefits influenced the changing family structure by increasing the number of female-headed households. Although welfare benefits rose in the 1960s, they declined in the 1970s and 1980s by almost 25% as eligibility rules were tightened. "Indeed, since 1973 the fraction of all children in single-parent homes grew from 12% to over 20% but the fraction of all children collecting Aid to Families with Dependent Children (AFDC) . . . benefits was unchanged" (p. 1051). Also, the highest rates of unmarried mothers were found in states with the lowest benefits, and vice versa.

Providing child care is a problem for the 70% of mothers who work, especially for those in poor and/or single-parent families. Bane and Ellwood (1989) estimated that a single mother must earn at least 6 to 7 dollars per hour and also obtain inexpensive day care in order for her work to be profitable. Many working mothers cannot afford child care; consequently, the care of a 2- or 3-year-old child is often left to an 8- or 9-year-old sibling. Such a situation is not conducive to the healthy development of either. Also, the working single mother usually is anxious about job security, because she knows that she will have difficulty staying home with a sick child or even leaving work to take the child for medical care. Bane and Ellwood (1989) concluded:

> Changes in family structure have not come about in isolation. They took place at a time when the country witnessed massive increases in labor force participation of women, an unprecedented stagnation in the real earnings of men, worsening employment patterns for many young people (especially young black men), considerably greater birth control availability and use, the legalization of abortion, important changes in social policy, and altered attitudes regarding the roles of women, work, and family. (p. 1051)

Family poverty, homelessness, and the exploitation of children raise disturbing questions. Perhaps the most distressing is whether we are again in an antihumanistic era in which the unfortunate, the disabled, and the disadvantaged are at the mercy of an unchecked economic system, a time reminiscent of Dickens's haunting descriptions of the poverty and distress in the crowded streets of London in the 1850s and the plight of the poor and homeless in London exposed by Jack London's (1904) photographs and words in *People of the Abyss*. Are we entering an era such as that described by Marx (1952) in *Das Kapital*, when the English working class was subjected to appalling exploitation? Industrialization and unbridled capitalism resulted in a declining standard of living for the working class in Great Britain during most of the nineteenth century.

Michael Harrington's death in 1990 may have marked the end of an era of concern and compassion about poverty, sentiments that began to wane in the early 1980s as they were being replaced by the triumph of style over substance and the proclamation "greed is good." Harrington's (1963) *The Other America* awakened the conscience of our nation by describing the extent of poverty in the 1950s and the "twisted spirit" it produced. His work shook a sensitive nation and led to the development of programs that reduced the number of the poor. The recent change in sentiments includes the turning away from the homeless, regarding them with looks of disdain, if not contempt, and shunning them as nuisances who should be out of sight. In their celebration of "family values" during the 1992 Republican National Convention, neither Vice President and Mrs. Quayle nor President and Mrs. Bush once mentioned homeless families.

By the end of the 1980s, the problems were climbing the socioeconomic ladder; increasing numbers of middle-class families were experiencing financial distress. Working wives as well as husbands became a middle-class norm, especially for the often elitist, consumer-oriented yuppies. In *Fear of Falling*, Ehrenreich (1989) described the anxiety of many in the middle class who could see their economic status and their dreams of greater upward mobility being crushed by staggering national (and personal) indebtedness and by financial scandals, the rising cost of living, increasing white-collar unemployment, and the chronic recession. Downward drift, previously associated in psychiatry with decline in socioeconomic status after mental illness, also became a threat for many who had viewed themselves as upwardly mobile.

"Fear of Falling" is realistic, not imaginary. In *America: What Went Wrong?*, Bartlett and Steele (1992) described the "changing face of America," the "dismantling of the middle class . . . whether blue-collar, white-collar, middle-level manager, or professional" (p. xi) and labeled them "the forgotten Americans" (pp. xvi, 1). As a percentage of all families, the core middle-class group—those with adjusted gross incomes between $20,000 and $50,000 (median family income was $34,213)—dropped from 39% in 1980 to 35% in 1989. Bartlett and Steele pointed out: "The wage and salary structure of American business, encouraged by federal tax policies, is pushing the nation toward a two-class society. The top 4% make as much as the bottom half of U.S. workers" (p. ix). Thus, families' worries about falling behind financially, of having to work extra hours to stay even, or of never being able to buy a house are all too real. And they are augmented by family members' concerns about being dumped by their company for younger employees, restructured out of a job, or deprived of their pensions when they retire. Bartlett and Steele asserted: "You are right. Keep worrying" (p. 2).

A view of the complexity of the problems of families and children requires consideration of our society's values. Sylvia Hewlett (1991) stated that, at the end of the 1980s, children in all social classes "deal with risk and neglect on a scale unimagined in previous generations" (pp. D1, D4). Since 1970 there has been a 21% increase in children living in poverty; 12 million have no health insurance; and 15 million have been deserted by their fathers. She concluded that "over the past 25 years . . . American society has been tilting in an ominous new direction—toward the devaluation of children" (p. D4). The federal government spends only one fifth as much money on children as on those over age 65; less than 5% of the federal budget has been devoted to children, only one third to one half as much as in Canada, Great Britain, and Italy. Children living below the poverty line are a common sight in the United States but a rarity in western Europe.

The conservative retrenchment, with its policies, sentiments, and economic changes that dominated life in the United States during the 1980s, affected the family. The economic changes, including increased poverty, lower incomes for the undereducated and the unskilled, and the necessity for more mothers to enter the work force, produced problems of overwork, stress, and inadequate child care that ravaged family life. Thus, we can see that the antifamilism expressed by "the CEOs second wife" (Connelly, 1989) reflects sentiments at upper levels of business and government and places the well-being of many children and families in jeopardy. Throughout history, changes at one level of society, especially at the top, are paralleled by changes at other levels.

To assess the extent of the changes in the United States in the past dozen years that have influenced the stability of the family and the character of our society, it is necessary to look at fundamental factors. The two major ones are economic forces and prevailing sentiments.

ECONOMIC FACTORS AND ANTIFAMILISM

Kevin Phillips (1990) pointed out that the extent of the upward distribution of wealth in the 1980s had occurred only three other times in our history: in the 1790s, the 1870s, and the 1920s (pp. xix–xxi). Phillips, who had presciently written *The Emerging Republican Majority* in 1969 and who had a position in the Reagan government, emphasized the growing income inequity. The gap between the highest and the lowest 20% of the population was considerably greater (at least 25%) than in France, Britain, and Canada, and about 50% to 60% greater than in Germany, Sweden, the Netherlands, and Japan (p. 9). The accumulation of wealth during the 1980s shocked even billionaires such as David Rockefeller. In 1985, the family income of the top 1% of the population was 11.6% of the total national income, about a 30% increase in 8 years, and was predicted to climb to 12% in 1990 (p. 214). Phillips emphasized that "easy money at the top with loss of hope and faith at the bottom," along with conspicuous consumption and "short-term 'non'-values" (p. 217) were associated with small-town decay, urban crime, and weakened families. He attributed the problems to excessive individualism in American society and to the encouragement given business "to seek its rewards regardless of the social cost" (pp. 214, 217, 220). Will Durant (1927) similarly described some of the effects of excess wealth in a society:

> A leisure class . . . [is] adept in the arts of luxury. Leisure begets speculation. . . . Thought, adventuring in a labyrinth of analysis, discovers behind society the individual; divested of its normal function it turns inward and

discovers the self. The sense of common interest, of commonwealth fades; there are no citizens now, there are only individuals. (p. 397)

Such trends are indicators of antifamilism. We have presented some of the social history of the United States in the 1980s because general living systems concepts of the family position it between the level of the individual and that of the wider society. Consequently, the family influences and is influenced by what is happening in the society and also by its individual members' character structure(s) and values. Substantial evidence shows that antifamilism surfaced in the early 1960s with such protests as youth revolts, experiments with so-called alternative lifestyles, and communal living. But during the 1980s, it became national policy, as evidenced by the drastic reductions in funding for social programs and for families that were announced (somewhat righteously) by the Reagan and Bush administrations. For example, in 1991, President Bush vetoed the Family and Medical Leave Act, a law (since signed in altered form by President Clinton) that guaranteed unpaid leave and job security to men and women when they were confronted with family emergencies (*The Courier-Journal*, "Wayward votes," 10/8/91, p. A8). The antifamilism of the 1980s was both practiced and praised by many of our nation's social, economic, and political leaders, some of whom were in a position to gain materially from the harvest of the "greed is good" ethic of the decade.

"Greed is good" is a hallmark of individualism and thus conflicts with familistic codes that place the group's interests and well-being ahead of the individual's. The increasing antifamilism in this century culminated in the 1980s with attacks by the Reagan administration, which blamed the family first (and schools, to a lesser extent) for the delinquency, crime, and most of the social ills of the era. The endorsement of antifamilism by the upper class and the national leadership, the delays in marriage in the middle class, and the problems in the lower social class (with its many single-parent families) may signify that antifamilism has reached its cyclic crest—or perhaps that its forces have triumphed.

Antifamilism and the American Character

The concerns about the family that have become so manifest ultimately pivot around the nature of the American character. The foremost of the two basic functions of the family is the nurturance and development of the children (the other is the meeting of the adults' sexual and emotional needs and stabilization of their personalities). In 1835, Alexis de Tocqueville (1945) compared the new nation and its people with its western European counterparts and praised Americans for their vigor, liberal attitudes, and strength of character. His two major reservations were the disgraceful slavery problem and the extreme individualism that could impair community life. As will be discussed in Chapter 3, Charles Pearson (1894) expressed concern about whether the changes in the family that were appearing and the increasing individualism that accompanied the conquests by capitalism during the nineteenth century would affect the character of the young. In 1915, Goodsell (1934) decried the difficulties of family life that he saw and feared that they and the growing individualism would affect children's character adversely and lead to further family disruption. Riesman, Denney, and Glazer (1950) described the changing American character, especially the disappearance of the inner-directed character type and the emergence of the other-directed, peer-oriented type (about which they had forebodings). Friedenberg (1964) cited the endorsing of enemy propaganda by American prisoners of war (POWs) during the Korean War as an indicator of change in the American character, inasmuch as American POWs had never before collaborated with the enemy.

At the end of the 1980s, some of those concerns about the American character appear to have materialized. To what extent were the changing allegiances of some of Friedenberg's POWs analogous to the divorce-remarriage shifts in the American family? The August 12, 1991 issue of *Time* magazine asked, "Busy-Bodies and Crybabies: What's Happening to the American Character?" In the cover story (Morrow, 1991), the young were pictured as "fashioning some odd new malformations of American character" (p. 14): The "busy-bodies" were overly zealous, exhibited a nasty intolerance, and could be bullies, whereas the "crybabies" tended to be abject and manipulative and to blame others, not themselves, for anything that was wrong. Morrow used a psychoanalytic metaphor to analogize the "busy-bodies" and the superego, and the "crybabies" and the id; both were squeezing the ego, the executive apparatus of the mind. He explained that both the puritanical need to regiment others and the passion for blaming others smacked of the "immobility of addiction," and he described the "busy-bodies" and the "crybabies" as "two moral defectives of the schoolyard jumping up and down on the social contract. . . . (America is) not entirely a society of grownups" (p. 15).

These descriptions appear to be applicable as well to the nation's leaders. In discussing President Bush's 1992 trip to the Orient with wealthy business leaders, which was aimed toward increasing U.S. exports, George Will (1992) stated that "blaming Japan, particularly, for our problems is a national pastime" (p. A21). The generally conservative

Will described the president "and his equally whining entourage . . . as the crybaby of the Western world" (p. A21). He further identified the former commerce secretary and then-current Bush campaign manager as "Robert 'Alibi' Mosbacher" (p. A21). We emphasize such glaring parallels because, in accord with concepts of general living systems theory, we see the family as being influenced by and as influencing both the character of its members (especially the young) and the wider society.

Blaming the family for the nation's social pathologies began in the 1980s, when the Reagan administration almost defiantly abdicated responsibility for poverty and other social problems. It blamed the poor, the unemployed, and homeless individuals—many of whom were ill or disadvantaged—and their families. In so doing, it increased polarization between the classes and abandoned the Founding Fathers' dream of a classless society. Also, it raised the fundamental question formulated by Plato in both of his great dialogues on utopian societies, *The Republic* and *The Laws*—namely, does the individual "make" the community (i.e., determine its health and well-being), or does the community make the individual? William J. Bennett, secretary of education in the Reagan administration, took a firm stand. He announced that children would be held to "higher standards" (Kozol, 1990, p. 52) and that their parents could be blamed for having a "lack of values" (p. 52).

Blaming reached a height as the 1992 election campaign heated up and our society's social problems thundered through the nation from its riot-torn epicenter in Los Angeles. The White House announced that the riots "were a result of social welfare programs that Congress enacted in the 1960s and 70s" (Wines, 1992), especially Lyndon Johnson's Great Society legislation—the War on Poverty, the Civil Rights Act of 1964, the Model Cities Act, and even Head Start, an "unqualified success, that at one time was opposed by Reagan" (Wines, 1992).

Vice President Quayle attacked a "poverty of values," asserting that "the lawless social anarchy which we saw [in Los Angeles] is directly related to the breakdown of family structure, personal responsibility, and social order in too many areas of our society. . . . For the poor the situation is compounded by a welfare ethos that impedes individual efforts to move ahead in society" (Keen & Harney, 1992). Quayle supported Moynihan's (1965) controversial view that the breakdown of the family was responsible for America's social problems. This view has been opposed by many social scientists and political figures who insist that strengthening the family requires first providing an economic and educational base for it via jobs and improved schools. Quayle stated that the "social breakdown" was "reaping the whirlwinds of decades of changes in social mores" and could not be blamed simply on either the Great

Society programs or on the "growth and success most Americans enjoyed during the 1980s" (p. 2). With a twist of logic, Quayle stated that "marriage is probably the best anti-poverty program" because the poverty rate in families headed by two parents is less than in single-mother headed families. But damning the social programs of 25 years earlier can have some degree of logic when viewed in terms of Jonathan Swift's great 1729 satire *A Modest Proposal*, in which he proposed that eating the young babies in Ireland would relieve starvation and also prevent them from "being a burden to their parents or the country." Had the millions of poor people in the United States not been helped by social programs, many would have died early deaths from the malnutrition, disease, and violence that accompany poverty.

In "A Crisis of Character," Daniel Coats (1991), a Republican senator from Indiana, indicted the popular youth culture, the educational system, and the family for a loss of values and for social pathologies, especially increased crime, family abandonment, child neglect, and "an exponential growth of drug and alcohol abuse" (p. 1). He emphasized that "this is an economic golden age" (p. 1) and blamed the social problems on the media, rap music, "relativism," the "lack of firm values," and the culture's setting "itself against moral restraint" (p. 3). In addition, he deplored "the breakdown of moral instruction through school and the family" (p. 3). He charged the schools with not having standards and also of having been transformed into correctional institutions, but he said nothing about past reductions in their funding.

Recently the senior author of this book consulted on the case of a 32-year-old schoolteacher who was suffering from both anxiety and depression. In his special education classroom in which adolescents were to learn about computers, there were only two small computers for the 30 students. The instructor attempted to assign two students every 20 minutes to the computers, but could not teach any pair because he had difficulties keeping the others from fighting. After 6 weeks, he had to seek psychiatric care. In *Savage Inequalities*, Kozol (1991) described the problem: In the first term of the "education president" (Bush), "most children are getting second-rate educations in third-rate schools, and the government isn't doing much about it" (Mitgang, 1991, p. A19).

Critics such as Senator Coats do not point out that reductions in funding for family and educational programs during the past 12 years have been accompanied by the widespread financial corruption described in Stewart's (1991) *Den of Thieves*. Also, the preference for style rather than substance, and such scandals as the illegal sales of arms by government officials, government officials indicted for lying to Congress, and the savings and loans atrocities (which involved a president's son and at least one senator and increased the debt burden for all Americans) influence character formation. In such a situation, when there seems to be a collapse of moral leadership at the top, blaming the schools and the family is not helpful and is an additional indicator of executive irresponsibility. This shifting of blame obviously "trickles down" to influence the ordinary parents and children who are the strength of the society and who often strive for humaneness and honesty. The Republican presidents alone should not bear all the blame for the excesses, corruptions, and carelessness that characterized the political and economic leadership of the United States in the 1980s; many Democratic members of Congress voted for the programs that wasted billions of dollars and for the spending cuts that disregarded the needs of children and their families. But the president is expected to epitomize the values that are the beacons of light to the people, and we ask: Is it possible that the character of Senator Coats's "golden age" and its social pathologies were two sides of the same coin and possibly were producing each other?

Morrow (1991) stated that Americans are subscribing wholeheartedly to the "pursuit of happiness—their own happiness . . . [the idealized rugged individualism and frontiersman's self-sufficiency and stoicism] belong now in some wax museum of lost American self-images" (p. 15). He quoted Marianne Glendons's statement that "the language of responsibility is meager: 'A tendency to frame nearly every social contract in terms of a clash of rights (e.g., a woman's right to her own body vs. a fetus's right to life) impedes compromise, mutual understanding, and a discovery of common ground'" (p. 15). Also, Morrow pointed out that our social contract changes rapidly and is postmodernist inasmuch as our society is ever changing. He concluded with the poignant statement that "when old coherences break down, civilities and tolerances fall away as well. So does an ideal of self-reliance and inner autonomy and responsibility" (p. 15).

The overlitigation that Morrow and others see as a characterological problem may be a manifestation of decadence, especially the decadent individualism and materialism that became prominent in ancient Greece and
Rome during their decline. In late twentieth-century America, families and community integration have been stressed by the self-righteousness, self-indulgence, and the excesses of the 1980s, which included fierce attacks on the family and concomitant family disruption. Self-indulgent excess did not just trickle down, it cascaded through our society.

In an incisive article, Joe Klein (1992, pp. 19–22) focused on some of the basic issues in the "family values" controversy—namely, economics and job loss, the need for two parents to work, consumerism, unlimited personal freedom, and "rampaging materialism" (p. 19). Quoting Fred

Siegel, he noted that "we have conducted a 30-year experiment in desublimation" (p. 19). Klein saw both the self-actualizing liberals obsessed with personal freedom and the predatory conservatives obsessed with "commercial freedom to the point of pillage" as being self-indulgent. He equated the "greed is good" ethos of the 1980s with the "do your own thing" mantra of the 1960s and the "you can have it all" ethos of the 1970s.

The American family is at the center of the debate, which boils down to community and family versus individualism and personal rights. Klein (1992) cited both the familiar and new data: In psychiatric hospitals, 80% of the adolescents are from broken families; higher rates of single-parent households are associated with higher violent crime and burglary rates; and children "living apart from a biological parent are 20% to 40% more vulnerable to sickness" than those living with both biological parents (p. 21). He concluded that our culture is centrifugal, especially as embodied in advertising, marketing, and diversity of cable television programs. The centrifugal force disrupts the home and family, fragments the community, and splinters the society often into divisive, antagonistic groups. The blurring of standards and the marginal character of the upper levels of our government, along with the splintering centrifugal character of our society, have become clinically manifested by the great increase and even popularity of the diagnoses of borderline and multiple personality disorder.

From many viewpoints, the nature of the American character appears to be in jeopardy. Throughout this book, we will be noting the influences of family structure and composition, community life, and the prevailing political and cultural trends on character formation and development and, in accord with principles of general living systems theory, the reciprocal influences of individual-family-community interactions.

CONCLUDING REMARKS

The family crisis of the 1980s appeared 100 years after the first rumblings of concern about the stability of the family were heard in the 1880s. The speed at which the problems of the family grew increased greatly during the 1960s and erupted in volcanic fashion during the Reagan and Bush presidencies. The most obvious concern was the family disruption evidenced by the divorce rate, which reached an all-time high in the early 1980s but declined slightly toward the end of the decade. Glick (1988) reported that since 1974, the "majority of marriages [are] ending in divorce," the percentage remarrying after divorce had declined to about 80%, and "61% of divorced men and 54% of divorced women end their second marriage in redivorce" (p. 869). The serial monogamy first mentioned by Goodsell (1915) has been rapidly becoming the dominant marriage type. It brings to mind the Marquis de Sade's utopian study "Aline et Valcour," in which the boys and girls on the mythical South Seas island would live with each other for a trial week before making a decision about marriage, but once married they were allowed only two divorces (Bell, 1980, p. 93). The second major concern is the children's problems. These include the large number living in poverty, mental illness rates of at least 12% (20% for the disadvantaged), delinquency, drugs, violence, and suicidality. Hewlett (1991) declared that "an anti-child spirit is loose in the land" (p. D4).

Family scholars and other social scientists maintain that the causes of the marriage and family problems are complex and involve many social forces. Extreme individualism is blamed for much of the distress. In their penetrating analysis of American society in the mid-1980s, *Habits of the Heart*, Bellah, Madsen, Sullivan, Swidler, and Tipton (1985) emphasized that the paramount problem is that of individualism and the self versus commitment and community. Individualism has been a strong feature of the American character since the settling of the colonies, and in the 1830s, de Tocqueville expressed concern about its long-term disintegrating effects on our society. Throughout the century of concern about the family, from Pearson in the 1890s to Goodsell in 1915 and Kevin Phillips in 1990, individualism has been seen as a growing threat to the family, and family problems have frequently been depicted as conflicts between individualism and familism.

In his masterful essay, "The Fall of Community, the Ruins of Sex," the Kentucky poet Wendell Berry (1992) described a community as a commonwealth with a mutuality of interests that lives by the common virtues of trust, goodwill, and respect. It has power to influence behavior and also is

> a set of arrangements between men and women. These arrangements include marriage, family structure, divisions of work and authority, responsibility for the instruction of children and young people. These arrangements exist, in part, to reduce the volatility and the danger of sex— to preserve its energy, its beauty and its pleasures; they preserve and clarify its power to join, not just husband and wife to one another, but parents to children, families to the community, the community to nature; to assure . . . that the inheritance of sexuality, as they come of age, will be worthy of it. (pp. D1, D4)

But Berry maintains that the community is being destroyed by private and public exploitation and lack of community interests and respect. Communities have deteriorated as a result of the "external predation and private disaffection," and the arrangements between men and women have become those of "sexual politics, instinct and polity without culture" (p. D4). The resulting "culture of liberated sexuality" is free of courtesy, ceremony, and responsibility; restraint is dependent on the advice of experts, litigation, or arrest. The consequences are pathologies, some of which are child molestation, sexual harassment and abuse, unwanted pregnancies, venereal diseases, and AIDS. To protect women from "the terrifying advances of obsessed men," a law against stalking (defined as the willful, malicious and repeated following and harassing of another person) was passed in California in 1990 and an additional 18 states by the first half of 1992 (Landsberg, 1992).

Berry (1992) described the economic brutality that leads to sexual brutality, and he expressed hope that the "current revulsion against sexual harassment may be the beginning of a renewal of sexual responsibility and self-respect"(p. D4). He concluded that "humans who wish to be treated and to treat others (as human beings and living souls made in the image of God) must understand that this is not a kindness that can be conferred by a public economy or by a public government or by a public people. It only can be conferred, upon its members, by a community" (p. D4).

In the early 1970s, Zimmerman (1972a,b) predicted that the turning point for the family crisis would come shortly before the turn of the century, and he expressed optimism because the family has survived for millennia despite seemingly overwhelming adversities. But the antifamilism of the 1980s, along with the crime, reckless national indebtedness, and the control exercised by the military-industrial complex (which Zimmerman apparently did not foresee) may have impeded restorative processes. If the family does not reinstitutionalize, some new form of family life probably will emerge early in the twenty-first century. Based on demographic data, Hagestad (1986) has suggested that if there is a continuation of current divorce and remarriage rates, fertility patterns, and of the male/female mortality differential, the most stable social system in our aging society early in the next century will be the vertical grandmother-mother-daughter axis, not the horizontal male-female axis.

Finally, the overarching concern is about the effects on character formation of the prevailing social and political processes, antifamilism, the antichild spirit, and disruption of the family. Strauss and Howe (1991) have maintained that there will be an "inner-driven era" between 1991 and 2003, with those entering adulthood being "reactives" who will clash with the older "boomers." The reactives will be financially burdened and threatened by the AIDS epidemic. Some of them have returned to their parental homes, and many appear to be prolonging their years of dependency; they may be the first generation in many years "to reach age 40 with a lower standard of living than their parents had enjoyed at like age" (p. 410). Strauss and Howe predicted alienation and dire economic need for the reactives, but that they will seek "stability in family life as a result of the economic risk-taking and cultural aberrations" (p. 413). To avoid their parents' divorces and because of family pressures, these individuals will marry late, live in dual-income households, become more conservative in their private lives, and make "a great effort to shield their offspring from the less pleasant facts of life" (p. 413).

Thus, we can see that social scientists and other family scholars have been making somewhat different forecasts about the future of the family. To evaluate family research and the current family crisis and to place them in a meaningful perspective, it will be helpful to look at the history of the family, as we will proceed to do in the next chapter.

CHAPTER 2

History of the Family

> We in our time need to recover the past in order to obtain fullness. But this is not so much because history has meant decline, as because the fullness of meaning isn't available with the resources of a single age.
> —Taylor (1989, p. 465)

As we have seen, the family crisis of the 1980s stimulated interest in the family and concerns about its well-being. To grasp the meaning of the changes in the structure and functions of the family that have been occurring, as well as the concerns and pathologies, it will be helpful to look at the history of the family. We shall do so not in terms of Santayana's famous aphorism—that a person who does not learn the lessons of the past is doomed to repeat it—but more in accord with Benedetto Croce's (1960) thesis that the past has contemporary significance because it is within us.

ANCIENT TIMES AND MYTHS

The Beginnings of the Modern Family

How families began has been a subject of intense interest throughout the ages. Families, even as we understand them today, are prominent in the ancient myths. Zeus and Hera, Jupiter and Juno, and Wotan and Fricka are the fathers and mothers in the Greek, Roman, and Teutonic myths, respectively; their domestic quarrels and problems with their children have a surprisingly modern ring. Even earlier, in Egyptian mythology, the supreme deity was the sun god, Amon or Ra, the creator who "fertilized Mother Earth with rays of penetrating heat and light" (Durant, 1935, p. 198). About 5000 B.C., the Egyptians worshipped

Amon (to whom the great temples of upper Egypt were dedicated), his consort, Mut, and their son, Khonsu, god of the moon. The parallel between that family of three (perhaps the first trinity) and the modern nuclear family supports Zimmerman's (1947) view of the family as "a cultural necessity."

The myth of "the great mother," Isis, is particularly appealing. She made the earth fecund and found the first wheat and barley, which she gave to her husband/father, Osiris, the god of the Nile and of death and resurrection. In the earliest story of sibling rivalry, Osiris was slain by his brother, Set, who hacked the corpse into small pieces and scattered them throughout the land, where they made the earth green. When Horus, son of Osiris and Isis, came of age he slew his uncle, Set. Isis then brought the pieces of Osiris's body together and nourished them back to life. This myth recounts classic family struggles of violence and vengeance that later became some of the essential features of such fifth-century B.C. Greek tragedies as Euripedes's *Alcestis* and *The Oresteia*, and the sibling rivalry was retold in the story of Cain and Abel. According to Durant (1935), Isis was

> the symbol of that mysterious creative power which had produced the earth and every living thing, and of that maternal tenderness whereby, at whatever cost to the mother, the young new life is nurtured to maturity. She represented . . . the originative leadership of women in tilling the earth . . . [and annually, at the winter solstice that coincided with the rebirth of the sun, she was shown] in holy effigy nursing in a stable the babe that she had miraculously conceived. (pp. 200–201)

Was this the prototype for the many depictions of Mary with the infant Jesus in her arms?

Durant (1935) conjectured that "it is highly improbable that the first human beings lived in isolated families" (p. 30), because such families would have been relatively defenseless; early human beings survived by developing some type of group solidarity. He regarded the family as the "most deep-rooted of all historic institutions" (p. 30). Kinship and clan were eventually succeeded by more complex levels of social organization: "The government took over the problem of maintaining order, while the family assumed the tasks of reorganizing industry and carrying on the race" (p. 30).

Anthropological research during the past two centuries has supported these views. The isolated family is nonexistent; even Arctic groups of as few as 30 persons consist of an extended family or several related families. Also, the human being's innate aversion to isolated living is well known. Solitary living is a punishment in prisons, and Carstairs (1969) conjectured that the immense appeal of *Robinson Crusoe* is that it describes the challenging yet frightening fantasy of aloneness.

In his classic study of the institutions of ancient Greece and Rome, Fustel de Coulanges (1901) maintained that neither generation, kinship, nor natural affection was the basis of the ancient family; instead, it was "a religious rather than a natural association" (p. 42). Although religion did not create the family, it gave the family its rules. The first institution established by domestic religion probably was marriage: "The institution of a sacred marriage must be as old in the Indo-European race as the domestic religion; for the one could not exist without the other. This religion taught man that the conjugal union was something more than a relation of the sexes and a fleeting affection, and united man and wife by the powerful bond of the same worship" (pp. 59–60).

Nowhere have the origin and necessity of the family been described more poetically than in Lucretius's (1952) 74 B.C. classic, *De Re Naturem*, which has inspired philosophers and other scholars for 2,000 years:

> And Venus would join the bodies of lovers in the woods; for each woman was gained over either by mutual desire or the headstrong violence and vehement lust of the man or a bribe of some acorns and arbute-berries or choice pears. . . . Next after they had got themselves huts and skins and fire, and the woman united with the man passed with him into one domicile and the duties of wedlock were learnt by the two, and they saw an offspring born from them, then first mankind began to soften. For fire made their chilled bodies less able now to bear the frost beneath the canopy of heaven, and Venus impaired their strength and children with their caresses soon broke down the haughty temper of parents. Then, too, neighbors began to join in a league of friendship mutually desiring neither to do nor suffer harm; and asked for indulgence to children and womankind, when with cries and gestures, they declared in stammering speech that meet it is for all to have mercy on the weak. (pp. 73–74)

As we can see, Lucretius based the development of humanity's noblest sentiments and enduring institutions on the relationship between man and woman: They had children, and their emotional life was enriched. Language developed, and families formed clans, communities, and eventually societies. In 1771, John Millar of Glasgow, in a long-overlooked study, gathered information about the family from the classics and from the writings of seventeenth- and eighteenth-century explorers and missionaries. Millar (1960) argued that emotional and social attachments as well as biological necessity perpetuated the extended unions of men and women that became culturally institutionalized. Sexual passion led to parental affection, and the familiarity that developed over time began to include care in old age. Thus, the life course of the human, with its prolonged childhood and extended senescence, required personal attachments and group cohesion.

To substantiate his arguments, Millar pointed out that some sort of marriage or permanent union between men and women had been established early in prehistory. Some birds and other animals have reasonably monogamous attachments that provide for the care of the very young. For humans, the prolonged helplessness of infancy and the dependency of childhood that allow for learning over time and the transmission of the cultural heritage require protracted care. Two other biological factors that contributed to the development of the family as an institution were the almost 1:1 male-female birth ratio and the necessity to regulate sexual activity to ensure survival of the group.

The central importance of children to the family was emphasized by Millar (1960) who cited Cicero to point out that marriage among the early Romans developed by "use" (i.e., by the man and woman living together for about one year and having children), and the early Greeks married in "the same simple manner" (p. 186). Millar reported that vestiges of what was in his time considered a rather primitive custom could still be found in some parts of northern Scotland, where a marriage could be dissolved after a year and a day if a child had not been born. Cicero's marriage by "use" has been common in many societies, including Jamaica (McLaren, 1992) and also in the middle-class United States in recent years. Are we witnessing reversion?

Some type of divorce was common among preliterate people as well as in modern societies. According to Goodsell (1915), evidence indicates that divorce may be almost as old as marriage itself. Many societies elaborated rules about the status of the divorced wife, the care of the children, and the disposal of property. Often she was required to return to her own people; in some societies, the children were divided between the parents. A wife's adultery or childlessness, for example, has been an acceptable ground for divorce in many societies, possibly in prehistoric groups and certainly in Egypt as long ago as 2000 to 3000 B.C. Divorce was relatively common among the Hebrews, especially in the four to five centuries before Christ.

The Egyptian Family

It is likely that social organization and its institutions began in the Nile valley around 5000 to 10,000 B.C., but Aryan or Mongol groups also may have established societies in ancient Sumeria about the same time. In Western civilization, the Egyptian is the earliest family about which we have a reasonable amount of information. It is surprising that well-known histories give the Egyptian family little attention or overlook it altogether, inasmuch as it is more ancient than the Old Testament family (which is usually cited as a forerunner of the modern family). Numerous Egyptian documents and wall sculptures from as early as about 2700 B.C. attest to the importance of the family. The tombs at the famous pyramid of Sakkara (about 2500 B.C.) contain paintings that show agricultural and other economic activities, fishing, early industrial work, and amiable families.

In the second and third millennia B.C., the Egyptians had large, stable families. Divorce was rare until the era of the decadent dynasties (about 1000 to 300 B.C.). If a husband divorced a wife for a reason other than adultery, he was compelled to give her a substantial share of the family property. Brother–sister marriages were customary even among the common people as late as 200 to 300 B.C. As Durant (1935) explained, "Men married their sisters not because familiarity had bred romance, but because they wished to enjoy the family inheritance, which passed down from mother to daughter" (pp. 164–166).

The status of women in Egypt was much higher than in other societies, according to authorities cited by Durant (1935, p. 164). The great queen Hatshepsut reigned from 1501 to 1479 B.C.; her magnificent tomb on the west bank of the Nile near Luxor is a major tourist attraction. Durant pointed out that the Greeks were amazed at the freedom and status of both married and unmarried Egyptian women, who walked unattended on the streets, ate and drank in public, took part in industry and trade, and bequeathed property in their own names.

It was acceptable to women to take the initiative in courtship, and they spoke openly about sexual affairs. They married at a young age, and "premarital morals were free and easy" (Durant, 1935, p. 166), although adultery was a serious crime. Infanticide was rare; "parents guilty of infanticide were required by law to hold the dead child in their arms for three days and nights" (p. 166). Women's status declined late in Egyptian history—after the Assyrian occupation in the sixth century B.C. and the conquest by Alexander two centuries later—although Cleopatra ruled between 51 and 30 B.C.

In *The Dawn of Conscience*, Breasted (1933) emphasized that the Egyptian family was "the primary influence in the rise and the development of moral ideas" (pp. 116–117) and traced the development of character to about 3000 or 3500 B.C. As early as 2900 B.C., sentiments had extended from the family to the community; one tomb inscription read, "'I gave bread to all the hungry. . . . I speak no lie, for I was one beloved of his father, praised of his mother, excellent in character to his brother, and amiable to [his sister]'" (pp. 123–124). A 2200 B.C. landmark in the development of moral order, about 1,000 years before Mosaic law, is an Egyptian king's writing for his son: "More acceptable is the virtue of the upright man than the ox of him that doth iniquity" (p. 356). Breasted stated that the pharaoh and his priests decreed what was right or wrong, and that gradually such ideas were "humanised and socialised to become a great social force introducing the age of conscience and of character, many centuries later" (p. 42).

Those developments were followed by two other Egyptian "firsts." One, the maxims of Ptahhotep, governor of the city of Memphis and prime minister of the king of Egypt about 2000 B.C., may be a prototype for the Ten Commandments:

> Take to thyself a wife as the heart's mistress;
> Fill her body, clothe her back;
> Make her heart glad as long as thou livest;
> Have children; rear them right; that is correct living;
> Be not avaricious toward thy kin;
> Treat other families as if they were yours;
> Conjugal infidelity means death;
> Never practice the corruption of boys. (Breasted, 1933, p. 133)

Durant considered these maxims to be the oldest work in philosophy, and Breasted (1933) concluded, "The thing which was long called the moral consciousness of mankind has grown up with each generation out of the disciplines and emotions of family life, supplemented by the reflection and teaching of experienced elders" (pp. 133–134).

The other first is the earliest monotheism, dating from between 1362 and 1400 B.C., when Amenhotep III and his son, Ikhnaton, triumphed over the priesthood and established the one God who had "fatherly solicitude" (p. 272) for all cultures and was the source of eternal light. Freud (1939) maintained that monotheism, like paternity, was one of human beings' first great abstractions. Breasted (1933) pointed out the human aspects of Ikhnaton's new religion that Moses would eventually adopt. A statuette has been found that shows Ikhnaton holding his little daughter on his knee and kissing her, and there is a scene on Tutankhamen's famous chair (about 1350 B.C.) that shows him relaxing and Queen Nefertiti touching him with "drops of fragrance" from a perfume jar: "For the first time in the history of art, we have here a scene, the subject of which is *human relationships*, and interpretive art is here dealing with human life as its subject" (p. 295; italics added).

Thus it can be seen that many of the moral and institutional bases for the family have been derived from Egyptian civilization. We speculate that little has been written about the history of the Egyptian family for two reasons. One is that little was known directly about Egypt, relative to the vast amount of information about ancient Greece and Rome, until Napoleon's invasion in 1798 and Champollion's deciphering of the Rosetta stone in 1822. The other is that, in their efforts to assert the primacy of their religions, the Judaic-Christian church fathers deliberately overlooked early Egyptian social organization and institutions. The Egyptian contributions were transmitted to our modern era via classical Greece and Rome. Durant (1935) emphasized that "Greece did not begin civilization. . . . It was the spoiled heir of three millenniums of arts and sciences brought to its cities from the Near East by the fortunes of trade and war. Our own European and American culture derive by a continuous succession through the mediation of Crete and Greece and Rome" (p. 116).

Most information about the history of the family in Western society comes from three major sources. One is the Judeo-Christian tradition described in the Bible. The second is the scholarship of antiquity, especially the myths, histories, philosophies, and drama of classical Greece and Rome. The third is the Anglo-Saxon heritage of the Western family that was passed down through the generations by myth and by saga and later by writings.

EARLY SOCIAL SCIENTISTS' VIEWS OF THE FAMILY

A number of developments early in the nineteenth century stimulated scientific inquiry into the origin of the family. They included the emergence of the social sciences, advances in the biological and physical sciences, and the discovery by archaeologists of "early man." Those developments were succeeded by the stimulus given to scientific inquiry by Darwin's *Origin of Species* in 1859 and the concepts of evolution. Also, the modern idea of progress that had emerged during the Enlightenment surged throughout the nineteenth century and complemented evolutionists' views of the family as a developing institution. For many years in the late nineteenth and early twentieth centuries, scholarly work on the history of the family was pursued by specialists in jurisprudence, anthropology, sociology, and other social sciences.

Opposing views about whether the early family was matriarchal or patriarchal were quickly advanced, and their adherents continued the controversy for decades. It began after the Swiss scholar J. J. Bachofen (1954) published *Das Mutterrecht* (mother-right) in 1861. He maintained that legal evidence indicated the family had been an evolving institution. Early human beings had lived in hordes like gregarious animals, and sexual promiscuity prevailed. Children belonged to the group, and inasmuch as fatherhood could not be determined, descent was reckoned through the females. Consequently, a matriarchal form of social organization was common. In several of his criticized speculative works, such as *Totem and Taboo* (1927), Freud subscribed to the concept of the primal horde and asserted that the development of the concept of paternity was one of humanity's first great abstractions. With domestication of animals and private ownership, eventually the patriarchal family became the dominant type in Western society.

Lewis Henry Morgan (1908), America's first great anthropologist, and John McLennan (1865) supported Bachofen's views about the primal horde early in the development of social organization. Morgan is credited for his pioneering 1830–1860 field studies of Indian groups in North America. To obtain firsthand data, he lived with Indian tribes; the Seneca made him an honorary tribe member to reward him for his legal efforts on their behalf. Morgan theorized that both civilization and the family had developed through three successive but interrelated stages: savagery, with dependence on hunting and gathering; barbarism, with pottery, domesticated animals, and iron tools; and civilization, with the alphabet and writing. Also, he conceptualized five stages in the development of the family, from a promiscuous horde to the "monogamian" family of the nineteenth century. Morgan's schema—the associations between postulated stages of the development of civilization and of the family—is almost panoramic in its scope and obviously has to rely on analogy and inference rather than on facts. But Harris (1968) stated that Morgan's work was unprecedented because it emphasized "movement from systems based on sex and kinship to those based on territoriality and property," included meaningful concepts of family form and kinship terminology and their associations with the technoculture of different periods, and foreshadowed "the role of property in the development of stratified groups" (pp. 182–187). An example of Morgan's (1908) views is that because citizenship in the United States depends on a mixture of territorial and kinship principles, every child born in the country is entitled to U.S. citizenship, and a child of a U.S. citizen is a U.S. citizen wherever he or she is born. Morgan sympathized:

> We should value the great institution of the family, as it now exists, in some proportion to the expenditure of time and of intelligence in its production; and receive it as the richest legacy transmitted to us by ancient society, because it embodies and records the highest results of its varied and prolonged experience. . . . The question at once arises whether this form [the "monogamian" form of the family] can be permanent in the future. The only answer that can be given is, that it [the family] must

advance as society advances, and change as society changes, even as it has done in the past. *It is the creature of the social system, and will reflect its culture.* . . . Should the monogamian family in the distant future fail to answer the requirements of society, assuming the continuous progress of civilization, it is impossible to predict the nature of its successor. (p. 499; italics added)

The fieldwork that Morgan had begun in the 1830s when he lived with various Indian tribes was praised by Marx and Engels. In 1888, after Marx's death, Engels (1972) compiled Marx's notes on the family and added substantially to them, emphasizing that "the determining factor in history is the production and reproduction of immediate life . . . of the production of the means of subsistence, of food, clothing and shelter and the tools requisite there . . . [and of] the production of human beings themselves, the propagation of the species" (p. 8). According to Engels, monogamous marriage developed from matriarchal groups that had lived in communistic fashion with neither ownership nor private property. He agreed with Bachofen that women in such situations must have found the conditions of life oppressive, if not dangerous, and therefore sought to develop permanent relationships. With the domestication of animals and early agriculture, women's labor became increasingly more valuable and, along with increased ownership and private property, men began to accept some type of monogamous relationship. "This advance could not have originated from the men, if only for the reason that they have never—not even to the present day—dreamed of renouncing the pleasures of actual group marriage" (pp. 87–88).

To correlate his cultural-materialist views with the research by Morgan (1908) and Tylor (1958), Engels (1972) postulated that there had been group marriage (such as that described by Caesar in his account of the conquest of Britain) during the savagery period; the pairing family arose during the stage of barbarism; and the monogamous family, along with adultery and prostitution, became dominant with civilization. Engels maintained that ownership and private property led to the concentration of wealth in some men's hands and their wishes to pass the wealth on to their children. To Engels, as well as to Marx, bourgeois marriage in the nineteenth century meant oppression, if not slavery, for most wives. Engels envisioned a bright fourth stage in the development of social organization: the classless society, without private property but with peaceful community living and a single standard for sexuality to ensure monogamy. As Plato had advocated, the care and education of the children would be a public matter. Engels agreed with Morgan that the family would advance as society advanced and also change as society changed. Both of them foresaw progressive changes and viewed history and social development in evolutionary, not cyclic terms.

But opposing views about the origin of the family were put forth quickly by an articulate group. In 1861, the English scholar Henry Maine reported that studies of legal customs showed that the patriarchal was the earliest form of the family, at least in ancient India and early Rome. Maine's most important contribution, according to Harris (1968), was his thesis that kinship was the basic principle of organization of early groups. Maine (1861) envisioned the preeminence of individualism, stating that "the unit of an ancient society was the Family, of a modern society the individual" (p. 121). According to Harris (1968), Maine regarded a family-organized society as being one with fixed status, in contrast to the more individual-organized society, which could be a free-contract society (p. 192). Also, in the family-organized society, property is held in common, whereas in the individual-organized society there is private ownership as well as contracts; Maine's views appear to be some of the fundamentals of Sorokin's (1941) contractual relationships in society.

About the same time, John McLennan (1865) advanced his views about the origin and development of the family, emphasizing totemism, exogamy, and wife capture. He conceptualized the family as developing from a horde that had no marriage rules and considered itself descended from an animal ancestor; according to Harris (1968), this concept was the origin of totemism as we understand it (p. 193). McLennan maintained that the harsh conditions of life experienced by early humans in their struggle for existence were responsible for infanticide (especially of females), for polyandry, and for the capture of wives from neighboring hordes, which led to exogamy (marrying a person from another tribe). Wife capture was described in early Roman literature and has been portrayed often in such great art as Reubens's "Rape of the Sabine Women." Wife capture led to polygyny and the wife purchase that was common in Anglo-Saxon groups until the tenth century; vestiges of it are dowries, bridal gifts from the groom, and in a sense, the now-popular prenuptial agreements. With the recognition of private property, matrilineal descent was replaced by the patrilineal, and as property and power became more centralized, the importance of the tribe and other kinship groupings lessened considerably (Harris, 1968, pp. 194–195).

For many years, the most popular history of the family was Edward Westermarck's (1922) *History of Human Marriage*, which was first published in 1898, revised several times, and presented in an abridged volume in 1922. Westermarck argued vigorously for the evolution of the monogamous, patriarchal nuclear family. He defined marriage as a social institution, a relationship of a man to a woman that is recognized by custom or law and that involves certain rights and duties for those entering into the union and the children born of it. Westermarck maintained that marriage developed out of a "primeval habit, that a man or woman would tend to live together and rear their offspring, in common" (p. 20). Like earlier writers, especially Millar, Westermarck based his opinions on concepts of evolution. He maintained that certain species of birds had monogamous unions and that some male and female anthropoid apes remained together for long periods of time after the birth of the offspring. Thus, there had been evolutionary progression from the "highest monkeys to human beings in which the family consists of the father who was the protector and supporter of the mother and the children" (p. 21). Some of those views about monogamy are being refuted by contemporary research, which indicates that there is little or no validity for the contention that some birds, chimpanzees, and other primates have monogamous relationships. Also, it is perilous to generalize from other species to the human.

The power of male jealousy was another force that, Westermarck (1922) argued, would not allow for female sexual promiscuity. Jealousy could be observed in anthropoid apes as well as among "existing races of men" (p. 21).

> That masculine jealousy is a general human characteristic may be inferred not only from the direct statements of the observers but from the customs or laws concerning adultery, which makes the seducer or the unfaithful wife or both libel for punishment of some sort, inflicted either by the injured husband himself or by the society of which he is a member, or in all events give him the power to divorce his wife. (p. 18)

Also, Westermarck rejected the reckoning of descent through the mother as evidence either of sexual laxity or of a matriarchal period in society. He saw it instead as a natural result of the mother-infant tie and of matrilocal marriage, in which the husband lived with the wife's family.

To support his insistent views of monogamous marriage and to counter notions about an early stage of promiscuity, Westermarck (1922) explained that many of the sexual activities of so-called primitive groups had been misunderstood by Western observers. The apparent prenuptial freedoms that had been observed were not promiscuity but "very frequently a preliminary to the marriage. They may be a regular method of courtship, or they may be a trial before establishing more permanent relationships" (p. 9). Westermarck's views of premarital sexual activities as courtship behavior or as "a trial before establishing more permanent relations" (p. 9) are strikingly similar to sexual relationships in the United States in the 1980s.

Some of Westermarck's arguments for patriarchal marriage have only partial validity. For example, he would have difficulty supporting his contention that jealousy was a masculine attribute not shared equally by women. Westermarck concluded his discussion of the origin of marriage with the assertion that "we may truly say that marriage is rooted in the family rather than the family in marriage" (p. 30). He emphasized that an adult male and female lived together for the benefit of the young and, as Millar (1960) had pointed out, "Sexual relations which happen to lead to pregnancy or the birth of a child are, as a rule, followed by marriage or make marriage compulsory" (p 30).

The views of the original family as being matriarchal or matrilocal that were advanced by Bachofen, Morgan, Engels, and others are again receiving attention. Letty Pogrebin (1983) and Marilyn French (1985) asserted that the domination of institutions, including marriage and the family, by men has resulted in hardship and oppression for women. They, and other feminists, have been citing Briffault's (1927) scholarly but long-neglected masterpiece, *The Mothers*. Briffault's appealing thesis was that the maternal instinct is the fundamental basis for all positive emotions, especially love and caring. The mother's selfless devotion, along with the relatively long dependency of humans, fostered caring and love that gradually developed into romantic love. Such dedication is exemplified by Alceste and Orpheus, as well as by the thirteenth-century troubadours' songs.

ECONOMIC INFLUENCES ON THE ORIGIN OF THE FAMILY

Most authorities on the origin of the family agree that a society's economic basis has been a powerful determinant of its marriage, family, and kinship types. Polygyny is closely associated with the division of society into classes based on wealth; generally, only the wealthier males can afford more than one wife. And polyandry, the rare family type in which two or three men (often brothers) share one wife, is found only in starkly poor, often remote societies. Among the Toda in southern India, the men sharing the same wife are often brothers, and in Tibet and Nepal, where men work as guides or bearers for Himalayan expeditions and are away from home for many months, polyandry can involve one husband's being at home to take care of domestic matters while the other is away. It has been postulated that polyandrous groups have an excess number of male births, but it is more likely that the number of females is limited by infanticide. Obviously, polyandry itself keeps the birth rate low.

The almost 1:1 male-female birth ratio (about 104 male to 100 female births) combined with a slightly higher infant mortality rate in males, strongly favors pair marriage and at least a semblance of monogamy. Also, infanticide, practiced in many poor societies and probably more common in Western societies than we realize, is generally directed toward females. The killing of infant females helps to compensate for the loss of males in war or other violence and to maintain a reasonable male-female parity in numbers.

Since early times, the family has been an economic unit. Our word *economy* is derived from the Greek term for the practical administration of household affairs. A division of labor developed within the family; women began to plant seeds and thus made the stride toward civilization that came with agriculture. Women also are credited with inventing the first primitive household implements, such as the mill for grinding seeds. Children were seen as property, and they often had (and still have) little status. In harsh economic situations, the period of childhood is short; children are expected to care for themselves as soon as they can gather berries or other food. Anthropologists' descriptions of the deprived lives of children in, for example, Tierra del Fuego and the Fiji Islands remind us of the terrible conditions of life for many children in the United States today.

THE FAMILY AND THE INCEST TABOO

Morgan maintained that the realization that inbreeding had negative biological consequences led to the incest taboo (Harris, 1968). In contrast, McLennan (1865) theorized that the incest taboo was socioculturally, not biologically, determined, and his views were supported by such prominent anthropologists and sociologists as Spencer. But it was Edward Tylor (1958), the father of modern anthropology, who emphasized as early as 1881 that there was an obvious link between exogamy and the incest taboo. Tylor stated that exogamist marriages created alliances between groups of early human beings and thus advanced social organization, and he stressed that early human beings had either to "marry-out" or be "killed-out" (Harris, 1968). Levi-Strauss (1985) supports Tylor's thesis: "The incest prohibition succeeded in weaving the web of affinity that sustains societies and without which none could survive" (pp. 54–55). Still another view, which appears to be more secondary than basic, is Westermarck's (1922) insistence that there was a universal dread of incest and an almost instinctual repulsion to sexual relationships with those with whom one has grown up. It is likely that cultural factors and, to a lesser degree, biological factors led to the development of the incest taboo.

According to Harris (1968), Starcke pointed out in 1889 that marriage within the family endangered the father's authority. Both Malinowski (1927) and Murdock (1949) agreed with this viewpoint, which was at the heart of Freud's often-criticized *Totem and Taboo* (1927). Whatever its origin, incest destroys the nonsexual affectional bonds in the family and in most instances, the family itself. Thus, the incest taboo sustains the family. Furthermore, according to Levi-Strauss (1985), "It established an interdependence between biological families and forces them to produce new families; and through these only will the social group succeed in perpetuating itself" (p. 53).

CURRENT VIEWS OF THE ORIGIN OF THE FAMILY

Harris (1968) stated that the lengthy argument between the proponents of the matriarchal and patriarchal origins of the family was

> one of the most heated and useless discussions in the history of the social sciences.... Both groups were wrong, constituting one of those rare cases of diametrically opposed positions about which it is impossible to say that either contained a grain of truth. Descent rules [often used to support views of the origin of the family] ... reflect residence patterns; and residence patterns are primarily a matter of local techno-environmental and techno-economic conditions. (p. 187)

In that spirit, Goodsell (1934) had insisted that "the family has a psychical as well as an industrial basis. Feelings of responsibility and rudimentary affections for dependent offspring created the family, and these feelings, beyond question, have operated in part to maintain it" (p. 15).

Social scientists who attempted to ascertain the origin of the family had only limited information on which to base their opinions. Often, they extrapolated from data gathered by explorers and missionaries on so-called primitive groups in Africa and Polynesia to speculate about the origins of the modern family. Such speculations have questionable validity, however, because observations of various groups' marriage customs and family structure pertain only to the groups studied. Also, there is no evidence that the customs and forms observed represented stages in the development of the modern family. Viewing primitive groups as forerunners of more "advanced" types assumed that those groups were on a relatively low rung on the evolutionary ladder, if one exists. Nevertheless, the extensive field studies showed that there were families in all societies, and they increased knowledge of the family as an institution. The studies were so fruitful that for many years more was known about families in the South Seas than in the United States.

In *The View From Afar*, Claude Levi-Strauss (1985) criticized the evolutionary view of the development of marriage and the family popularized by many social scientists in the latter part of the nineteenth century. Facts accumulated during the last few decades, he argued, indicate that the family appears to be a

> universal phenomenon, present in every type of society. . . . We do not know anything important about the types of social organization that prevailed in the very early stages of the history of humanity. . . . All that can be said . . . is that the conjugal family occurs frequently and that it seems absent, in general, in highly evolved societies and not, as one might have expected, in the most rudimentary and simple ones. (p. 43)

Levi-Strauss (1985) maintained that the previous existence of a society of some type is a prerequisite for the family and that it is unlikely that we will ever know how human beings were first socially organized. Survival probably depended on social organization, of which marriage and family were basic elements. Marriage created bonds between groups; in many ways, it was the means for "exchanging women" (who will produce children) in order to maintain social organization and survival through human interdependence.

Levi-Strauss (1985) concluded that there were only three distinctive characteristics about families that could be stated categorically:

1. The family originates in marriage. (Westermarck saw the opposite sequence.)
2. It includes the husband, the wife, and the children born of their union, forming a nucleus around which other relatives can eventually gather.
3. The members of the family are united among themselves by:
   a. Legal bonds.
   b. Rights and obligations of an economic, religious, or other nature.
   c. A precise framework of sexual rights and prohibitions, and a variable and diversified group of feelings, such as love, affection, respect, fear, and so on. (p. 44)

THE BIOLOGICAL AND SOCIOCULTURAL BASES OF THE FAMILY

Scientific advances have uncovered the biological and sociocultural bases of the family. The biological bases are (a) the sex drive and the need to reproduce; (b) the extended dependency of the human infant and child that requires the care of parents for its survival and that of the species; (c) the almost universal 1:1 male-female birth ratio; and (d) the absence of the estrus period, thus allowing for sexuality throughout the year. All four of these were conducive to permanent attachments. The sociocultural bases include the inherent gregariousness, if not herd instinct, of the human being; the incest taboo, which solidified the family structure; the advantages of kinship; and the need for social ties gained by exogamy to reduce aggression.

George Murdock's (1949) ethnographic study of 250 societies showed that the nuclear family is universal and that, "Nowhere on earth do people live regularly in isolated families" (p. 79). Community organization enhanced chances for survival in many parts of the world and provided social life and group control of behavior as well as protection. Variations in family type, such as polygyny (which reflects affluence) or polyandry (indicative of scarcity), are economically determined. The nuclear family is able to fulfill the essential family functions.

THE THREE ROOTS OF THE MODERN FAMILY

The Classical Root

As we have seen, the family has firm biological and sociocultural bases and, as the oldest institution, apparently was well established in prehistoric times. The development of the modern family, however, was influenced by the social organization that began in Egypt 10,000 to 12,000 years ago when, as Budge (1969) has described, the compression of the people by the encroaching desert and the annual flooding of the river made social organization mandatory for survival in the narrow Nile valley. Contemporary historical research is just beginning to overcome the arrogance and prejudice that were barriers to understanding the influences of the ancient Oriental and Egyptian cultures on our society and its institutions. We can hope that this increasing knowledge will deepen our understanding of the modern nuclear family and, as we shall see, the relationship between the vitality and integrity of the society and the stability and well-being of the family at various times in history.

The Greek Family

The early Greek family was a religious organization. Fustel de Coulanges (1901) emphasized that religion "established marriage and paternal authority, fixed the order of relationship, and consecrated the right of property, and the right of inheritance. This same religion, after having enlarged and extended the family, formed a still larger association, the city . . . from it came all the institutions, as well as the private Law, of the Ancients" (p. 13).

According to Goodsell (1934), in ancient Greece, "marriage was regarded as a contract entered into for 'family ends' and as such was arranged for by the parents with small attention to the preferences of their children" (p. 89). Marriage was a highly esteemed and sacred ceremony that was performed at home, where the domestic god presided. It took place before the "domestic hearth" (p. 44); the Greek word for *family* meant "that which is near our hearth" (p. 42). The ceremony itself consisted of three acts. In the first, at the bride's home, her father gave her away or separated her from the paternal hearth. In the second, the young, veiled woman, preceded by the nuptial torch and accompanied by heralds who sang the hymeneal, was carried to her husband's house; after a feigned struggle, the husband carried her through the doorway with great care so that her feet did not touch the sill. The most sacred part of the ceremony was the third, which consisted of the new husband and wife approaching the hearth, where they shared a wedding cake.

Several of our wedding ceremonies are derived from Greek customs. The groom's carrying the bride over the threshold symbolized her having no rights in her new home until her husband had placed her in it by force (possibly a vestige of wife capture). Also, the modern wedding cake can be traced to the Greek custom of giving each guest a cake made of sesame seeds and honey.

Marriage detached the woman from her family of origin. Thereafter, she belonged entirely to her husband's family and to his religion and worshiped at the sacred fire at his hearth. His authority was based on his being the trustee of the family estate as well as the priest of the domestic worship of his ancestors. As described by Homer, the Greeks traced kinship through males. The early Greek patriarchal family differed from the Hebrew family because, in Greece, the family was the unit of power, whereas the Hebrew father could be likened to an absolute monarch who patterned his family after Jehovah (Goodsell, 1915, p. 79).

Although Greek families were in theory monogamous, concubinage was common, and with the development of Greek civilization in such cities as Athens and Corinth, a class of young women (the hetaerae) were trained to be courtesans. The husband had the right to divorce his wife for barrenness or for adultery. The wife, however, could divorce her husband only if he grossly neglected the family or was cruel to family members. Divorce was looked upon as a family rather than as a state matter.

In 440 B.C., in his famous oration at the funeral for Athenian soldiers who had died in battle early in the Peloponnesian War, Pericles praised the ancestors and the families of the fallen soldiers. He claimed that their ideals, virtues, and traits—passed through successive generations—had been responsible for the greatness of the city with its constitution and democratic way of life. He emphasized the stability of the Athenian family and declared that the parents, widows, and children of the fallen warriors would be supported at public expense (Thucydides, 1954, pp. 143–151).

Greek women, especially in Athens, were considered to be inferior to the men and often were confined to their homes with Oriental strictness. The wife's functions were to bear children and to manage the household. Infanticide, usually by exposure, was sanctioned by law. In *The Republic*, Plato discussed the care and education of children in detail and maintained that women should have the same education, rights, and obligations as men. The position of women in Sparta seems to have been higher than in Athens. Even as late as about 330 B.C., Aristotle (1952) stated that the "male is by nature fitter for command than the female" (p. 453).

Millar (1960) cited an old myth that explained the marriage and social sex roles in Athens and accounted for women's inferior status. After the city was built during the reign of the legendary king, Cecrops, Athena and Poseidon competed for the honor of naming it. Cecrops called a public assembly to determine the winner. As expected, the women favored Athena and the men Poseidon, with the women winning by one vote. Shortly afterward, a tidal wave swept over the city. The inhabitants believed that Poseidon had punished them; to appease the god, it was ruled that children could not be given their mothers' names, and women were not allowed to participate in the public assemblies.

Although Greek wives were accorded few rights, they were not powerless. Significant evidence indicates that by 400 B.C., and especially after the end of the Peloponnesian War, the status of women in Athens improved. In his satiric drama *Lysistrata*, Aristophanes (1987) fantasied an alliance between the Athenian and Spartan women that would bring the internecine Peloponnesian War to an end: The women would not have sexual relations with their husbands until the men opted for peace rather than war. Also, in his late satires, Aristophanes (1917) portrayed the Athenian women as intelligent, courageous, and certainly not powerless. *The Trial of Euripides* described the Athenian women taking over the public assembly for a day and passing laws. Aristophanes's dramas, written less than a century after Pericles' famous oration, depict the decline of both Athenian society and the Greek family.

The Roman Family

Excellent records have supplied descriptions of the Roman family and the immense changes that took place in it between the founding of the city about 750 B.C. to the fall of the Western Empire in A.D. 476. As Maine (1861) showed, in the early years, marriage and divorce were regulated. For about five centuries, until the end of the Punic Wars in 202 B.C., the Roman family, according to Goodsell (1915), was the "most complete example known to history of the patriarchal type" (p. 112). It was a religious, legal, and economic unit under the control of the father, who was the patriarch and priest of the family cult. The home had a sacred hearth fire for ancestor worship. The family often consisted of the husband, wife, children, grandchildren, and slaves. In early Rome, the ideals of family life were "stern, simple and wholesome, although harsh and rigid" (Goodsell, 1915, p. 112). The husband's authority (*patra protestas*), as laid out in the Law of Twelve Tables (450 B.C.), extended even to life and death over his wife and other members of the family. Although the status of the Roman matron was higher than that of the Greek wife, in early Rome she had few rights.

Marriage required formal consent by both parties. The marriage rites were elaborate: The bride was carried in a brilliant procession from her father's home and lifted over the threshold into her husband's house, where she was brought under the hand (*manus*) of her husband to symbolize the sale of the woman to the man. Goodsell (1915) stated that this formality was probably the last relic of purchase marriage in Western civilization (p. 120). Until the end of the Punic Wars in 202 B.C., monogamous marriage was praised as the ideal, although concubinage was recognized. Divorce was one of the husband's rights, but it was a private matter.

The end of the Punic Wars marked a change in the Roman family. The power of women increased greatly during the fifty years the Romans had fought in Italy, Spain, and North Africa. The victory over Carthage enlarged the Roman Empire, and there was an influx of wealth and people. The easy conquest of Greece in 146 B.C. led to the recruitment of Greek scholars and teachers to Rome and to the adoption of many aspects of Greek culture. By the second century B.C., the simplicity and celebrated virtue of the family in Rome's early centuries had given way to complicated property rights and frequent divorce. Increased wealth enabled women to bring dowries to the marriage, and as their wealth and power grew, their social status rose. Fathers began to endow their daughters with money and property for their personal use during marriage. Marriage increasingly became a matter of mutual consent; Goodsell (1915) maintained that by the second century A.D., the Roman matron was largely "a free agent" (p. 133). Also, celibacy increased, and especially in the upper classes, contraception, abortion, and infanticide limited the number of children for whom the women had to care. Divorce increased greatly in the first centuries B.C. and A.D. Marriages were easily contracted and quickly dissolved. Among the rulers, divorce was common; Caesar divorced Pompeia, and Cicero repudiated his wife, Terentia. (Such developments bring to mind the modern CEOs mentioned in Chapter 1.)

The consolidation of the empire in the first and second centuries A.D. was accompanied by many changes in Roman life. Peasants flocked to the cities, which became huge urban centers. From Asia Minor to Britain, wealthy citizens maintained country villas as well as city homes and were cared for by large groups of servants. Churchill (1956) stated that the British people had a higher standard of living in the second and third centuries A.D. under Roman rule than at any time until about 1914.

The literature of the first and second centuries A.D. contains many references to parents turning over the care and education of their children to servants. Marriage and rapid divorce became commonplace, and even the sacred hearth was moved from its central position in the home to a private place (Goodsell, 1915, pp. 146–148). In *Germania*, Tacitus (1911) contrasted the Roman family unfavorably with that of the Germanic tribes, which was characterized by chastity, late age of marriage, and monogamy. Zimmerman (1947) pointed out that by the second century A.D. there were two forms of marriage—the traditional (*dignitas*), and the less binding and presumably less enduring (*concubinitas*). Wives and children of the latter marriages had few legal, property, or other rights.

During the last few centuries of Roman hegemony, a third form— marriage without the transfer of authority (*in sine manu*)—allowed a woman to maintain membership in her father's *familia* and retain her inheritance rights; the husband received only the bride's dowry. Such arrangements led to independent marriages that were arranged not by families but by the man and woman involved. In the upper classes, divorce was so common that according to Seneca, wealthy women recalled dates not by the name of the incumbent consul but by that of a first, second, or succeeding husband (Goodsell, 1915, p. 142). The government took steps to stabilize marriage and the family. Augustan legislation in A.D. 50 rewarded marriage and children, penalized the childless and the unmarried, and emphasized that the family was a social unit that belonged to the state.

Goodsell (1915) compared the status and activities of Roman women during the last centuries of the empire's greatness (from A.D. 200 to 476) to that of American women during the early decades of the twentieth century. In both situations, women sought outlets for their social, intellectual, and political activities, and the decline of marriage and the birthrate among the middle class in Rome was paralleled by a similar decline among the American upper class. Goodsell maintained, however, that social consciousness was at a higher level in the United States than in Rome during its last few centuries.

Much of our information about marriage and the family in Rome refers only to the upper classes. In Volume I of *A History of Private Life*, Veyne et al. (1987) point out that much of the decadence and moral laxity for which the decline of the Roman Empire is noted prevailed mainly in the upper classes. Some evidence indicates that many ordinary citizens, even in the third and fourth centuries A.D., had stable marriages. In some ways, we would regard their sexual activities as conservative; ordinary citizens frowned on nudity, and even in marriage, sexual intercourse was deemed to be a nighttime rather than a daytime activity.

The Judeo-Christian Root

The Hebrew Family

The development of the early Hebrew family is sketched in the Old Testament, especially the Pentateuch and the Book of Ruth. The traditional Hebrew patriarchal family appears to have been preceded by a maternal kinship system. The "generations of Esau" are traced through his wives in Genesis, and Jacob's first wives, Leah and Rachel, are referred to later as the women who "did build the house of Israel" (Ruth 4:11).

The domestication of cattle and the development of agriculture led to private ownership and property rights that, according to Marx, Engels, and others, resulted in paternal kinship and family systems with dominance of the husband/father, who had authority over his wife as well as the children and others in the household. According to Goodsell (1915), in the Talmud, "Women are frequently grouped with slaves and children" (p. 52).

Old Testament marriages were not monogamous. Sarah, Leah, and Rachel gave their personal servants to their husbands as concubines, and David, Solomon, and other leaders between 900 and 1000 B.C., as well as Abraham and Jacob earlier, had many wives. Generally though, polygyny was practiced only by the wealthier men. Although Malachi in the fifth century B.C. praised marital fidelity, Josephus and Justin Martyr reported in the second century A.D. that Jewish law permitted a man to have four or five wives (Goodsell, 1915, pp. 57–58).

The Hebrews regarded marriage and large families highly. The legal age for contracting marriage was puberty—age 12 for females, and 13 for males. The consent of both the man and woman was necessary. Goodsell maintained that in such ancient societies "*families*, not individuals, were in a far truer sense than today the units of society" (Goodsell, 1915, p. 61).

In 600 B.C., the Mosaic law stated that a husband could write a bill of divorcement and give it to his wife if he found "some uncleanness in her" (Deuteronomy 24:1, 2). Over the centuries, divorce changed from being a relatively private concern (as indicated by the "bill of divorcement") to a religious and social act controlled by the religious authorities. In the centuries immediately before Christ, various prophets expressed their disapproval of divorce and especially of the School of Hillel's broad interpretation of the term *uncleanness*, which gave men a great deal of freedom to divorce. In the first few centuries A.D., rabbis tended to disapprove of divorce unless it was on the grounds of adultery, refusal to cohabit for a year or more, refusal to carry out the ritual laws of the household, other wifely deficiencies, leprosy, or barrenness.

Goodsell (1915) concluded that the Hebrew family was

> a school of great moral and social value. Representing as it did a strongly knit organization with well-defined social, religious, economic, and educational functions, the Jewish household offers a contrast little less than startling to our modern individualistic homes, which have long relegated many of these duties to specialized social agencies such as the school, the church and various clubs and organizations for children. (p. 76)

Christianity

By the third century A.D., Christianity was influencing marriage and family life among the Romans. Early Christians regarded sexuality as dangerous, if not sinful; they valued virginity and chastity and praised celibacy. During the first and second centuries A.D., ascetic precepts limited the birthrate of early Christians. Some groups refrained from bathing to dampen sexual appetites, and celibate cults began to grow. But, most early Christians heeded Paul's admonition that "It is better to marry than to burn" (I Corinthians 7:9).

The influence of Christianity on marriage and the family is shown by the declaration of the church fathers (Jerome, Basil, and Chrysostom) that the marital union of a man and a woman was for life. The Christian church denounced abortion and attacked the fairly widespread practice of infanticide. There is controversy about the status of women, but early Christianity recognized the "spiritual equality of women and men" (Goodsell, 1915, p. 163). By the ninth century, marriage in the church rather than at home had become fairly common. But according to Goodsell (1915), even in twelfth century England, the marriage ceremony often was performed in front of the church rather than in it (pp. 188–194).

Jesus opposed the common views of his time when he recognized no right for divorce except adultery (Matthew 5:32). Divorce among Christians in the Roman Empire, however, was permitted as late as the age of Justinian (A.D. 527–565) when one partner wished to enter a monastic order, when the husband had been five years in captivity, or when there was no prospect of having offspring. The church fathers lamented the frequency of divorce. In the ninth century, in the Eastern Empire, divorce was pronounced invalid by Emperor Leo the Philosopher. In the twelfth century, when marriage became a sacrament, divorce was prohibited in western Christendom (Goodsell, 1915, p. 174).

The Anglo-Saxon Root

The third major root of the modern family reaches back to the marriage and family customs of the Teutonic tribes that invaded the Roman Empire in the second and third centuries A.D. and swept over western Europe during the fifth through eighth centuries. In his "Gallic Wars," written about 50 B.C., Caesar described group marriages in British tribes in which a child was considered to be fathered by the man who had first married the woman, although some authorities have questioned the validity of these observations. In the first century A.D., Tacitus praised the strength of the matrimonial bond among the Germans; almost always, one man had only one wife (p. 308). In most Anglo-Saxon groups, the fundamental unit of social organization was the large extended family grouping—the great family, or *sippe*—and until the ninth or tenth centuries A.D., wife purchase was common. Consequently, kinship relationships were important. Kinship was traced through both the mother and the father; a child born out of wedlock had no rights of inheritance.

The Franks and Burgundians had strict laws about marriage and the family. The father was the protector of the family. He could send a son or daughter to a monastery or a convent, but could not sell a child. A child received partial emancipation when he or she came of age. Folk laws and customs allowed for divorce, but it was uncommon because the regulations were elaborate and there was fear of a blood feud with the spouse's relatives or of fines that might be levied. The church, meanwhile, strengthened the regulations against divorce.

During the Middle Ages, the Christian church slowly influenced the age-old established marriage and family customs. Christian doctrines advocated higher status and improved condition of life for both married women and girls and a lessening of the often harsh authority of the husband and father.

The earliest English betrothal ritual extant, which dates to the reign of Eadmund of Aethelstan (about A.D. 900), contained seven provisions:

1. If a man desire to betroth a maiden or a widow, and it so be agreeable to her and her friends, then it is right with the bridegroom, according to the law of God, and according to the customs of the world, first promise and give a "wed" (O.E., pledge or stake) to those who are her "foresprecas," that he desire her in such wise that he will keep her, according to God's law, as a husband shall his wife: and let his friends guarantee that.
2. After that, it is to be known to whom the "fosterlaen" (wine money) belongs: that the bridegroom again give a "wed" for this: and let his friends guarantee it.
3. Then, after that, let the bridegroom declare what he will grant her, in case she choose his will, and what he will grant her, if she live longer than he.
4. If it be so agreed, then it is right that she be entitled to half the property, and to all, if they have children in common, except she again choose a husband.
5. Let him confirm all that which he has promised with a "wed"; and let his friends guarantee that.
6. If they then are agreed in everything, then let the kinsmen take it in hand, and betroth their kinswoman to wife and to a righteous life, to him who desired her, and let him take possession of the "bohr" who has control of the "wed."
7. But if a man desire to lead her out of the land, into another Thane's land, then it will be advisable for her that her friends have

an agreement that no wrong shall be done to her; and if she commit a fault, that they may be nearest in the "bot" if she have not whereof she can make "bot." (Howard, 1904, pp. 269–271)

In addition to wine money for the wedding celebration, the groom gave the bride a *morgengifu* (morning gift) "in case she choose his will"—a present of money the morning after the marriage was consummated (Howard, 1904, p. 271). Also, the wedding contract called for a *weotuma*, a monetary provision for the wife in case her husband died before she did. Between the sixth and ninth centuries, the *withum* (purchase price) began to be paid to the bride rather than to her kinsman, and she was promised the *weotuma* after the death of the husband.

In the first century A.D., in *Germania*, Tacitus described a *beweddung*. He was surprised that the wife did not bring a *dos* or dowry to her husband, but that the husband gave one to the wife. The wife did bring arms (sword, shield, etc.), however, that signified the mysterious *sacra* or the gods of marriage. There is widespread evidence of sale marriage among Teutonic groups in the first few centuries A.D., but by the time of Eadmund at the beginning of the tenth century, the *beweddung* had become merely a "formal contract" (Howard, 1904, p. 268).

The nuptial ceremony consisted of three parts: the solemn gift or tradition of actual giving of the bride to the husband, the joyous bringing home of the bride, and the festal initiation into wedded life in the bridegroom's house (Howard, 1904, pp. 271–272). The *gifta* or tradition was the most important part of the ceremony; the father or guardian acted as a priest or magistrate who surrendered the bride to the husband's protection. On receiving the bride, the bridegroom paid the *weotuma*, delivering the charter providing for the morning gift or for other allowance if she became a widow. The third part of the ceremony consisted of his treading lightly on her foot, which eventually was symbolized by the delivery of a shoe or slipper. The betrothal was of greater legal significance in ancient than modern times (p. 275).

Changes in the ceremony depict the changes in the Anglo-Saxon marriage and family. In the prehistoric era, the betrothal was a binding contract that required both sides to fulfill certain obligations—mainly a payment to the guardian or family of the bride and the delivery of the bride, all of which went hand in hand. In the second stage, from the time of Tacitus in the first century, there was still a real contract, but it was one-sided; the purchase price was paid to the guardian but the "tradition" (sexual intercourse) was postponed until after the wedding. The *weotuma* was given to the bride at the time of the nuptials (it appears to have been an early form of a dower). The *beweddung* was still a contract, but not a contract for sale. Later, nothing was paid and nothing transferred at the betrothal, which consisted of promises and sureties.

In the eleventh century, marriage became freer. The power of the bride's father was weakened, and the woman's consent was necessary for the contract to be binding; still later, the father had only veto power. By 1000, Canute forbade the marriage of a maiden against her will. The contract usually was sealed by a *hand schlag* or hand clasping; the *arrha* was paid to the bride in the form of a ring that we know as the engagement ring. The ring, the bridal wreath, and the bridal veil have Germanic origins (Howard, 1904, p. 278). Howard maintained that, according to Henry Adams, the wedding ring originally was the earnest money that bound the marriage contract. Later, the ring proved that the marriage was a civil contract, "not that women were deprived of rights, but that their rights were secured to them in marriage by the most careful provisions known to early society" (Howard, 1904, p. 280). To some, the ring symbolized the fetters with which captive maids were bound; the exchange of rings was a custom only among the aristocracy and at the court. The kiss at the betrothal was borrowed by the Christians from an older pagan custom and was given legal importance by Constantine: In case one party died before the nuptials, if there had been a kiss at the betrothal, the other party could inherit half the espousal donation. During the twelfth and thirteenth centuries the bride gained the right of self-betrothal and the right of self-*gifta* (i.e., of contracting herself).

THE NUCLEAR FAMILY

Gies and Gies (1987) described the modern family as a direct descendant of the European Middle Ages, the product of the Roman family and society, the Anglo-Saxon "barbarian" clan organization, and the developing Christian religion. They maintained that marked changes in the family had occurred in the thousand years from the fall of Rome to the beginning of the modern era: "Both Romans and barbarians would have found marriage and the family in 1500 radically different from what they had known" (p. 295). The most important change was a reduction in the functions of the family. The influence of the church had grown so that it, not the family, was responsible for religion, and the legal system had developed to the point that justice was not controlled by the families (as it had been during much of the Middle Ages) but was again in the hands of the courts (as it had been in the Roman Empire). Likewise, education passed from the family to the school and the university. The home was the center of industry, however, as well as of family life.

The status of women improved, and a few began to be accepted into the guilds that started in the twelfth and thirteenth centuries. In the thirteenth and fourteenth centuries, the influence of chivalry further improved matters, and during the Renaissance, the status of women rose with the increase in learning and in wealth in western Europe. By the twelfth century, even daily work had begun to be regulated by custom, and the crafts and guilds had established rules. The increasing centralization of power by the new national governments in the fifteenth and sixteenth centuries impinged steadily on family functions. Where the power of the state increased, that of the great family or clan diminished; conversely, where central authority was weak, the clan or kin group exercised power.

The development of the nuclear family was associated with the development of capitalism in the late Middle Ages in northwestern Europe. According to MacFarlane (1986), a selective marriage pattern had developed in England between the tenth and thirteenth centuries. Marriage became optional and did not have strong kinship or class controls, but

> *the one hard and fast rule was that the young couple should be able to form an independent unit at marriage.* . . . Marriage was viewed as something one "saved up for," which one could only "afford" at a certain point. . . . The major purpose of marriage was to satisfy the psychological, sexual, and social needs of the individuals concerned. . . . *To be "married friends" was, for many, the ideal.* Ultimately, therefore, marriage was based on a blending of, or compromise between, economic necessities on the one hand and psychological and biological pressures on the other. . . . The heart of the matter was the deep attachment of one man to one woman. (pp. 321–322; italics added)

Thus, marriage was not "embedded in kinship or status" (p. 322) but became a matter of choice.

Engels (1972) associated capitalism with modern marriage. He maintained that in antiquity and in medieval society, family interests determined marriages, but by the late fifteenth century, capitalism had created a new world:

> By changing all things into commodities, it dissolved all inherited and traditional relations and replaced time hallowed custom and historical right by purchase and sale, by "free" contract. But to make "contracts," people must be "free" and "equal," and hence 'the creation of these "free" and "equal" people was precisely one of the main functions of capitalist production.' (MacFarlane, 1978, p. 325)

Romantic marriage, MacFarlane (1978) agreed, was a "by-product of the rise of capitalistic, contractual and individualistic societies" (p. 325). He quoted Max Weber, who emphasized that the increasing bureaucratic and rational characteristics of Western society had to be balanced by "an impulsive, irrational and non-capitalistic emotion at the level of the individual" (p. 326). MacFarlane (1978) further quoted Gerth and Mills on Weber: "Standing in radical opposition to functionality and rationality is the boundless giving of oneself (in romantic love and marriage) . . . the unique meaning which one creature in his irrationality has for another" (p. 326). MacFarlane pointed out the parallel between purchasing objects in a market and "the desire to completely 'own' or 'possess' another human being. . . . The 'selling' of consumer goods through mass advertising, and the passions between people, are used to reinforce each other. . . . Both romantic love and capitalistic activity are based on individual choice, possession, property and 'free enterprise'" (p. 327).

MacFarlane (1986) stated that Marx and Engels's views about capitalism producing the nuclear family are attractive; however, modern conjugal marriage and the nuclear family system emerged earlier than capitalism. In England, it arose from the tendency for the Germanic people to marry late and to be monogamous, as Tacitus (1975) had described. The bride "enters her husband's home to be the partner of his toils and perils, that both in peace and in war she is to share his suffering and adventures" (MacFarlane, 1986, p. 330). By the thirteenth century, Christianity had greatly reinforced monogamous marriages and the nuclear family.

In the fourteenth century, Anglo-Saxon marriage consisted of four main elements. First, it was based on the mutual consent of the man and woman, a doctrine that was present in the tenth or eleventh century in the Laws of Canute (Howard, 1904, vol. I). Second, marriage was considered second best to celibacy. Third, marriage was "above all to be entered into for companionship's sake, as a partnership of mind and body. . . . The husband-wife bond is the strongest of all relationships; this new contract overrides all the relations of blood—with parents, with siblings, with children—which in many societies are more powerful than the marital relationship. . . . Certainly the companionate view of marriage was accepted formally and informally, by the fourteenth century, and probably before" (MacFarlane, 1986, p. 330). Fourth, love was the basis for marriage.

For many years, numerous writers have maintained that romantic love developed in the twelfth or thirteenth centuries when it began to be celebrated in song by the troubadours in southern Europe. Even Marc Bloch (1962), in his highly regarded two-volume history, *Feudal Society*, held that opinion. But it is difficult to believe that such a strong sentiment as love and the emotional bond between a man and a woman could have developed only a thousand years ago.

Bloch mentioned the "idea of amorous relationships" (MacFarlane, 1986, p. 331) as being new, but 2,000 years earlier Longus wrote about them in the story of Daphnis and Chloe, and passionate as well as spiritual and dedicated love between a man and a woman were prominent features in such Greek dramas as *Alcestis* and *Medea*. MacFarlane cited early Anglo-Saxon and Celtic love poetry and studies by Trevelyan indicating that love matches were common among the peasantry in the Middle Ages but not among the aristocracy, who generally arranged marriages for economic and political purposes. Since the thirteenth century, however, marriage for love has been moving up the social ladder.

The existence of the two-generation nuclear family in England by the fourteenth century is also evidenced by the economic system, which involved children and youth becoming servants, apprentices, or wage laborers. The separation of the children and parents "led to a situation where the family no longer acted as an undivided unit of production and consumption. . . . These separate, nuclear, neolocal patterns appear to have been established quite early, probably becoming widespread by the 14th century, if not long before" (MacFarlane, 1986, pp. 334–335).

MacFarlane raised the interesting point that if capitalism did not produce the modern marriage and family system (as suggested by Malthus, Marx, and Engels), it is possible that "the individualistic family and marriage system, and its consequent 'rational' demographic pattern, was a necessary, if not sufficient cause of capitalism" (p. 335). Thus, the marital system, capitalism, and individualism seemed to come together in England in the twelfth and thirteenth centuries in an extraordinary fit. MacFarlane praised the nuclear family pattern and individualistic philosophy associated with capitalism and the emphasis on equality of the sexes, physical comfort, and responsibility for one's life. But, there were costs, including "the destruction of wider groups and communities, the corrosion of loyalties, the calculative, rational view of life, that 'alienation' which Marx documented, (and) the 'anomie' that Durkheim analysed" (p. 344).

We can see that the views of the history of the nuclear family in Western society that were advanced from the 1930s to the 1960s by such family scholars as Burgess and Nye are being challenged, especially the view that the nuclear family, as represented by the typical American family in the middle of the twentieth century, was largely a product of the Industrial Revolution. Research by the Cambridge Social Science Research Council has supplied data indicating that the Industrial Revolution in Great Britain did not create the modern conjugal family system. According to Wrigley (1977), it was the result of changes in rural society in England even earlier than the fifteenth and sixteenth centuries, and it is quite likely that the Elizabethan Poor Laws of 1603 (which transferred responsibilities from the family or the kin to the parish) were a response to changes in the family unit that had been occurring over a few centuries.

Even before Elizabethan times, the "co-resident family group" in England consisted mainly of husband, wife, children, occasionally a grandparent, and some servants in more affluent families. Men and women married late; the mean age of the first marriage in sixteenth century England probably was in the middle or late 20s, and there is some evidence that late marriage was common even in the fourteenth century. Also, according to McFarlane (1978), Hajnal reported that since at least the sixteenth century, 15% or more of women did not marry. Thus, fertility was determined more by social than by biological factors, inasmuch as there was a gap of 10 years between sexual maturity and marriage. "As Wrigley pointed out, the work of Hajnal and Laslett had suggested in the 1960s 'the possibility that the pre-industrial West European family pattern—late marriage for women, a large proportion of women of child-bearing age remaining unmarried, a separate household at marriage, small households comprising only a single conjugal family—was unique among all traditional societies'" (MacFarlane, 1986, p. 28). Wrigley (1977) concluded that "many features of the 'modern' family have been the norm for many centuries before the Industrial Revolution" (p. 77).

Little change occurred in the structure of the family between Tudor and Victorian times, although mean age at marriage became younger and family size smaller. Thus, it is possible that the existing "complex of marriage and co-residential patterns helped to produce the radical economic changes of the Industrial Revolution" (Wrigley, 1977, p. 77). In preindustrial Europe, family life "spanned virtually the whole range of human activities" (p. 71). The family had a wider range of functions than it does today and was, to a considerable extent, "the chief unit of reproduction, production, consumption, socialization, education, and, in some contexts, religious observance and political action" (p. 72). Often membership in society was attained only through membership in the family.

THE EMOTIONAL BASIS FOR MARRIAGE AND FAMILY

Since the early 1920s, some family scholars have maintained that, in the past, emotional ties in the family were of less significance than in this century, when the companionate marriage emerged as the dominant type. In his widely heralded volume *Centuries of Childhood*, Phillippe Aries (1962) asserted that there had been relatively little emotionality in medieval family life. Later, Lawrence Stone (1973) and Edward Shorter (1975) supported that view. Opinions about restricted affection in the family in earlier times are based mainly on the frequency of arranged marriages in the upper classes and the view, discussed earlier, that romantic love did not flower until the twelfth and thirteenth centuries. More recently, however, Frances Gies and Joseph Gies (1987) pointed to evidence indicating that medieval families had not led impoverished emotional lives:

> A twelfth-century missal of Cahors instructs the priest to "firmly inquire as to the relationship of the couple and whether they love each other... If ... they are in love (and no impediment is found), let them be married." ... Familial affection was present among Romans, Franks, Anglo-Saxons, thirteenth-century English peasants, fifteenth-century Italian merchants, and other members of the large caste of medieval people (pp. 297–298)

Substantial data affirming the significance of emotions as the basis for marriage and family in Elizabethan England are presented in Michael Macdonald's (1981) analysis of Dr. Richard Napier's records of 2,036 medical patients (1,286 females, 748 males) with emotional problems. Napier was an astrological physician who practiced in a small town north of London between 1597 and 1634. The emotional content of the records is reflected by the title of MacDonald's book, *Mystical·Bedlam: Madness, Anxiety, and Healing in 17th-Century England*. Napier's patients came from various social strata. Only 5% belonged to the nobility, and only 20% were a master or mistress; the remaining 70% were farmers, craftsmen, servants, ordinary working people, and paupers. Of the 2,036 with emotional problems, about 800 reported stressful events and circumstances; 23.6% described troubled courtships; 17.6% had marital problems; 17.5% suffered from bereavement; and 12.9% had financial difficulties.

Finding that about 40% had problems stemming from courtship or marriage is seen by MacDonald (1981) as making "nonsense of historians' confident assertions that romantic love was rare in 17th century England, or that it was unimportant in choosing marital partners" (pp. 88–89). Stressful courtships, lovers, quarrels, unrequited love, seduction and rejection, grief, and threatened suicide because of lovers' quarrels indicated that "the young people suffered the unmistakable pains of romantic love" (p. 89).

Most of Napier's married female patients expected affectionate ties with their husbands, but marital problems were common. Wives complained that their husbands were not financially responsible, not sober, physically violent toward them, and unfaithful. There was little that a wife could do to escape her husband's behavior; the patriarchal character of Puritan life kept the status of women low. Obedience and fidelity were major wifely virtues, and wives were financially dependent upon their husbands, who had control of even their wives' inheritances or other properties. The case records also contained poignant accounts of the grief expressed by bereaved spouses. Death ended many marriages prematurely; almost one third of the mental illness episodes among Napier's bereaved patients were precipitated by the death of a spouse.

The Puritans emphasized the importance of marital intimacy. MacDonald (1981) stated that

> the aim of Protestant pamphleteers was to persuade their readers that marriage should be built on a foundation of religious, psychological compatibility. . . . The idea of an emotional autonomous marriage founded on sentiment rather than on economic and social advantage resembled the consensual union of the very poor. Cajoled by Puritan Moralists and pressured by changing economic conditions, the middling and upper strata of society gradually reduced the sizes of their households and embraced the emotional intensity small families fostered. Companionate marriages spread gradually up the social ladder. The ascent, however, was very slow. (p. 98)

MacDonald's (1981) work also showed that the nuclear family, as we know it, was well established by 1600. Such findings support the thesis that the nuclear family emerged in England in the thirteenth or fourteenth century and that husbands and wives, as well as parents and children, depended upon each other for emotional satisfaction (p. 98). MacDonald cited MacFarlane's opinion that the late age of marriage, mobility, and inheritance customs limited kinship ties and increased the importance of the nuclear group.

These case records present valuable data about families in England in the early seventeenth century and about the stresses and strains of everyday life that culminated in illness. The accounts of distress are similar to those that we hear and see today. It has been postulated that parents at that time could not allow themselves to become excessively emotionally invested in their children because of the precariousness of life; the frequent deaths of children and spouses would have produced overwhelming grief. The lack of fifteenth and sixteenth century portraits of children (except occasional royal figures) is cited as evidence for the opinions about limited emotional attachments, but such opinions run counter to common sense. As professionals who work daily with individuals' and families' emotions, it is difficult to believe that those powerful inner forces could have changed significantly within a few hundred years. In the classic Greek dramas, Alceste (who voluntarily sacrificed herself for her husband) is a model of marital love, and Medea's killing of her children was the cruelest vengeance that she could inflict on her unfaithful husband, Jason. From studies in neurobiology and clinical experience, we do not see how human beings could have changed emotionally during the 5,000 years of recorded history. Also, MacDonald's data on the English family around 1600 are applicable to the Anglo-Saxon family type that was brought to Massachusetts by the Pilgrims in 1620 and served as a model for many other colonial families.

From Napier's notes, there are indications that common people had often married for love and had greater freedom than those in either the propertied classes or the nobility. Historians' descriptions of arranged marriages and limited courtships devoid of romance usually depict only what was happening to the nobility and to those in the upper classes; in contrast, marriage for love and companionship was the norm among the common people in sixteenth and seventeenth century England. However, romantic love often was not associated with marriage in the upper classes until the eighteenth or nineteenth centuries. Before then, it was not rare for the man and woman not even to have seen each other until a day or two before the wedding or even the wedding day, and peace treaties frequently included provisions for arranged marriages. The Hapsburgs became notorious for their use of marriage as an instrument of national policy. The proxy marriage in 1500 of Ferdinand and Isabella's daughter, Juana la Loca, of Spain and Philip the Handsome of Burgundy, the future parents of Charles V, included the Burgundian ambassador's going through the ritual with the young bride at her father's court. After the priest conducted the ceremony, she and the ambassador lay down next to each other on her bed, and in the presence of the assembled priests and nobility, he placed his leg over hers to symbolize the consummation of the marriage.

According to de Maulde (1911), the upper-class sixteenth- and seventeenth-century marriage was a business partnership that involved a union of interests and social responsibilities. "To mingle with it love, the absolute, great enthusiasm of heart or intellect, was to lay up for oneself disasters, or at least certain disappointment. No passion can survive the humdrum, the monotony, the dead weight of matrimonial experience, and what marriage can hold against passion?" (Goodsell, 1915, p. 255).

THE REFORMATION AND THE INDUSTRIAL REVOLUTION

With the Reformation, marriage came to be regarded as a civil contract as much as a sacrament. Goodsell (1915) stated that Luther viewed marriage primarily as "a civil matter to be regulated and perhaps celebrated by state authorities" (p. 252). A decisive move of the Catholic Counter-Reformation was the 1545 Council of Trent declaration that to be valid, a marriage had to be celebrated by a priest and noted by two or three witnesses. The declaration was made to prevent the clandestine marriages (e.g., Romeo and Juliet) that had become a problem. Also, the language used in the vow compounded the increasing church-state struggles for control of families and community life. When the vow contained the Latin words *per verba praesenti* ("I take thee," etc.) the marriage was valid; in contrast, when the future tense, *sponsalia per verba de futuro* (I will take thee, etc.), was used, the vow was not binding. So many men declared their marriages invalid on the basis of the wording of the vow that the Swiss legislated against such marital disruptions. In the sixteenth century, Luther stated that "a regular fool's game" had been played with the verbs (Goodsell, 1915, pp. 246–248).

Thus, in the sixteenth and seventeenth centuries, Protestantism as well as Catholicism emphasized the importance of the family. Luther stated that "God established three hierarchies—the state, the Church and the family—and the family was the basis of the other two. . . . Family government is the basis of all other governments and . . . parents should appreciate profoundly the responsibility resting upon them, 'to train up their offspring for society and the church'" (Goodsell, 1915, p. 283).

Cottage industry flourished in England until the late 1700s. In his celebrated 1748 tour of Great Britain, Daniel Defoe described the land as being "divided into small enclosures from two acres to six or seven each. . . . We could see at every House a Tenter and on almost every Tenter a Piece of Cloth, Kersie or Shalloon which are the three Articles of this countries Labour. At every considerable House was a manufactory" (Goodsell, 1915, Vol. III, pp. 137–139). Defoe saw women and children carding or spinning and men working at the looms or at the dye vats. Families raised grain and vegetables on their small plots and manufactured cloth at home, usually on commission.

The Industrial Revolution had a major effect on the family. The improvement of the shuttle by John Kay in 1738 and the invention of the spinning jenny by Hargraves in 1767 marked its beginning, but even in the late 1690s, groups of 10 to 20 men and women were being employed as weavers or cloth manufacturers in the cities. Throughout the eighteenth century, there was an increasing migration of people from the countryside to the cities that Goldsmith (1909) described in the poignant lines of "The Deserted Village." The invention of power machinery in the early 1800s led to the development of the factory system in England and in the United States. By 1805 to 1810, early psychiatric epidemiologists noted a high prevalence of mental illness in certain London boroughs or districts. Only a century after Goldsmith, in the 1840s, Dickens (1958) described the terrible working conditions in the sweatshops and the ghastly distress of the slums of the English cities, and Wordsworth (1850) described "the close and overcrowded haunts of cities where the human heart is sick." In England, by the mid-nineteenth century, Wrigley (1977) declared: "Life contained uncertainties far greater even than those forced upon agricultural societies by the vagaries of weather and harvest. Both mortality and fertility rates were high and in the newly industrialized cities the dependence on wages for survival produced massive uncertainty" (pp. 81–82). A network of relatives and friends was needed to provide a buffer against disaster.

Family life for the poor deteriorated as many women and children were recruited for work in the new factories, where they could be hired at lower wages than men. The resulting social evils were described as late as the 1870s by Karl Marx. In England, the form of employment called "the family system" was especially pernicious: Mother, father, and children (including those aged 4 or 5) worked in factories at starvation wages, obviously to the detriment of the family and to the health of all. Tuberculosis and alcoholism became terrible scourges. Goodsell (1915) cited Gibbins's *Industry in England*:

> "A curious inversion of the proper order of things was seen in the domestic economy of the victims of the cheap labor system, for women and girls were superseding men in manufacturing labour, and, in consequence, their husbands had often to attend, in a shiftless, slovenly fashion, to those household duties which mothers and daughters hard at work in the factories were unable to fulfill. Worse still, mothers and fathers in some cases lived upon the killing labour of their little children, by letting them out to hire to manufacturers who found them cheaper than their parents" (p. 423).

Between 1841 and 1891, the percentage of women working in textile factories increased 221%, in contrast to only 5% for men. The appalling conditions in England existed until World War I, when women's wages increased; the dreadful poverty seen by Shaw and other social critics was alleviated somewhat by the rise of the unions and the Labor party's coming to power in the 1920s. But the Great Depression led to many families having to go on the dole in the 1930s, to subsist on little more than bread, margarine, and tea.

THE EARLY AMERICAN FAMILY

The type of family that was brought to North America by seventeenth century British settlers was a strong, often self-sufficient unit that had developed over the course of five centuries along with individualism and capitalism. The Puritan fathers believed in faith, family, and firmness. Community control of behavior supported the monogamanian family, and the Protestant ethic prized thrift, work, finance, and fidelity. The early women settlers worked with their husbands to clear the land, build cabins, and defend against the attacks of hostile Indians.

Firsthand accounts indicate that the arduous work done by the women during the settling of the English colonies resulted in some loosening of their traditional inferior status. In the seventeenth century, the status of women in the American colonies was higher than in England, even though the prevailing English common law gave women few legal rights. According to Goodsell (1915), in the colonies a man was not permitted to beat his wife, although he was permitted to do so in England (p. 348). Also, the scarcity of white women, especially in the Virginia colony, led to their being held in high esteem. In the early 1970s, a radio program described the discovery of a gravestone in a remote tidewater area in eastern Virginia. The words on the stone were: "Here lies the body of my wife. She set her foot upon this continent and the wilderness became a home."

Marriage was a civil contract for most of the British settlers. Large families were desirable in view of the vastness of the land and the scarcity of the population; bachelors were considered selfish and sometimes were taxed at a higher rate than married men. Attitudes toward marriage differed in the various colonies. In Puritan New England, the father was the absolute authority. In Pennsylvania, William Penn's liberal policies prevailed, and in Maryland, the first Roman Catholic colony, there was recognition of both religious and civil marriages. In Virginia, the law upheld the Church of England's views of marriage. By the time of the American Revolution, however, in many colonies there was increasing tolerance and recognition of civil marriages.

Family life emphasized work. The women and children, as well as the men, worked at weaving, repairing, and farming. According to Goodsell (1915), "The colonial family restricted its education of the young very largely to moral, religious and industrial training, relegating such intellectual education as was deemed fitting to dame school, the town, church or private school, and, in the Southern colonies, to tutors brought in from the mother country" (p. 404). In the South, the plantation became a relatively self-sufficient economic unit. The wife/mother generally was the overseer for the household workers and slaves and also was in charge of the health of the family members and of the slaves.

There was a steady emigration, mainly of the poor, from England to the American colonies in the early 1700s, and later in the century the so-called Scotch-Irish emigrated following the unsuccessful military attempts of the Stuarts to regain the British throne. Many young British boys came to America as indentured servants; they worked, usually on farms or plantations, for 7 years to repay the cost of their voyage to America. Criminals, prostitutes, and other undesirables often were given the choice between going to America or to prison; some were not given a choice, but were simply deported. The increasing number of poor and "the dregs of humanity" that were coming to America alarmed Benjamin Franklin, who as early as 1759 feared that they would have a deleterious influence on life in the colonies.

Early in the nineteenth century, many young unmarried women (but only a small number of married women) worked in factories, mainly in New England. But, as Calhoun (1917-1919) explained, the Civil War resulted in many women beginning to work in factories in the North and also in Richmond, Virginia, and other Southern cities. The highly romanticized life of women in the antebellum South evaporated during and after the Civil War. By the 1880s, many women in the North and the East were working in the sweatshops and industries of the new large urban centers. In the mill towns of the Carolinas, work in the cotton mills paid so little that pellagra was epidemic, and the conditions of life were those described by Erskine Caldwell in *Tobacco Road* and *God's Little Acre*. According to Goodsell (1915), in 1900, one fifth of the women employed in the cotton mills were married or widowed. The widespread acceptance of child labor in the factories may have stemmed from—or perhaps just was rationalized by—the Puritans' views of idleness as a grave sin. Goodsell cited an English woman's 1829 reproach: "In your manufacturing districts you have children worked for 12 hours a day . . . and you will soon have them as in England, *worked to death*" (p. 426).

But the nineteenth century saw some social progress. By the end of the century, laws provided protection for working women in Great Britain. In the United States, women began to obtain some legal and property rights. In both England and the United States, educational opportunities were extended to women. In 1848, Queen's College in London was opened to offer higher education for English women, and in 1862, a limited number of women were admitted to the University of Cambridge. In the United States, girls were first admitted to public schools in Boston in 1822; in the Midwest, Oberlin admitted women in 1833. Mount Holyoke Seminary for Women was opened in 1837, and after the Civil War, a number of women's colleges were founded.

Divorce laws and practices differed in the various colonies. In the 1700s, divorce was sanctioned in New England, where civil marriage was deeply rooted (Goodsell, 1915, p. 377). In the middle Atlantic colonies, the attitude toward divorce was conservative, and in the southern colonies, divorces or legal separations were rare. Divorce laws became more liberal during the nineteenth century than in the past, but still varied from state to state.

Phillippe Aries (1977) maintained that three major developments during the nineteenth and twentieth centuries had produced changes in the family. One was political and involved the increasing state scrutiny and control over many aspects of everyday life. The second was economic: the "division of space" or the separation of work and living areas. The third was psychological, as attitudes, emotions, and feelings that formerly had been directed toward church figures, family, nature, and the community became more specifically focused on the immediate family. Consequently, the family tended to be removed from the community and to become increasingly more private.

In preindustrial Europe, the family had been a less important determinant of the individual's fate than the community. "The role of the family was to strengthen the authority of the head of the household, without threatening the stability of his relationship with the community" (Aries, 1977, p. 228). In the nineteenth century, before the automobile "conquered space," such neighborhood meeting places as cafes, pubs, coffeehouses, and the parish church played vital roles in the lives of the inhabitants. During the twentieth century, however, there has been a marked decline of the socializing function of the city that has affected family life. With the increase in population, crowding in the cities, and the mass production of automobiles, middle-class inhabitants moved to suburbs to have more attractive living quarters. The spread of suburbia was at the expense of the cities, which became densely packed during the day but empty and dangerous at night. Aries concluded that the deterioration of urban life and its loss of vitality in the last few decades has been paralleled by an overexpansion of family roles and functions that has produced family strain.

By the early decades of this century, the American family showed evidence of the maladjustment that will be described in Chapter 3. The prevalence of divorce, the increase in desertion, and the effects of industrialization and urbanization on the family were evidence of its precarious condition. Goodsell (1915) stated that "it is a far cry from the closely knit, highly unified family organization of the ancient Romans or the Middle-Age Teutons to the more loosely organized household of modern times wherein each member tends to claim independence as an individual with a personality to be developed and respected" (p. 456).

In his comprehensive *Family and Civilization*, Zimmerman (1947) described three family types: the trustee, the domestic, and the atomistic. The trustee family was too decentralized and "localistic" to function significantly in a great civilization. The domestic family was the one that made the greatest contributions to civilization; it provided a fairly stable social structure and yet freed the individual for creative work. The transition period, when the domestic was changing to the atomistic family, often was one of great creativity because there was stability and also a loosening of dogma. The atomistic family, however, was too individualistic and fragmented to contribute significantly to the society and its culture.

According to Zimmerman, questions about the family and its future arise when the atomistic family is the dominant type. The great Greek philosophers' speculations about the family coincided with atomism in Greece (p. 802). In Rome, historians reported massive family decay in the third century. At about the same time, the church fathers "finally concluded that the trouble lay in the decay of human character. The Greeks perceived the relation between family and civilization only dimly; the Church Fathers saw the connection far more clearly" (p. 802). Zimmerman attributed the cyclic history of great civilizations to changes in the family. He associated the greatness of the Renaissance to the stability of the family that had been developing in the eleventh and twelfth centuries in western Europe, and he credited the humanitarianism of Roman society for adopting the "ethical documents of Christianity" that humanized the trustee family of the barbarian invaders (p. 803).

Zimmerman (1947) asked whether only a major change in the law or the development of a new religion could stop the decay of a civilization. He gave Solon's laws (c. 600 B.C.) credit for resolving the many problems of the preceding century and for the greatness of Athens during the next two. Analogously, Christian doctrines probably sustained Roman civilization for an additional two centuries and transmitted it across the Dark Ages to the medieval period. In drawing a parallel between those examples and our family crisis, Zimmerman expressed concern abut the then-current fascination with popularity and style and the avoidance of the "real issues." He insisted that "the forces of both rejuvenation and decay are well armed. . . . We are again in one of those periods of family decay in which civilization is suffering internally from the lack of a basic belief in the forces which make it work" (p. 805). In accord with the rapid change in Western society, the family is

> already so completely atomized that it produces no stable social body in which to solidify. Its human products, children, are not sufficient to reproduce the society of which it is a part. Its psychological product, the human stuff of society . . . seems insufficient to give the society a workable, stable moral code widely enough accepted to enable the great society to hold together. (p. 806)

Zimmerman advocated "a recreated conception of familism and its basic meaning to society. . . . The making of familism and child-bearing [are] the primary social duties of the citizen. This will have to be voluntary—not compulsory. The solution will prove to be not in *fides* alone but in the strong unit of *proles-fides* children and familism" (p. 810).

THE BLACK FAMILY

The uniquely tragic history of the black family in the United States requires special attention. A discussion of it is complicated by the terrible history of slavery and the biases about it. Apologists maintain that many of the problems of the black family during the past few decades are a continuation of problems basic to the social organization of the blacks in Africa prior to their being captured or purchased. They attribute the high rates of illegitimate births, teenage pregnancies, and single-parent households with absent fathers to their opinion that the black family in Africa had existed only in a "primitive form." It has even been averred that slavery was a necessary stage for the development of black social organization. Also, slavery was rationalized on the basis that it had been practiced and approved by the authorities in the Old Testament, and that slavery was needed to Christianize the blacks. The support that some Christian churches gave to slavery and the conditions of life for slaves is a despicable chapter in church history.

In contrast, there is a mountain of evidence indicating that slave traders and the white slaveholders did everything possible to eradicate the slaves' African heritage. According to Adams (1971), Elkins analogized slavery in the United States before the Civil War with the Nazi concentration camps during World War II. In both cases, the oppressors' actions often led to the victims' viewing each other through the master's eyes. The master disciplined, and the slave adopted the role of the child who respected the master and, in some instances, identified with him. Such identification with the captor or with the aggressor leads to mistrust of or cruelty to one's fellows rather than the needed meaningful relationships. Personal relationships were tenuous among the slaves because they usually were sold one or more times, their conditions of life were horrible, and their struggle for survival had dire emotional consequences.

There is a dearth of information about the black family in Africa prior to slavery, and many misconceptions and distortions about it during the slavery years. Most slaves came from West Africa, about which little was known until the middle of the nineteenth century, even though the young Scottish surgeon Mungo Park explored the Gambia and Niger rivers in the mid-1790s and died there on his second expedition in 1806. Park, who "is the outstanding name in the early European exploration of inland West Africa" (Lupton, 1979, p. xxii) hoped to explore the length of the Niger River. Park's (1800) *Travels, in the Interior of Africa* is a classic.

According to Lupton (1979), Park "agreed that Africans 'are not to be considered as an uncivilized race.' He rejected any notion of their living, as the pro-slavery writers maintained, in lawless savagery, rife with witchcraft . . . or cannibalism . . . or nakedness. . . . 'The author found . . . what has been found in all countries, a mixture of good and evil'" (p. 113). Park reported that African societies lived under moral codes just as people did in other countries. Life for most Africans offered limited opportunities, but "it was lived out in an intelligible, dignified, and humane way . . . and for the women in particular he had nothing but praise: ' . . . I found them uniformly kind and compassionate. . . . The Negroes of these districts are not to be considered as an uncivilized race; they have religion, established governments, laws, schools, commerce, manufactures, *wars!*'" (pp. 112–113; italics added). Lupton considered that Park's "greatest single achievement was to get across convincingly that between Africans and Europeans no difference existed 'in the genuine sympathies and characteristic feelings of our common nature'" (p. 114).

Park's book became a best seller; it was interpreted variably by British groups favoring and those opposing the slave trade. Park's young life and adventures had a tragic ending. In 1806, at age 35, on his second expedition to the Niger, his party was decimated by disease and the last few of them, including Park, drowned after their boat struck rocks while trying to escape from hostile natives. In 1827, his younger son, Thomas, died in West Africa while searching for information about his father.

In *Democracy in America*, the first comprehensive study of our social and political institutions, Alexis de Tocqueville (1945) presented his analysis of the society in the early 1830s when he visited the United States as a French government official. He expressed special concern about the divisions between the three races inhabiting the country. Those of European descent were superior, whereas for "the two unhappy races, the Indians and the Negroes, [the] only resemblance lies in their misfortunes. . . . Both suffer from tyranny" (p. 344). He emphasized the degradation, described later by DuBois and Frazier, that the slaves had endured: "Oppression has at one stroke deprived the descendents of the Africans of almost all the privileges of humanity" (p. 344).

Early Christianity had suppressed slavery, de Tocqueville noted, but it had been reestablished by the Christians "as an exception, indeed, to their social system" by the nineteenth century. Slavery was a calamity, "the most formidable of all the ills that threaten the future of the Union" (p. 370). Prejudice and racism would be perpetuated, he foresaw, because "the real inequity . . . is always succeeded by an imaginary inequality that is implanted in the manners of the people. . . . Slavery recedes, but the prejudice to which it has given birth is immovable" (pp. 371, 373).

In the North, de Tocqueville noted that although the Negroes were free, there was no intermarriage, and the schools, hospitals, churches, and even the cemeteries were segregated. He recounted meeting an elderly white slaveholder in the South who had lived illicitly with one of his Negresses and had several children by her. He wanted to free their children and bequeath some property to them but had to overcome legal obstacles for years to do so. He told de Tocqueville that he was now close to death and was in anguish because "he pictured to himself his sons dragged from market to market and passing from the authority of a parent to the rod of a stranger" (p. 396).

In America, de Tocqueville saw the condition of slaves as "not far removed from that of the brutes" (p. 388), and the legislation in the southern states as perverting the laws of humanity: "The Ancients kept the bodies of their slaves in bondage, but placed no restraint upon the mind . . . (whereas southerners) have forbidden them . . . to be taught to read or write" (p. 395). He contended that the influence of slavery "affects the character of the master" (p. 378) and that the slavery in the South involved three prejudices: "that of the whites, that of the slaves, and that of color." He concluded that the events taking place in the South "appear to me to be at once the most horrible and most natural results of slavery. . . . I see the order of nature overthrown. . . . I hear the cry of humanity. . . . I reserve my execration for those who, after a thousand years of freedom, brought back slavery into the world once more" (p. 397). His observations portray the tragedy of slavery in unforgettable words and have validity—he was a noted French historian and was in a position to be objective.

In 1891, English author William Clowes (1970) was commissioned by the *London Times* to report on black America. He found "a state of affairs that is without parallel in the history of modern civilization, and which is, no doubt, destined to exercise a momentous, and possibly a terrible influence upon the future of America" (p. viii). He described the history of slavery and reconstruction, cited examples of white tyranny, emphasized the excess mortality among the "coloured," and deplored the moral conditions evidenced by the few Negro families that were "legally married." He quoted black ministers' railings against the many divorces.

Clowes (1970) agreed that blacks had made considerable educational progress in the 25 years since the end of the Civil War. Also, he recognized the "ignorance [that] was imposed by law upon the slaves . . . [by] the South Carolinian statute of 1834: 'If any person shall hereafter teach any slave to read or write, or procure any slave to be taught to read or write, such person, if a free white person, shall be fined not exceeding one hundred dollars for each offence and imprisonment not less than six months'" (pp. 116–117). Notwithstanding such handicaps, by 1890 almost 50% of the Negro population of 4,358,000 in the south was literate.

Clowes (1970) viewed the racial problem in the United states pessimistically. He noted that the "half-breed of the south . . . is no more the friend of the black than he is of the white" (p. 213). Thus, he saw the problem of marginality that Park (1950) and Stonequist (1937) would describe in the 1920s. Clowes concluded that the Americans owed the Negroes an immense debt but that white prejudice would persist. The solution was a separate nation: "Only when the Negro shall have departed will the name of the United States truly represent anything more than a magnificent aspiration" (p. 214).

In his classic *The Negro American Family*, W. E. B. Du Bois (1908) stated that it was "exceedingly difficult and puzzling to know just where to find the broken thread of African and American social history" (p. 9). Available information was contradictory: "It is difficult to get a clear picture of the family relations of slaves, between the Southern apologist and his picture of cabin life with idyllic devotion and careless toil, and that of the abolitionist with his tale of family disruption and cruelty, adultery and illegitimate mulattoes" (p. 9). He cited Ratzel's comments on West Africa, that "marriage is concluded by purchase. . . . A man's wealth is measured by the number of his wives. Polygamy is usual whenever there are means to support it" (p. 10). In his *History of the Yoruba*, Ellis described some groups in which the girls were betrothed as "mere children" (Du Bois, 1908, p. 13), but the marriage was not consummated until they were pubertal. Antenuptial chastity was important; in many groups, family relationships were traced through the female line. Du Bois quoted Ellis:

> When we consider the extraordinary vitality the system of descent through mothers possesses . . . it seems probable that the acknowledgement of a father's blood-relationship to his children was brought about by the intercourse of the northern Yorubas with the Mohammedan tribes. . . . It is no doubt in consequence of the change from kinship in the female line to

kinship on both sides of the house that the family has become, to a certain extent, disintegrated. (pp. 14–15)

In Africa, parental affection was strong; the tie between the mother and the children was stronger than that between the father and the children. In some families, certain aspects of ancient Roman law could be found, as the wives, children, and servants were under the power of the *paterfamilias*. In most of the tribes, adultery was infrequent and divorce rare, complicated by "the business thread which runs through the band of wedlock" (Du Bois, 1908, p. 15) and appearance before a tribunal. According to Du Bois, during the slavery years (from 1619 to 1863) the law recognized some "*quasi* family rights—forbidding . . . in some cases, the separation of mothers and very young infants . . . [but] the great body of field hands were raped of their own sex customs and provided with no binding new ones. Slavery gave the monogamic family ideal to slaves but it compelled and desired the most imperfect practice of its most ordinary morals" (pp. 21–22).

Three main features of slavery were no legal marriage, no legal family, and no legal control over the children. Du Bois quoted slave laws as follows:

> A slave cannot even contract matrimony. . . . A slave had never maintained an action against a violator of his bed. . . . No slave can commit bigamy because the law knows no more of the marriage of slaves than of the marriage of brutes. . . . No law exists [except in Louisiana] to prevent the violent separation of parents from their children, or even from each other. . . . Slaves may be sold and transferred . . . without any statutory restrictions, as to the separation of parents and children (except in Louisiana). (p. 22)

Some descriptions of the separation of mothers from their children are searing. In 1835, the Presbyterian Synod of Kentucky asserted: "Brothers and sisters, parents and children, husband and wife, are torn asunder and committed to see each other no more. These acts are daily occurring in the midst of us. The shrieks and agony often witnessed on such occasions proclaim, with a trumpet, the iniquity of our system" (p. 25).

The white masters and sons' sexual exploitation of their female slaves is well documented. Du Bois noted President Madison's sister's statement that "we Southern ladies are complimented with the name of wives; but we are only the mistresses of seraglios" (p. 25). Evidence of slave breeding is shown by the census data. In 1850 there were 405,751 mulattos, and in 1860 there were 588,352. Unbelievably, in his *History of Slavery in Virginia*, Ballagh defended slave breeding because it prevented continued importation of slaves, which was cheaper (Du Bois, 1908, p. 26).

In 1908, Du Bois emphasized the progress as well as the problems of blacks since the Civil War. In the South, only bad housing was available to blacks. During slavery, the slave dwellings were so poor that the conditions necessary for family life were absent or deficient. Against overwhelming odds, however, the black family had made some progress. A 1900 study of housing in Atlanta revealed that there was severe crowding; about 35% of black families lived in homes of one or two rooms. In 1890, in the southern states, about 55% of black males and females were married, a percentage close to that of whites. The excess number of females that resulted from the black males' high mortality rate, though, was responsible for the "sexual immorality [that] is probably the greatest single plague spot among Negro Americans, and its greatest cause is slavery and the present utter disregard of a black woman's virtue and self-respect, both in law court and custom in the South" (p. 41).

Du Bois (1908) concluded his historic work with the question: "Judging from family life and other conditions, how far, is it fair to conclude, has the Negro American emerged into twentieth century civilization?" (p. 151). In 1900, 10.7% of Caucasians were illiterate, 46.5% owned homes, and about 2% of births were illegitimate; the comparable figures among blacks were 44.5%, 28.3%, and 25%, respectively.

The pioneer social worker and founder of Hull House, Jane Addams, spoke at the end of the 13th annual Conference for the Study of the Negro Problem at Atlanta University on May 26, 1908. She emphasized that many among such immigrant groups as the Italians had retained the folkways of their ancestors for many years. But, "I take it, your difficulties are quite unlike that. The habits that you might have had from your ancestors were all broken into, they were all scattered, and especially the habits connected with family life" (Du Bois, 1908, p. 152). An advantage would be that the past would not hinder adaptation, but the disadvantages were primarily that "you lack some of the restraints of the traditions which the people I have mentioned bring with them" (Du Bois, 1908, p. 152). Reverend E. L. Henderson, the Episcopal archdeacon of the diocese, ended the conference with an expression of concern: "What is home without a father? . . . If there would be further transitions from ignorance, poverty, and moral darkness to enlightenment, thrift, industry, and improvement of the individuals and the Negro family, the Church and the Home must unite in a more vigorous warfare to reduce to a minimum the prevailing evil of divorce" (Du Bois, 1908, pp. 152–153).

A third classic early study, following those of Mungo Park and W. E.

B. Du Bois was E. Franklin Frazier's (1966) *The Negro Family in the United States*, first published in 1939. Frazier described the heritage of "forgotten memories of Africa and the lack of a 'social organization to sustain whatever ideas and conceptions of life the Negro slave might have retained of his African heritage'" (p. 23). Slavery stripped the African-American of his cultural heritage and exposed him and her to the attitudes and sentiments of the dominant white masters and mistresses. Thus, the slave, who had been dehumanized in the slave caravans in Africa and during the terrible middle passage, "acquired a new personality on American soil. . . . The Negro mother remained the most dependable and important figure in the family" (p. 41).

According to Frazier (1966), the exploitation of the blacks for lust and breeding included "a traffic in mulatto women especially for prostitution [that] became a part of the regular slave trade in Southern cities" (p. 64). White masters who became attached to their "colored mistresses" (p. 60) often were considered to be mentally ill. Heirs-at-law attempted to define as insane the white men who bequeathed estates to their "colored mistresses and mulatto children" (p. 75).

After the Civil War, the Negro family generally followed one of two courses. Those that were fairly well organized during slavery made the transition without significant disruption, especially when the father's authority was established and the "woman in the role of mother and wife fitted into the pattern of the patriarchal household" (p. 106). The other course was followed by those who had been held together by loose ties or only nominal marriages; many of the men cut their family ties and wandered about the country, and the deserted women were "responsible for the maintenance of the family group. . . . Thus motherhood outside of institutional control was accepted by a large group of Negro women with an attitude of resignation as if it were nature's decree" (p. 107).

According to Frazier (1966), the black family was established on an institutional basis first by the Negroes who had been free before the Civil War. They provided a model for the ex-slaves, many of whom stayed on their plantations after the war and worked under an indentured system as sharecroppers for their former masters. Emancipation had brought only limited freedom; ex-slaves could not vote and were bound in "serf-like" fashion to the land because of their limited economic opportunities, but they did have freedom to move about. Many Negro families and large numbers of "roving men and homeless women" left the plantations to live in the cities of the South. During World War I, at least a half million Negroes left the South to work in such Northern cities as Chicago, Detroit, and New York. Frazier termed the migration "the flight from feudal America" (p. 291). Unfortunately, the migrants overwhelmed the already deteriorated slum areas, and "family desertion" increased greatly (p. 341).

Frazier (1966) described the Negroes' development of their own institutions after emancipation and their consolidation of a folk culture, even though the masses were "illiterate and propertyless [and] forced to become croppers and tenants under a modified plantation system" (p. 483). The urbanization after 1900 had produced the most tremendous changes in the Negro's family life since emancipation. But modern urban civilization along with economic disadvantage increased family disorganization, although there was some occupational differentiation and the development of a small black middle class. When those in lower socioeconomic status had regular work in industry, the family structure tended to become stronger, and the father became the responsible head of the family. Frazier feared, however, that "the travail of civilization is not yet ended" (p. 487). He was concerned about the crowding of migrant blacks into the urban centers that was occurring, and he deplored the destructive forces of urban life that disrupted families, increased illegitimacy and crime, and often left the families poverty-stricken. Frazier concluded that the "process of assimilation and acculturation" had been proceeding but that it "will be limited by the extent to which the Negro becomes integrated into the economic organization and participates in the life of the community" (p. 488).

"Race relations" began to receive the attention of sociologists in the 1920s, as evidenced by the work of Robert Ezra Park (1950) and Everett Stonequist (1937) on marginality. Gunnar Myrdal (1944) presented a survey of race relations and emphasized that caste, not class, was at the heart of the serious racial difficulties affecting the United States. He considered the biracial system pathological inasmuch as it affected the personalities of both blacks and whites adversely (pp. 461–462). Lynchings epitomized the ghastly brutalities.

During and after World War II, black ghettoization continued at an accelerated rate, especially in the cities of the North and East. By the mid-1950s, in New York, sections of Harlem were "off-limits" to whites, and during the 1960s, the overcrowded slums of Chicago and other major cities were crime-ridden areas where drug wars and gang battles were waged openly. Moynihan (1965) declared that the United States was "approaching a new crisis in race relationships" (p. i). The fundamental problem was the family structure: "The Negro family in the urban ghettos is crumbling. . . . So long as this situation persists, the cycle of poverty and disadvantage will continue to repeat itself" (p. i). The quality of life in the Negro community had been deteriorating and the black-white gap was widening.

The root of the problem, according to Glazer, was American slavery, which was "'the most awful the world has ever known'" (Moynihan, 1965, p. 15). Tannenbaum had described the differences between slavery in Brazil and the United States. In Brazil, the legal traditions based on Roman law and the Napoleonic Code gave the slave "a place as a human being in the hierarchy of society. . . . In contrast, there was nothing in the tradition of English law or Protestant theology which could accommodate to the fact of human bondage—the slaves were therefore reduced to the status of chattels" (p. 15).

Moynihan described a "tangle of pathology" as well as a cycle of disadvantage. The pathology included the frequent reversal of the husband-wife roles and prominent matriarchal features, the lesser educational attainments of the black males compared to females, the economic dependence of many black men upon women, and the absence of the father from the home. Other major pathologies were delinquency, crime, drug use/abuse, and alienation. Moynihan concluded that the serious problem that included lack of employment and educational opportunities might be "out of control" (p. 47). He called for "a national effort toward the problems of Negro Americans (that) must be directed toward the question of family structure. The object should be to strengthen the Negro family so as to enable it to raise and support its members as do other families" (p. 47).

The view of the black family as matricentric has been disputed by some authorities. In 1966, Rainwater pointed out that many white as well as black lower-class families are matrifocal, especially when compared with middle-class families. Generally, in lower-class families, the wife makes most of the decisions, keeps the family going, looks to female relatives for support and counsel, and does not consider the husband as being interested in everyday problems. But Rainwater insisted that those matrifocal characteristics are determined more by social class than by race (Adams, 1971, p. 122).

In contrast, Billingsley emphasized that racial discrimination produces the problems of the black family and of blacks as a minority in a white-dominated society. But, black families have considerable strengths and "act as a buffer against the debilitating effects of white racism and discrimination. It is the strength of the black family and its social network which makes possible upward mobility and stable relationships among the majority of blacks in a society calculated at every turn to hold these individuals down and to weaken relationships" (Adams, 1971, p. 128).

Adams stated that the problem for blacks in America is different from the problems encountered by European immigrant groups that became incorporated into the wider society over two or three generations. In contrast to those immigrants, the blacks, *"after incorporating much of the dominant culture, have not been allowed into the dominant society"* (p. 130). He concluded that the majority of black families are nuclear family units, that the black family has serious problems but is also a resource, and that many of "the crucial issues revolve around white attitudes and behavior" (p. 130).

Collins (1985) pointed out that the often widely held view of the black family as having many problems (e.g., broken homes, the cycle of poverty, illegitimacy, delinquency, unemployment, and living on welfare) is somewhat faulty. He criticized Moynihan for emphasizing that weakness of the black family structure was the central problem, that the broken homes, absent fathers, and power wielded by the women led to boys' developing a low self-concept and consequent low school achievement, high school dropout rates, delinquency, and unemployment. Collins emphasized that such a view "overlooks the large number of black families that do not fit the stereotype" (p. 85), noting that more than 60% of all black families have two parents in the home and 80% of adult black men support their households. The most important factor appears to be social class, and specifically lower socioeconomic status for many blacks. Wilson (1978) argued that increasing numbers of blacks were moving into government and corporate positions and that "Moynihan mistook a social class problem for a problem of black culture" (p. 86).

According to Collins (1985), some barriers to discrimination had been broken down, and the major problem for the black population was its low social class position. Also, the black community was split between the affluent and the poor and uneducated, the disadvantaged underclass that constituted one third of the black population. Collins cited Wilson's view that Moynihan had mistakenly seen the problem as one of the black culture rather than of social class. C. V. Willie, a black sociologist, insisted that racial discrimination was a continuing problem, arguing that blacks were paid about 15% to 20% less than white persons in equivalent positions even when matched for education and occupation.

A significant fact for the family in the 1990s is that the gap between white and black family incomes increased during the 1980s. Phillips (1990) reported that in 1987, the income of the typical black family was $18,098, about 56% of that of a typical white family—the lowest comparative percentage since the 1960s" (p. 207). Also the income gap between the upper- and lower-class black families had increased, and "'income inequality is now significantly greater among black families than among white families'. . . . The unskilled and uneducated underclass was coming undone, but sociologists could legitimately point to 'the first secure generation of middle-class blacks'" (p. 207).

Among middle-class blacks, Collins (1985) maintained that "distortions in employment patterns owing to discrimination—the role of the black woman and her earnings often exceed those of the male—are played out in family relationships" (p. 87). In contrast to the white upper-middle-class family in which the father's career is of paramount significance, the black family is required to work together as an economic unit in order to achieve middle-class status. Collins cited Willie: "The affluent black family has held together more firmly than the comparable white family . . . [but] both adults and children of such [black] families pay a price in subordinating their individualism and spontaneity to their achievement" (p. 87). It appears that racial discrimination has produced cohesion for middle- and upper-middle-class black families; cohesive black middle-class families have been termed "affluent conformists" (p. 89). Collins reported that studies as early as 1945 showed that black working-class families were much more like black middle-class families than their white counterparts. In *The Mark of Oppression*, Kardiner and Ovesey (1962) emphasized the strivings of many blacks for middle-class status and the resulting stress disorders, especially peptic ulcer and hypertension.

There are continuing arguments about the relative significance of the effects of discrimination and poverty on the black family. Demos (1990) reviewed 283 data-based articles on black families that were in the *Journal of Marriage and Family* from 1939 to 1987. The "culture of poverty" thesis, which minimizes the effects of racial discrimination, was a frequent topic in the 1960s, but the percentage of articles devoted to it in the 1980s decreased greatly. Demos raised questions about possible methodological biases influencing family studies; there are many more quantitative than qualitative studies, even though the qualitative have greater exploratory power.

Collins (1985) discussed the effects of black female power in the family. Many social and behavioral scientists have expressed concern about the female-headed family not being able to provide adequate role models for the children, particularly the boys, and studies have shown associations among broken homes, female-headed households, poverty, and juvenile delinquency, although definite cause-and-effect relationships have not been established. Collins pointed out that females tend to have more power in lower- than in middle-class white and black families, but "black women rate themselves as having more power than white women, and black husbands attribute more power to their wives than white husbands do" (p. 88). According to Collins, female dominance in the lower-class families probably helped hold those families together. The black women carved out "a protected sphere for themselves as women in a world of chronic poverty and under the threat of considerable male violence" (p. 91).

The comparative marital status of white and nonwhite women during the past few decades deserves further comment. In 1950, 82% of white women were married and had a husband present in the home, in contrast to 66% of black women of the same age. By 1979, the percentages had dropped for both, but to a much greater extent for blacks than whites; the percentage of women aged 25 to 44, married, and with a husband present in the home was 77% for whites, but down for blacks to only 45%. The percentage of never-married white women aged 25 to 44 years was 10% in 1950 and also in 1979, whereas that percentage rose for blacks from 9% in 1950 to 23% in 1979 (p. 91). Although blacks used to marry at a younger age than whites, since about 1950 they had been waiting longer than whites. Blacks had a higher divorce rate than whites, and more blacks than whites never married. Collins stated: "The female-headed lower-class black family of today represents a *relatively recent type of family structure.* . . . Black women may simply be less willing to enter into marriages from which they derive so little" (pp. 92–93).

Collins concluded his discussion by emphasizing that recent black family trends have been followed by similar trends in the white family. In the 1950s, black women were delaying marriage even as white women were marrying at the youngest age in this century; in recent decades, however, white women, too, have been delaying marriage. Also, higher divorce rates, avoidance of marriage, and "deliberate illegitimacy" are more common in the white community than previously. He noted Scanzoni's 1977 suggestion that "black marriages may represent the image of the future for everyone" (p. 93).

Hampson, Beavers, and Hulgus's (1990) recent study of cross-ethnic family differences that assessed interactions in white, black, and Mexican-American families found three distinct types of black families: (a) the matriarchal, (b) the egalitarian two-parent, and (c) the patriarchal-affluent. Their results suggested that healthy black families, compared to the white and the Mexican-American families, were less verbally explicit, generally expressed a warm feeling tone, discouraged dependency in their offspring, and were apt to include extended kin or nonrelated individuals in the nuclear family unit.

Lewis and Looney (1983) replicated the research on family competence in volunteer upper-middle-class white families described by Lewis, Beavers, Gossett, and Phillips (1976) by studying 18 working-class black families. They hypothesized that the most competent working-class black families would be rigid and that their organizational structure would be characterized by a dominant parent, usually the mother, who would be the core of the family's strength. But the results of their study showed that "the most competent working-class black families are much more like than different from the most competent middle- and upper-middle-class white families studied 12 years earlier. The parents share power and together provide effective leadership for the family" (p. 100).

The chronic recession of the early 1990s was accompanied by a heightening of racial tensions. Widespread unemployment in the cities of America (especially for minority youths), black males' terrible homicide rate, and unrest erupted as a flow of red-hot problems on the surface of an already worried, weary society. The Bush-Quayle administration insisted that the main cause of the distress, and even the violence in Los Angeles in 1991, was the social programs of the 1960s. There was a renewal of the arguments about whether the family, especially the black family, was responsible for such problems. Despite the glossy appeal of this opinion, clearer voices asserted that the problems were twofold: (a) lack of economic opportunities and secure jobs for many of the poor, especially minority youths and males, and (b) racial discrimination. William Raspberry (1992) insisted that violence was widespread because it was the only behavior that boosted the self-esteem of the deprived and demoralized inner-city inhabitants, and because it was profitable. Relief for the situation could be furnished by providing jobs and housing that would strengthen the black family's efforts to increase educational and social opportunities for its members.

CONCLUDING REMARKS

We have looked at the history of the family not just as a chronicle of events and customs but as a way to deepen our understanding of the American family at the end of the twentieth century. From the past, we have seen the rise and decline of great civilizations, notably ancient Egypt, classical Greece, and the grandeur of Rome. At their height, the foundation of each was a social order based on strong domestic family units. The decline of those civilizations was paralleled by a corresponding instability of the family. Whether one preceded the other or whether there were cause-and-effect relationships are complex questions for which there are a few opinions, but no simple answers. But ignoring the lessons of history is a special type of ignorance; it substitutes the pretense that "it cannot happen to us" for the fact that no civilization has escaped the cycle of history—growth and vitality have been succeeded by decline and fall. Studies have revealed what appear to have been some of the constituent forces of decline. They included militarism and war, unrestrained drives for power and wealth accompanied by greed and corruption, increasing inequality of income and property, and the growth of secularism at the expense of religion, all of which have been accompanied by family disruption.

What is our destiny? As Spengler (1929) intimated, can we accept our fate, enjoy the autumnal pleasures, and hope that the new civilization that succeeds ours will be wiser and more enduring? Or will we be saved from the inevitable cycle of decay by the vitality of an ethic or of resurgent Christianity, as Toynbee (1934) hoped? But we need to stop and think: Will a Phoenix arise from the ashes of nuclear destruction? Will any life be possible? Why have we squandered our wealth and jeopardized our children's as well as our nation's health? Perhaps more in-depth studies of the family will bring at least partial answers. In Chapter 3, we look in detail at the American family during the past 100 years in order to trace the development of conditions and problems that culminated in the crisis described in Chapter 1.

CHAPTER 3

A Century of Concern

> Perhaps the characteristic of the twentieth-century family that most sharply challenges the attention of the student of family history is its instability.
> —Goodsell (1915, p. 456)

Many of the concerns about the family described in Chapter 1 have mounted during the past century. In 1889, Commissioner of Labor Carroll D. Wright shocked the nation with his report that the number of divorces had increased from 10,000 in 1867 to 25,000 in 1886, a rise of 157% compared to the population increase of 100% from 1870 to 1890 (Ellwood, 1910). Ellwood stated: "Already in 1885, this country had more divorces than all the rest of the Christian civilized world put together" (p. 114). By the 1880s, desertion and divorce in the cities were major social problems. The first family organization, the National Divorce Reform League (later called the National League for the Protection of the Family) was the forerunner of some current family organizations.

BACKGROUND: THE LATE NINETEENTH CENTURY

Charles Pearson (1894) described the changes in family life resulting from desertion and emigration, the increasing role of the state in the control of children, the increase in women's rights, the industrialization that enabled women to find jobs to support themselves, and a weakening of religious sanctions. He feared that there would be a diminution of filial piety and dilution of family bonds. "Individualism is bound to gain as family obligations are weakened . . . [the drastic changes will produce] a decay of character" (p. 267).

Changes in the stability of the family have profound implications for society. According to general living systems theory, the family is positioned hierarchically above the level of the individual and just below that of the community. Inasmuch as one of the main functions of the family is the socialization of the young, parental influences determine a child's character and thereby the nature of the society in which he or she will live.

The society-family-individual interactions and influences have been recognized for at least 2,500 years. Parallels between the vitality of the society and the quality of the family were emphasized by Tacitus (1975) when he described the increasing moral laxity of Roman life in the first century A.D. and contrasted it unfavorably with the strength and virtue of the encroaching Germanic tribes. About 1,500 years later, the Puritans emphasized the relationships between the family and the state and the necessity for each to be disciplined, firmly governed, and principled, inasmuch as the well-being of one depended on the well-being of the other. A look at the history of Western society over 2,500 years reveals that if the current flood of pessimistic reports about the family has validity, it is reason for concern because of its far-reaching consequences.

A necessary question is why concerns about the family in Western society became so prominent in the last few decades of the nineteenth century. Some plausible answers are that the rapid social and cultural changes—the stream of inventions and innovations—were changing ways of life. The development of sanitation in the 1860s and 1870s and the concurrent discoveries in bacteriology and parasitology led to safe drinking water. Pasteurization and plumbing were followed by the emergence of hospital medicine and advances in the medical sciences, and life expectancy increased. The invention of the railroads and steam-powered vessels earlier in the century had increased the movement of peoples from more populated to less populated areas. The telegraph, which had been invented in the 1840s, and the telephone, invented in the 1870s, brought words and voices closer even as persons became more distant. The continued development of electricity, public transportation, and even the bicycle changed everyday life in the 1870s and 1880s.

Discoveries in the applied sciences and inventions were accompanied by rapid developments in the natural sciences and the growth of the new social sciences. Darwin's *Origin of Species* in 1859 marked, as its opponents foresaw, the spread of new attitudes toward both human beings and the heavens. Concepts of evolution included convictions about the inevitability of progress that had been enunciated a century earlier by Adam Smith, Condercet, Hume, and others. Traditions and institutions were attacked as reactionary, just as older scientific beliefs were shown to be useless and were discarded. As noted in Chapter 2, social scientists argued for decades about the origins of the family, even though little was known about it because it occurred in the foggy millennia of prehistory. Also, they examined the relation of the human being to society and looked for sociocultural influences on health and illness (both medical and social). In 1897, Durkheim's use of national statistics to reveal the anomic and alienative causes of suicide became a model study for social scientists. Intellectual traditions and the nineteenth century bourgeois aesthetics as well as customs became obsolete as modernity developed from its Schopenhauerian roots and the political transformations following the revolutions of 1848. The *fin de siècle* included both the optimism of the evolutionists and the pessimism of those who saw cynicism, anomie, decadence, and the limits of form in a world that was rapidly entering the era of relativity and uncertainty.

The developments in the sciences and changes in attitudes affected connections and relations within the family and, more profoundly, its structure and the institutional foundations. As the mysteries of life and the universe were unveiled by science, faith in the omnipotence of God weakened. The shoots of secularism grew while the trunks of religion withered or split into flimsy branches. Einstein's 1905 announcement of the theory of relativity tolled the death knell for Newton's *De Principia* and the scientific standards used by Western society since the 1690s. It foreshadowed the uncertainty principle that was to be outlined by Nils Bohr in 1927 and, after the horrors of the first half of the twentieth century, the "God is dead" thesis of the 1950s and 1960s that had first been pronounced by Jean Paul during the Enlightenment. The most immediate problem for the family in the 1880s and 1890s, however, was the rampant growth of capitalism, with its industrialization, urbanization, and class structure based exclusively on wealth. Although the growing middle class benefited, the exploitation of the poor and the impoverishment of the working class often was accompanied by deplorable conditions of work and a degraded family life.

The rush of concern about the American family in the early decades of this century contained many references to the turmoil of the 1890s.[1] The excesses of the unbridled capitalism of the 1870s and 1880s, the exploitation of immigrants and the poor, the slaughter of the Indians and the buffalo, and the accumulation of wealth by the new "captains of

---

[1] Evidence of concern about the family in the early decades of the century is reflected by the dates of the publication of the three most comprehensive histories of the family in English, those by Howard (1904), Goodsell (1915), and Calhoun (1917–1919). Also, what is apparently the first book on the black family, *The Negro American Family* by W. E. B. Du Bois, was published in 1908.

industry" led to widespread economic difficulties and the panic of 1893. Laborers, farmers, miners, and other workers gathered to form a new populist movement. Early labor unions struggled to be born, and the "Wobblies" (the International Workers of the World) attempted to organize workers in industrialized nations in order to counter the massive exploitation of people and, in the USA, of natural resources and the national treasury.

It is no accident of history that those events coincided with the "closing of the frontier" described by Frederick Jackson Turner (1920) in his 1896 presidential address to the American Historical Society. The United States had reached its continental boundaries; the good land and easily obtainable resources had been claimed and often wastefully exhausted. Internal unrest was manifested by a wave of strikes, the repression of unions (and sometimes murder of union organizers), crowding in the cities, and poverty on the farmlands as well as in the new and congested urban areas. On occasion, troops were used to control mobs and to patrol the streets, as well as to break strikes. The domestic turmoil became somewhat quieter only after the turn of the century when, as William Appleman Williams has described, the United States turned to a new frontier in Latin America. The Spanish-American War, probably instigated by this country and popularized by the Hearst and other newspapers, opened vast new areas and underprivileged populations to Yankee development and commercialization—often by force. The resulting externalization of aggression provided a needed safety valve for the release of tensions in the US, but some damage had been done as the turmoil of the 1890s reverberated throughout society, shook and loosened basic institutions, and stimulated a century of concern about the family.

In 1873, Marx (1952) described the terrible crowding, even of the rural population, in England: "Adult persons of both sexes, married and unmarried, are huddled together in single small sleeping rooms . . . and morality almost of necessity must suffer" (p. 754). He cited Hunter's public health investigation of 5,375 agricultural laborers' cottages of which 2,195 had only one bedroom: "Great depression and sometimes death are the lot of the female participation in the offence of incest. . . . They live like pigs, great boys and girls, mother and father all sleeping in one room in many instances" (p. 326). This massive distress of the poor and the degradation of family life by poverty, exploitation, and prostitution is documented in Marcus's (1966a, b) *The Other Victorians* and in that masterpiece of pornography, *My Secret Life*. In a review of *My Secret Life*, J. H. Plumb (1967) expressed outrage at the middle- and upper-middle-class masters and sons' preying on the helpless servant girls. The hypocrisy of the era, especially of late nineteenth-century English family life, is reflected by the efflorescence of pornography in London and its tales of incest and sadomasochism as well as promiscuity and prostitution.

Conditions had scarcely improved when Jack London (1904) presented an especially disturbing account of the deleterious effects of urbanization and poverty upon families in his long neglected classic, *The People of the Abyss*. In 1902, while waiting for an assignment as a journalist to South Africa during the Boer War, he "went down into the underworld of London with an attitude of mind which I best liken to that of the explorer" (p. vii) and lived there for a number of weeks. He described the poverty in words and photographs. At best, family life was mere existence; at worst, it was degradation. "When a father and mother live with three or four children in a room where the children take turn about in sitting up to drive the rats away from the sleepers, when those children never have enough to eat and are preyed on and made miserable and weak by swarming vermin, the sort of men and women the survivors will make can readily be imagined" (p. 277).

The outlook for the children was hopeless; they had no home life. One boy stated: "'at ten we 'ops the wag; at thirteen we nicks things; an' at sixteen we bashes the copper' which is to say, at ten they play truant, at thirteen steal, and at sixteen are sufficiently developed hooligans to smash the policeman" (p. 220). The women were slaves of their overworked husbands, who "become caricatures of what physical men ought to be. The men work long hours in miserable conditions and express their frustration, when possible, by drinking and often by wife-beating. The wives become screaming harridans or broken-spirited, doglike, lose what little decency and the self-respect they have remaining over from their maiden days and all sink together, unheedingly in their degradation and dirt" (pp. 223–224). Suicide was an everyday occurrence (p. 230).

London's book was a catalogue of human misery that included crowding, homelessness, the effects of alcoholism, "the wail of hunger," and the precariousness of life among the 25 to 30 percent of the 1,800,000 people in London who lived on or below the poverty line. He expressed concern about the materialistic nature of the society that was evidenced by the extension of the rights of property at the expense of the rights of the person. "To pound one's wife to a jelly and break a few of her ribs is a trivial offense . . . [and] the lad who steals a few pears from a wealthy railway corporation is a greater menace to society than the young brute who commits an unprovoked assault upon an old man over seventy years of age" (p. 186).

In the United States, Byington's (1910) study of families in a small steel mill city showed that family life was hard. The men worked long hours and for low wages. Deprivation as well as lack of family interaction and recreation had a debilitating effect on the family, and Byington concluded that in such circumstances industrialization diminished family solidarity.

THE TURN OF THE CENTURY AND THE EARLY 1900s

From our perspective near the end of the twentieth century, we can see that concerns about the family have been prominent in each decade of this century. Concerns stemmed from seven major sources. The most obvious were the changes in material culture and the inventions that were altering everyday ways of living. Others were the drastic social and economic change associated with industrialization, capitalism, and urbanization; women's struggle for rights, if not equality; growing individualism that increased the already existing tension between it and familism; the decline in religion which heralded the loss of the institutional basis for marriage and the family; the increasing power and everyday influence of the state; and the effects of wars.

The linkages between the family and society and the influences of events on the family are illustrated dramatically by a brief look at the effects of war. The American Civil War had four major impacts. First, it allowed the black family to emerge. Second, it, like the Punic Wars in the third century B.C., changed traditional roles. According to Calhoun (1918), the Civil War "had a great disturbing influence on the traditional functions of the sexes" (p. 375). Women went to the war as nurses in both the North and the South and practically "took over" work in the factories and war industries, often at lower wages than the men. Also, some women began to be admitted to the professional schools, especially in medicine. Third, the war speeded up women's long struggle for equality, which had begun in the 1690s with Mary Astell's (1970) pleas for their greater educational opportunities. Fourth, migration to the West and to the cities increased. Also, the war was blamed for increased juvenile delinquency, a loosening of sexual mores, and "immoralities." Calhoun (1918) concluded that "the Civil War helped to usher in the new era of city industrialism so pregnant with menace to the integrity of the family" (p. 366).

These interrelated sources of concern were described by family scholars during the decades of the twentieth century; they varied mainly in emphasis. As early as 1906, in her Barnard College lectures, Elsie

Clewes Parsons (1906) deplored the disintegration of family life. She attributed it to economic developments that entailed production outside the home, migration that loosened family ties, advances in science that weakened religion and custom, and the spirit of individualism that "undermined marital and paternal privilege" (p. 355). She feared the adaptations required by the complexity of the environment were producing juvenile delinquency. In view of the increased number of divorces and of the "legal causes for divorce" (pp. 330–331), she advocated reform of divorce laws to provide for two types of divorce—easy ones for couples without children and more formidable processes when there were children—in the hope that the simple divorces would encourage voluntarily childless marriages for those "not capable of prolonged monogamy" (p. 351). Also, she offered the radical suggestion that trial marriage be encouraged.

The 1909 third annual meeting of the American Sociological Association was devoted to the family. Sumner (1909) emphasized that even in primitive society, the family "became the arena in which folkways were formed and taught, traditions were handed down, myths were invented and sympathies were cultivated" (pp. 579–580). He pointed out that "the family has to a great extent lost its position as a conservative institution and *has become a field for social change*. . . . The changes in social and political philosophy have lowered the family. . . . [The parents] have constantly new problems to meet. They do not fear change and they do not shrink from it. So long as their own character is not corrupted it does not appear that there is any cause for alarm" (p. 591; italics added). Thus, Sumner recognized that the family was an institution that was linked to other institutions, a part of society and subject to its changes and influences.

Ellwood (1910) declared that "the Nineteenth century was . . . a great period of social change and unrest. Family life at the beginning of the Twentieth century [is] in a more unstable condition than it has been at any time since the beginning of the Christian era" (p. 113). In England, Helen Bosanquet (1906) extolled family life but expressed worries about the disintegration of the family "as a result of the loss of its economic foundations, child labor, the wreckage of the towns, crowding, and alcoholism" (pp. 220–240). Thus, she attributed changes in the family to changes in society.

Novelists, poets, and painters described the conditions of life. In 1910, in his great novel, *Howards End*, E. M. Forster wrote about the dulling effect of the new row houses and apartments on the middle class in London. To Forster, the new flats were colorless and impersonal, if not dehumanizing, and did not allow the home and the family to have the connectedness needed by human beings to give life richness and meaning.

In the United States, Chicago became the site of intensive study and research on the family. The University of Chicago, founded in 1892, developed world-famous academic departments. The city soon became the largest in the Midwest; people from farms and small towns of the Midwest and blacks from the rural South flocked to it for jobs, especially during the late 1880s and 1890s when the rural and mining areas were hard hit by depressions. A wave of immigrants swelled the population of the city that Carl Sandberg (1916) called the "Hog Butcher . . . Tool Maker, Stacker of Wheat, Player with Railroads and the Nation's Freight Handler" (p. 3). By the end of the first decade of this century, industrialization had yielded benefits but produced problems. Urbanization and the ills of crowding were exerting a centrifugal force on the family.

In the second decade, Willystine Goodsell (1915) described the difficulties of family life in the congested urban areas and the increases in divorce and desertion: "The social interaction of the ages abounds in reference to this instability of the modern family organization and foretells its extinction, at least in its present form. We are told that monogamic marriage is doomed" (p. 457). Goodsell expressed concern about the divorce and desertion and the "effect of modern industry in disintegrating the family" (p. 457). He feared the solidarity of the American family was being undermined by child labor, exploitation of women by industry, the growth of tenements, and the poverty resulting from irregular seasonal employment.

From 1890 to 1915 there were continuing concerns about the declining marriage and birth rates in the cities where women were being employed in factories (Goodsell, 1915, p. 481). The financial disasters of the 1890s were blamed for changes in the marriage rate, and family scholars attributed the declining birthrate in the middle and upper classes to voluntary restriction as a result of economic pressures, health problems, and the "unfavorable conditions of modern city life" (p. 495). The acceptance of Darwinian concepts of evolution and the new science of genetics led to the popularity of eugenics and to fears that the declining birthrate among the advantaged would mean a loss of leadership and even a lowering of intelligence in the future.

Reforms were demanded by radicals and moderate progressives and opposed by conservatives. Arguments between the two groups about marriage and the family pivoted on the liberalization of the divorce laws. Supporters of more liberal laws insisted that divorce was only a remedy, not the disease. But their opponents declared that although divorce might be the remedy for the individual, it could entail "sufferings of the social body" (Goodsell, 1915, p. 539).

The radicals, supported by social critics and dramatists, advocated women's rights and equality. They demanded realism and the ripping away of the Victorian veneer and the sentimentalized Edwardian superficialities that concealed the widespread poverty and exploitation. In 1908, H. G. Wells declared "women and children, just as much as men and things, must cease to be owned" (p. 59). In 1913, in *The Quintessence of Ibsenism,* Shaw called for women to repudiate their inferior status and their duties in order to obtain freedom. Critics of equality for women contended that it would eventuate in the acceptance and practice of free marriage and/or a sort of serial polygamy. Economic concerns were fundamental; opponents to the suffragettes feared that the professions would be open to women and that the wages of men and women would be "equal." But feminists such as Charlotte Perkins Gilman emphasized the need for women to work outside the home for "the sake of self-expression" as well as financial independence.

> In 1913, she described the desirable apartment-home of the future: The apartments would be without kitchens; but there would be a kitchen belonging to the house from which meals could be served to families in their rooms, or in a common dining room as preferred. It would be a home where the cleaning would be done by efficient workers, not hired separately by the families, but engaged by the manager of the establishment; and a roof-garden, day nursery, and kindergarten, under well trained professional nurses and teachers, would insure proper care of the children. . . . [Children who were brought up in nurseries by experts would learn the] peaceful lessons of equality and common interest instead of the feverish personality of the isolated one-baby household, or the innumerable tyrannies and extractions, the forced submissions and exclusions, of the nursery full of brothers and sisters of widely differing ages and powers. (Goodsell, 1915, pp. 516–517)

Such changes in everyday life, especially in child rearing, would eliminate domesticity and transform the family in ways that can only be imagined. But the notions of serial polygamy, the apartment-home of the future, and child care advanced early in this century appear strikingly modern in light of the extensive homelessness and ghettoization and the problems of divorce, child support, and child care that have been so prominent since 1980.

In contrast to the radicals' calls for women's rights and other reforms, the conservatives defended the status quo. Among their foremost arguments was that in many Christian religions, monogamous marriage was a divine institution, and that marriage was a religious and social rite as well as a contractual agreement. Another was that a child had a need for a right to have a mother and a father. According to Goodsell (1915), Foerster insisted that from a bio-sociological perspective, the paramount consideration for the individual, the family, and society was the woman's role as mother, as the person who carried the basic responsibility for the perpetuation of the species. He emphasized the importance of stable marriages and families for society, its institutions, and the social order: "A rigid form of marriage is essential to mankind; it represents his firm and lasting ego" (p. 523). He also stressed the importance for an individual's well-being of the linkage between the individual as a part and society as a whole: "He who breaks away from the whole and resigns his responsibilities ceases to be a whole: the economy of his personality goes to pieces" (p. 523). Feminism would be accompanied by "free love" and the destruction of society as well as the family.

The moderate progressives agreed that many of the prevailing economic and other social conditions were menacing family life but argued for reform by legislation and for education. They demanded social legislation, especially widows' pensions, protection of women from overwork in factories, maternity leaves, and child labor laws.[2] Attempts were made to pass legislation restricting the employment of 14- to 16-year-old children to 8 hours daily and no more than 6 days per week. Educational programs to reconstruct the family needed to include courses in schools on sexual hygiene and "the general laws of reproduction" (Goodsell, 1915, p. 549).

In his comprehensive study of the family, Goodsell (1915) foresaw the problems—divorce, serial monogamy, crowding, the conditions of poverty, and children at risk for mental and bodily illnesses—that have become such prominent recent concerns. Like Elsie Parsons (1906) and Charles Pearson (1894), he expressed forebodings about the effects of increasing individualism. The "modern household not infrequently presents the phenomenon of a group of clashing wills, an association of highly individualized persons. . . . The family of the twentieth century is markedly unstable. . . . For the independence of its members [the family has paid] the costly price of its very existence or its existence in a changed and incomplete form" (p. 457). He concluded that "the machinery of family life was out of joint" (p. 456) and pleaded with parents, teachers, and all citizens to regenerate the family.

---

[2]The 1910 census showed that 1,990,225 boys and girls aged 10 to 15 years—18.4% of the total number of the nation's children—were employed in gainful occupations, a larger percentage than in 1900 *(Goodsell,* 1915, p. 543).

When we recall what this institution has accomplished for the good of the social body in the past, we may well put forth our best efforts to preserve it. . . . What other form of organization so completely secures the proper maintenance and training of the young? What other type of sex relationship has done so much to nourish the more spiritual phases of sex and passion? (p. 550).

Cutler (1916) noted the current "pessimistic view of monogamous wedlock" and "the centers of concern" (pp. 226–227), mainly the disappearance of single-family dwellings in the cities, the rising divorce rate, and the lowered birthrate that reflected difficulties with family relationships and responsibilities. He distinguished between a dwelling and a home and pointed out that the loss of independent dwellings would lead to a loss of domesticity and splintering of family life, with women working outside the home, child labor, and a diminution of the traditional division of labor in the family; during the 1920s there was a marked increase in apartments. To Cutler, however, the American family was not disintegrating but in transition, going through "a period of essential and thoroughgoing readjustment" (p. 236). Too many, he averred, were focusing on symptoms—divorce and desertions—rather than seeking "a new basis for the stability of the family in accord with a higher status for women" (p. 236).

Although the clouds of war had been gathering in Europe for years, even as late as July 1914, humanists, other scholars, and the socialist-labor parties in Europe did not believe that there would be fighting, much less an apocalypse that would devastate Western cultural traditions and convulse the social order. (Ironically, the little known German gymnasium teacher, Oswald Spengler (1929), began his great opus, *The Decline of the West,* in 1911.)

With remarkable perspicacity, Goodsell (1915) feared the effects on the family of the war: "The terrible carnage and destruction now going forward in Europe will have disastrous effects upon all phases of the civilization so painfully built up in the past; and nowhere will the blight fall more heavily than upon family life for some generations to come" (p. 484). Unfortunately, his forebodings came to fruition. In the United States, the divorce rate rose 60% after World War I, from 1.0 per 1,000 in 1915 to 1.6 per 1,000 in 1920. During the 1920s, it plateaued at a higher level than before the war, and concerns about the family persisted throughout the decade.

World War I had to be romanticized in song and sentiment to soften the hardships, follies, and brutalities of the terrible trench warfare. Many churches in the United States even endorsed the slaughter in the name of "God and country." Brothels were made available to soldiers after they left the front for a few days' rest. Hundreds of thousands of women went to work in the profitable war industries. In Western nations there was a general relaxation of sexual restraints; one telling anecdote is about the madam of a prestigious New Orleans brothel closing her establishment because "the country club girls are ruining my business!" (Asbury, 1938, p. 455).

In 1915, Freud (1930) explained that only regression and the emergence of basic aggressive impulses could account for individuals allowing the group in wartime to murder, pillage, and rape—that is, to engage in forbidden behaviors. These were manifestations of the force that Freud later would conceptualize as Thanatos, the death instinct.

THE ROARING TWENTIES: SOCIAL CHANGE, CHANGING FAMILY FUNCTIONS, AND COMPANIONATE MARRIAGE

The already rapid rate of social change that had been quickened by the many inventions of the last quarter of the nineteenth century was given increasing momentum by World War I. With the passage of the Nineteenth Amendment in 1920, women obtained the right to vote, and increasing numbers went to work. American industry flourished, and confidence and consumerism surged through the "Roaring Twenties." America had changed. The Yanks, 1 million of them, had been to Europe. How could they be kept "down on the farm, now that they'd seen Paree?" A degree of American insularity, if not innocence, had been lost.

Family scholars attributed changes in the family since the 1880s to social change. Traditional views of social change had followed the ancient Lucretian description of evolution that had served as the basis in 1749 for Rousseau's famous *Discourse*, and in the same century Millar's (1960) study of institutions. The acceptance of Darwinian principles stimulated those evolutionary concepts of social change. Also, sophisticated views were advanced by the German sociologist Vierkandt in his studies of cultural history and ethnology. According to Martindale (1960), in 1906 Vierkandt anticipated Ogburn's theory of culture lag.

W. F. Ogburn (1922) maintained that the unprecedented rate of social change was bewildering and could be attributed to the increase in inventions. He advanced two major theses. One was that the rate of social change exceeded the human being's capacity to adapt because biological changes had been relatively constant, at least for 10,000 years. Thus, the "cave man in the modern city" was maladjusted. The second was the famous concept of culture lag: all parts of a rapidly changing culture did not change at the same rate, and the differential rates led to maladjustments (pp. 200–201).

As conceptualized by Marx and also Veblen, Ogburn (1922) defined culture as being both material (technology, homes, etc.) and nonmaterial (books, arts, institutions, etc.). The family was "part of the non-material culture that is only partly adaptive. . . . The material culture has gone forward while the adaptive culture has lagged behind" (pp. 203, 244, 245). The results were such social phenomena as delinquency and desertion and, for individuals, emotional and psychosomatic problems of adjustment.

Changes in material culture, led by the automobile, were producing changes in nonmaterial culture, especially family life. "The great size of material culture today, its rapidity of change, and its significance as a source of other changes in society make the material culture in modern society play a most important part" (p. 279). Ogburn foresaw an accumulation of lags in adjustments to the rapid changes in material culture and a consequent piling up of social maladjustments. "A highly developed accumulation of material culture . . . provides a wonderful opportunity for an apparently ruthless exploitation of selfish interests . . . [and] creates social problems in abundance" (p. 335). Both social problems and neuroses were indicative of a "lack of adaptation between human nature and culture" (p. 335), and the lack of adjustment also was evidenced by crime, sex problems, and the unequal distribution of wealth. But Ogburn was optimistic, maintaining that often relatively small social and cultural changes produced remarkably good adjustments.

In his 1950 edition, Ogburn made only a few revisions to his 1922 book but added the supplementary chapter, "Social Evolution, Reconsidered." He did not reject the biological lag theory of the gap between a Stone Age biology and twentieth-century technology. But he emphasized culture lag—the relatively slow rate at which nonmaterial culture (e.g., the family) was able to adjust to the inventions of material culture—and its resulting maladjustments and social problems.

Concern about the stability of the family stimulated research. Some family researchers undertook early studies of marital satisfaction and/or unhappiness. In view of the changes in sexual attitudes and behaviors that had been accelerated by World War I, along with the spreading influence of Havelock Ellis's (1903) and Sigmund Freud's (1927) ideas about sexuality, investigators began with a focus on sexual adjustment in marriage. In 1922, Katherine B. Davis (1929), general secretary of the Bureau of Social Hygiene, stated that "sex is scientifically an unexplored country" (p. 173). To learn about sexual activities and contraceptive practices, she sent questionnaires to middle- and upper-class married and unmarried women. Of the married women, 62% reported that their "sex relations" were pleasurable, 16% neutral, and 11.4% distasteful. About 68% had used contraceptives.

In 1929, G. V. Hamilton, a psychiatrist in New York, reported the results of his 5-year evaluation of marital adjustment in 200 middle- and upper-class spouses. Only about half of them had a reasonable degree of satisfaction with their marriage, whereas 14% "stated without hesitation" that they wished they had not married their spouses. Wives were less satisfied than husbands with their marriages. Factors related to satisfaction-dissatisfaction were frequency of "satisfying contacts with the mother during childhood" (p. 532), degree of harmony or discord in the parents' marriages, and degree of sexual satisfaction.

The institutional basis of the family appeared to be shrinking, and the nature of the family changing. According to Ernest W. Burgess (1926), many scholars were regarding the family as "*a collection of individuals* temperamentally compatible or incompatible, emotionally in harmony or in conflict" (p. 122; italics added). Burgess asked whether the modern family is any longer an institution, although historically it had been recognized as the original institution: "Is it now anything more than a mere *unity of interacting personalities?*" (p. 121; italics added). His words were quickly adopted by other social scientists and have continued to influence concepts of the family and family studies; 1926 can be viewed as the year in which family systems theory was born.

A view of the family as the transmitter of the cultural heritage and the molder of its members' personalities—two basic family functions—requires consideration of the interrelations between the family and the community. According to Burgess (1929), conflicts between families' standards and community values can lead to emotional disturbances and disturbed behavior. In the family, the growing child develops "slowly and painfully a conception of his role in society and a philosophy of life about which his impulses become organized and his character becomes formed. Thus, personality, family and society are tightly intertwined; the roles that constitute the family are, in fact, cultural patterns . . . that have a history and are subject to social change" (p. 132). The influence of the family on the children's personality development and character formation and on the adults' emotional stability is epitomized by W. I. Thomas's definition of personality as "'the subjective aspect of culture'" (Burgess, 1929, p. 122).

During the 1920s many family scholars, especially the University of Chicago family sociologists (W. I. Thomas, W. F. Ogburn, E. F. Burgess, H. J. Locke, L. S. Cottrell, Jr., and their colleagues) focused their studies on family functions, which they saw as changing, and also on marital adjustment. But as early as 1915, Goodsell had noted that "so many occupations have been taken away from the housewife" that even making clothing and preparing food were "extra-household pursuits . . . [and that] her responsibilities as a consumer rather than as a producer" (p. 481) should be emphasized. In 1928, Groves and Ogburn cited social indicator data showing that many traditional family functions—economic, educational, protective, recreational, and religious—were increasingly being taken over by the community and its agencies. In the same year, Mimi Knight (Ogburn & Nimkoff, 1955) introduced the term *companionate marriage* to designate a lawful marriage in which the husband and wife consciously chose not to have children.

Groves and Ogburn (1928) stated that throughout history, marriage and the family had included three basic elements: economic cohesion, regulation of sexual activities, and parenthood (p. 13). At different times in different cultures, these varied in proportion and importance and were changing, not static. In the 1920s in the United States, traditional attitudes were "disintegrating more rapidly than the new are being satisfactorily formed," as would be expected in a transitional era, when changes in the family would be indicative of "social maladjustment" (pp. 13–14). The element that "will emerge and receive greatest emphasis will be the subtle value which we call affection" (p. 16).

Accumulating data supported views of the new family as being connected by affectional bonds rather than being institutionally based. Groves and Ogburn acknowledged optimistically that the "new family" would encounter difficulties because it would be "maintaining higher standards that test character more severely, but it will offer richer fruit for the satisfying of human needs" (p. 16). They did not fear that affection, without institutional support, would be a weak bond; instead, they insisted that if affection were the basis for matrimony, marriage would tend to be "predominantly an expression of the profound need of men and women to find their highest happiness in the close, character-developing experiences of marriage and the family" (p. 29). They called for more research with normal and successful families, inasmuch as a great deal of attention was being given to "matrimonial failure" (p. 455).

In 1929, Ogburn was appointed by President Hoover to compile data about life in the United States during the 1920s and to forecast trends. In their massive report, *Recent Social Trends,* Ogburn and Tibbitts (1933) stated that the data on family life revealed two major trends: the gradual decline in the family's institutional functions, and the emerging dominance of its personality functions. The family's declining economic functions included the transfer of such activities as baking, canning, and the cleaning of clothes from the home to outside sources and shifts in women's occupations from home to factories. The number of married women working outside the home increased 60% during the 1920s, and about 90% of them contributed all or part of their wages to the home.

The family's educational, religious, and recreational functions also had been changing. Children were going to school at a young age, and schools started giving courses in manual training, industrial arts, and household activities. Family prayers "were apparently a declining practice" (Ogburn & Tibbitts, 1933, p. 674), especially in urban areas, where only about half as many children went to church (40%) as those in rural areas (85%). There was an increased number of public playgrounds, golf courses, and tennis clubs. Attendance at baseball and other sporting events jumped and millions of Americans began going to the movies (p. 675).

The second major trend, the personality functions, was defined by Ogburn and Tibbitts as

> those that provide for the mutual adjustments among husbands, wives, parents, and children and for the adaptation of each member of the family to the outside world. The family has always been responsible to a large degree for the formation of character. . . . The chief concern over the family nowadays is . . . how well it performs services for the personalities of its members. (p. 661)

Thus, with the decline in its institutional basis, the family could be seen as existing for the individual rather than for society.

Although there had been some loss in personality functions as a result of mothers working outside the home, urbanization, and some increase in peers' influence on children, smaller family size concentrated attention on one or two children. Members of the family were becoming increasingly individualized. Husbands and wives were being separated by changing occupations, business travel, and the growth of outside activities at, for example, clubs and the cinema.

The major problem foreseen by Ogburn and Tibbitts (1933) was that changes in the function and structure of the family would produce "some degree of instability." In the early 1930s, approximately one in every seven or eight families was "broken" (p. 689). The increasing divorce rate was attributed to "the weakening of the functions which served to hold the family together" (p. 708). But Ogburn and Tibbitts concluded optimistically that with the family's weakening institutional functions there would be a corresponding strengthening of other functions and bonds, especially the affectional bond, on which "the future stability of the family will depend" (p. 708).

Many of the new views of marriage were expressed dogmatically by the noted anthropologist Edward Sapir (1930), who stated that "the family is . . . no longer a self-sufficient castle in a semi-hostile world" (p. 147) and that the traditional institutional marriage did not "correspond to modern mentality" (p. 150). Also, the older marriage institution "tended to put an undue emphasis on the child because it looked upon itself as a holy institution rather than as a psychological necessity" (p. 150).

Sapir (1930) described four causes of the "weakening" of the family: (a) the multiplication of labor-saving devices, indicative of invasion of the family by large industry; (b) the cramping of family quarters, which led to members having to make sure of their individuality and "apartness from each other" by escaping into the streets and movie halls; (c) the automobile, which increased travel and made the family unstable in time as well as in space; and (d) the growing economic independence of women, which led to the home's losing its "character" and to husbands' disdain of domestic affairs as "things for women to worry about" (pp. 145–147).

Sapir extolled the new "psychological marriage," based on mutual affection and understanding, as the "cornerstone of the new family" (p. 150). The family was not being "killed off" but was developing "cleanly defined psychological patterns which have intimate relevance for the life of the individual at the expense of superimposed institutional patterns which take little or no account of individual psychology" (p. 151). He noted that "the psychological family is important not only for the maturing of the erotic relationship of the parents; it is important also as the background image for the development of the child's own future love life" (p. 150). The family was becoming "a little cleaner, a little more truthful, a little happier" (p. 151).

Sapir's views coincided with the end of an era of rapid social change that had gained increasing momentum from new inventions, the popularity of the automobile, the beginning of modern aviation, victory in World War I, by increasing prosperity, and the dizzying optimism of the decade. Also, the United States lost its isolation by involvement in World War I, by transcontinental travel (as evidenced by the acclaim given to Charles Lindbergh's transatlantic flight in 1927), and by such developments in communications as the radio. The changes influenced marriage and the family; the new "psychological marriages" were praised as being indicative of the American spirit of independence and freedom. Concern during the 1920s about the rising divorce rate was tempered by the optimism of the era. Just as that optimism blinded the society to the impending crash of 1929 and the Great Depression, those who asserted that the family was only in transition did not see the possibility that changes in the family—the loss of functions, lessening of parental influence, and high divorce rate—contained the seeds of instability and pathology. There were few, if any, questions about the effects of divorce on children.

One exception was August Aichhorn (1935), who reported that "the child who grows up without appropriate training does not fit into the social order and therefore comes into conflict with society" (p. 7). Aichhorn, who had cared for several hundred children in a school in Austria in the harsh years just after World War I, insisted that "we have only to recognize that shocking [childhood] experiences can lead to psychic traumas and thence to delinquency" (p. 61). He saw the adverse effects of childhood traumas and parenting problems; either delinquency or neurosis could be a result. His book title *Wayward Youth* referred not only to "merely delinquent and dissocial children but also [to] so-called problem children and others suffering from neurotic symptoms" (p. 3). A child's not having a good parent figure with whom to identify was a particular concern, but therapy could help those with superego deficiencies resulting from disturbed childhoods.

In the 1920s, developments in dynamic psychiatry paralleled the scientific and social changes of the post–World War I era. The evolution of the new analytic ego psychology began in 1921 (Alexander, 1927), and Otto Fenichel (1945) pointed out that two factors led to its development. One was the increasing necessity to analyze patients' resistances to therapy, resistances that often were the same behaviors that the individual used for defensive purposes in everyday life. Fenichel credited Wilhelm Reich's early writings in the 1920s (1972) for increasing understanding of resistance and for the ideas that led to "the first 'psychoanalysis of character.'" (p. 463).

The second was the change in neurotic patients' "clinical picture." As early as 1912, Karl Abraham suggested that personality disorders were likely to become more common and the classical neuroses less common. In 1945, Fenichel stated that for years more persons with less defined neuroses were being seen than previously, and that the problems were "sometimes less troublesome for the patients themselves than for their environment" (p. 464). Often the person was "patently torn or malformed, or at any rate so involved in the illness that there is no borderline between 'personality' and 'symptom'" (p. 464). The personality disorders primarily involved differences between the individual's behaviors and familial and societal customs and regulations. There was a concomitant shrinking in importance of the conflicts between the individual's id drives and the restraints imposed by the superego. Those developments, which reflected current problems and shifts in cultural norms for behavior, presaged changes in character types such as those that Riesman et al. (1950) would describe in *The Lonely Crowd*. The new ego psychology placed greater emphasis on the ego's executive function as the moderator between the person and society than on the ego as a somewhat passive stage on which the id and the superego struggled over personal conflicts. Changes in society and the increased complexity of patients' emotional distress were necessitating changes in therapeutic approaches. In 1934, Moreno introduced group therapy, another response to the new need for interpersonally and socially oriented therapies.

When we look back 50 to 75 years, we see that changes in psychoanalytic theory and practice mirrored changes in society. Unfortunately, in the past 30 to 40 years, there has been a marked increase in the number of patients with personality disorders (especially antisocial personality disorder) and of those whose symptoms and behaviors meet criteria for a diagnosis of what is all too descriptively termed borderline personality disorder. A major question is how the changes in the family in this century are related to such changes in psychopathology.

Changes in personality, interpersonal relations, and mental illness are reflected by modifications of existing therapies and the introduction of new ones. Changes in the psychotherapies have significance for our understanding of the family. During the twentieth century, parents have relied increasingly on experts in child rearing and on therapists for advice. By 1980, at least two generations of middle-class children had been reared according to child development specialists' precepts. By the mid-1980s, the therapist was a dominant figure on the American scene.

Concern about individualism and a loss of familism grew during the first three decades of this century. Many family scholars, especially Charles Pearson (1894), Elsie Parsons (1906), and Willystine Goodsell (1915) were wary of the trend toward individualism; a century earlier, de Tocqueville (1945) had feared the consequences of extreme individualism at the expense of a sense of community. Historically, individualism has been a major feature of American life. It grew from strong roots, including the process of selection that impelled early explorers to endure the unknown in order to break with the past, conquer the New World, find a haven for their distress and discontent, and build homes and lives in accord with their own principles and wishes. Their successes over three centuries, from Jamestown in 1607 to the rejoining with Europe during World War I in 1917, solidified Americans' often provincial views of their rightness, if not invincibility. Those views were fueled by inventions, especially of labor-saving devices, and by the prosperity of the 1920s. Apologists for capitalism usually emphasized that it stimulated individualism and achievement, which inevitably would result in a higher standard of living for everyone and thus compensate for the exploitation of labor and the disparities of a class society. But individualism also threatened familism, and the increasing polarization of the two concerned even the ardent advocates of the new modern family.

Although Karl Jaspers (1963) emphasized in 1923 that we should not underestimate the stability and security of Western society in the years before World War I, the rumblings of social and political movements—especially those of the socialist, communist, anarchist, and other workers' groups—were beginning to jar the social order before 1914. And the irrational aspects of life and culture were recognized by the acceptance of the unconscious even before Freud's (1955) publication of the *Interpretation of Dreams* in 1900. In 1905, Einstein's pronouncement of the theory of relativity foretold the era of uncertainty that already was evidenced by such extreme new forms in the arts as James Joyce's stream of consciousness, Schoenberg's 12-tone system, Stravinsky's dissonance, and by fauvism and cubism. Even nowadays it is a bit startling to realize that Yeats's prescient line in his poem "The Second Coming"—"The center cannot hold"—was written in 1921. As we look back 70 years at the splintering of nations and peoples, the horrors of World War II, and the paranoid politics of the ensuing 40 years, it appears that Yeats was this century's Cassandra.

By the late 1920s, Western culture had undergone a dramatic transformation. The advances in communications, along with the automobile and the airplane, led to increased travel and marked changes in customs and mores. The mass production of the Model T in the early 1920s probably did as much as any single development to modify the patterns of everyday life for the middle class, to change the family, and to alter cities and communities by providing for convenient transportation to, from, and within the suburbs. Sports, traveling, the cinema, jazz music, drinking in defiance of Prohibition, and speculation on the stock exchange dominated the social scene, and movie stars began to be idealized. The social changes included the lessening of formalities in relationships between men and women. The new outlook was manifested by changed fashions and, in the graphic arts, by surrealism and other movements. Ellenberger (1970) linked the surrealist movement with psychoanalysis through the painter Andre Bréton: "Emotional immaturity, irresponsibility, hopelessness, cynicism, and rebelliousness were the keynotes of this new melody, often as a cover for real but unavowed sufferings" (p. 834). The rejection of old moral standards and the all-pervading search for pleasure led the French to call the 1920s *les années folles* (the crazy years).

One of our major efforts is to relate societal events and forces to family life and well-being. Too often, it appears that the family is studied and recommendations made as if it were an isolated institution. But we can see that the dramatic changes in the 1920s in Western society, especially in the United States, led to or at least were paralleled by changing views of the family and changes within families. These rapid technological and social changes, along with a new outlook that included optimism as well as irrationality, probably stimulated social scientists to believe that there could be quick and drastic changes even in such an age-old institution as marriage and the family. The consciousness of the era included the belief that marriage based on affection, more than on traditional institutional functions, suited the modern mentality praised by Sapir (1930). Also, the optimism included confidence that affection and companionship would be sufficiently strong to ensure the stability of the family. Voltaire's famous maxim—the more things change, the more they are the same—seemed to have been forgotten.

THE GREAT DEPRESSION

An entire era came to a close with the collapse of the New York Stock Exchange in October 1929; within a year, the Great Depression convulsed Western society. In his incisive analysis of the beginning of the depression, Seligman (1982) emphasized that during the 1930s, many families were battered by unemployment and income loss. There was some renewed emphasis on the family's economic function. Social workers and family agencies were alarmed by the failure of many low income families to function well.

Angell (1936) focused on how families coped with economic adversity. His study of 50 culturally homogeneous families of graduate students showed that a high degree of adaptability on the part of the family members was more important than a high degree of integration for meeting adversity, provided that there was a minimal degree of family integration: "The essence of the problem consisted in the effect of the decrease in income on internal family relations" (p. 5). The depression played havoc with unintegrated families, especially those that reacted unpredictably and with quarreling to loss of income and the ensuing hardships.

At the end of the 1930s, Koos (1946) began a 2-year intensive study of a random sample of 62 tenement families in Manhattan to evaluate troubles that were occurring and the families' ways of resolving them. He found an inverse relationship between the adequacy of family organization and the occurrence of troubles, mainly financial and/or interpersonal. Among the families that were not reasonably well organized, financial and other troubles affected the home routine: It became more disorderly, there was a relaxation of rules, and the discipline of children was less consistent. Most couples reported decreased sexual activity, especially those with marginally satisfactory sex lives.

Overall, the most important change in these traditional families was the loss of the father's dominance, which had profound implications. The depression influenced character formation by changing roles and positions in the family and disrupting authority. Koos (1946) quoted Horkheimer:

> Of all the social institutions which make the individual receptive to the influence of authority, the family must be recognized as the most important. In its circle, the individual experiences the impact of social forces. Through it he gets his conceptions of their intellectual and moral content. . . . the patriarchal structure of the modern family serves by its very nature as an important preparation for the acceptance of authority in society. . . . The social relations which the family helps to preserve and strengthen, themselves constantly reproduce it. (p. 92)

Koos's analysis of the effects of trouble(s) on the families' relation to the outside world showed that "the poor and the unfortunate become progressively more socially lost as they encounter succeeding misfortunes" (p. 121). Although the below-average families (in terms of organization) often brazened "through their difficulties or . . . [sat] them out in taverns or in gossip sessions . . . [that] in no way alleviates the problem. An added indictment of our institutional system and our American middle-class ideology" (p. 121) was that the average and better-than-average families did not "face-down" troubles but undertook "a penalizing retreat in the face of the problem" (p. 121). Koos concluded, "Can the culture do anything about this destructive effect of trouble on the family?" (p. 121).

During the 1930s, the other major area of family study was the continuing search initiated by Davis (1929) and Hamilton (1929) in the 1920s for factors that predicted success or failure in marriage. Dickinson (1931) reported an analysis of 1,098 cases seen in his 40 years of practice of obstetrics and gynecology. During the preceding decade, compared to earlier years, there were fewer inhibitions and greater sexual freedom in marriage and increased "coital experimentation" before marriage. Extramarital sexual activity occurred in about 5% of the cases. Dickinson's conclusions were that (a) about half of his cases had marital and sexual difficulties, but only 4% led to separation or divorce; (b) the sexual difficulties had mental and emotional origins; and (c) physicians and educators needed to emphasize sexual education to foster success in marriage.

Adolf Meyer's discussion of Dickinson's study is of particular interest. Meyer (1931) emphasized that data from clinical practice could be more significant than survey data obtained from volunteers, because the former revealed the importance of psychobiology—of the totality of the mind, the body, and the social environment. He called for studies of normal sexuality (inasmuch as most attention had been devoted to sexual psychopathology) and pleaded for increased education about sexuality.

In 1933, Jessie Bernard (1933) developed an instrument for measuring "The Distribution of Success in Marriage" and tested it on 252 urban, well-educated young persons in 146 marriages. She concluded that 13% of the women and 18% of the men were dissatisfied with their marriages. Terman (1938) presented the results of his comprehensive California study of 2,484 urban, well-educated adults (1,133 married and 109 divorced couples) in which he had evaluated about 400 variables, mainly personality, background, and sexual adjustment factors. He found that there had been a cultural shift from the prudish sexual attitudes of the 1890s to the "liberal and forward" attitudes of the 1930s. Pleasurable sexual activity was related to marital happiness, but about 30% of the wives were sexually "inadequate"; in accord with Hamilton's findings, orgasmic sex was not likely if it had not been established in the first year of marriage. The most important sexual factors in marital happiness were the wife's orgasmic adequacy and the intensity of the couple's sex drive. Terman concluded that psychological and background factors were of prime importance in determining marital satisfaction but that "with every generation, new causes of marital unhappiness would become operative" (p. 378).

Burgess and Cottrell (1939) pointed out that marital adjustment had been recognized as a social problem in Western society only since individualism emerged during the Renaissance and the Reformation and since marriage was viewed as a contract rather than a sacrament. Their major findings from questionnaires distributed to young, middle-class, white urban dwellers were that about half of the respondents reported "very happy" marriages and that the wives made the significant adjustments in marriage. They concluded "that prediction before marriage of marital adjustment is feasible" (p. 349) and that affection, temperamental compatibility, and social adaptability were more important than biological or economic factors in marital adjustment.

These early studies of marital success, happiness, and/or adjustment reached about the same conclusion: the best predictor was the individual's emotional and psychological stability. Although they had severe limitations, those pioneer studies stimulated research on the family at a time when it was beginning to undergo changes that would extend throughout the century.

INDIVIDUALISM VERSUS FAMILISM

Not all family scholars agreed about the superiority of the new psychological family that became so prominent in the 1920s, nor were they confident that its concentration on affection and personality development would be beneficial when other functions were left to the state and its agencies. One of the chief dissenters was Carle Zimmerman, who feared an impending family crisis that was being played down as a product of "cultural determinism." Zimmerman's fears of the decline (if not decadence) of Western society and its institutions, especially the family, were based on his extensive historical orientation.

Zimmerman and Frampton (1935) expressed concern about the companionate hypothesis, especially its emphasis on "individualistic satisfaction" (p. 40). They maintained that in the companionate family, the individual's values would have a higher priority than family values; consequently, the family would be just a collection of persons, not an additional social system (p. 41). "Continued emphasis upon individualism in a society tends to weaken the family and to thwart the individual himself insofar as he needs family life" (p. 5).

Zimmerman and Frampton saw the major problem as individualism versus familism and the possibility that the companionate family would exist solely for the individual and not for society. "If society is functionally related to the family, as many observers since Confucius have contended, a change in the family may be associated with other changes in the social structure" (p. 9). The mid-1930s was a time of drastic change in American life that was bound to affect the family. The Great Depression and the economic and political disturbances could be seen as a result of World War I, or as "symptoms of a fundamental trend in the reorganization of the social system" (p. 4).

The significance of events and social processes can be variously interpreted depending on one's view of history. Since the latter part of the eighteenth century, when Adam Smith, Hume, and the *philosophes* of the Enlightenment forwarded the doctrine of progress, the history of Western civilization has been viewed in an evolutionary perspective that was enlarged by Darwinian concepts and advances in science and technology. In contrast, cyclic views, as enunciated by Spengler and Sorokin, are organic; the life cycle of a culture or civilization is analogous to that of an organism.

Zimmerman and Frampton (1935) subscribed to many of Sorokin's cyclic views of history. They feared that the changes that were occurring in the family and society were indicative of widespread societal malaise. What would be the long-term consequences of the widely praised "new family" based mainly on affection and also of the influential social changes that were occurring? Could the great increase in mobility made possible by the automobile lead to geographic mobility that diminished intimacy and increased anomie? Highly mobile individuals are compelled to turn to secondary groups to compensate for being distanced from their families. Sorokin, who maintained that mobility weakened a society, saw the United States as "a mobile society *par excellence*" (Zimmerman & Frampton, 1935, p. 22). During the depression, there was increased social as well as geographic mobility. Another influential change was the increasing specialization, primarily at work and in home activities, that tended to constrict human beings' capabilities.

The Great Depression and mobility had disintegrating effects on family life. Although many persons clung to or returned to their families for help, many others were not able to do so. America's homeless of the 1930s crossed the country by hitchhiking or often by "riding the rails"; in Steinbeck's (1939) *The Grapes of Wrath*, Mother Joad cried plaintively, "Our family is breaking up." According to Zimmerman and Frampton (1935), trends having adverse effects on the family included the continuing decline of the birth rate, the emphasis on consumption, urbanization, the anomie described by Durkheim, and especially secularism. "Beliefs tend to maintain the social order. . . . Human society differentiates itself from an amorphous horde by rules, regulations, beliefs, and attachments which give a limited amount of regularity, predictability, and systematization to behavior" (p. 14).

Zimmerman and Frampton called for studies of the family in relation to social processes. These could be based on the hypotheses and methods developed almost a century earlier in Europe by Le Play, who considered the family and the state to be interacting entities. An example was Zimmerman's research during the depression on rural Ozark "Highlander families." The families were small, their consumption of goods was low (indicative of cultural lag), and they were relatively isolated from commercial America. The major finding was that the native rural families were in better condition than urban families who moved to rural areas in an attempt to rectify some of the economic problems of the 1930s. The urbanized, industrialized family type was not prepared to make use of the potential advantage of decentralized industry in a rural area. Zimmerman and Frampton (1935) concluded that "if we decentralize industry without changing the family type, we may be in a worse situation than now" (pp. 73–85).

From a classical sociological tradition, Pitrim Sorokin (1941) described the three main classes of human relationships: (a) the *familistic*, "permeated by mutual love, devotion, and sacrifice"; (b) the "free *contractual* agreements of the parties for their mutual advantage"; and (c) "*compulsory* relationships imposed by one party upon the other, contrary to their wishes and interests" (p. 167; italics added). Sorokin wrote poetically about familistic relations among devoted family members or true friends: "The individual ego is merged in the sense of '*we*.' Joys and sorrows are shared in common. The individuals need one another, seek one another, love one another . . . [and] represent a single solidarity body. This is the supreme and noblest type of social relationship. . . . All-bestowing mutual devotion renders unnecessary any contract, with its limitations and reservations" (p. 167). In contrast, contractual relations are partial, limited, and specify each party's rights and duties. Each desires to gain some advantage, and each is "egocentric and individualistic" (p. 168). Relationships become compulsory or coercive, characterized by antagonism rather than love, by exploitation, and even at times by degradation.

Sorokin (1941) maintained that contractualism arose with capitalism and modernity in the fifteenth and sixteenth centuries and reached its height in the nineteenth and early twentieth centuries. Its downside was the economic exploitation of the poor and the terrible conditions of life that often accompanied industrialization, urbanization, and the profit ethic. At the same time, the achievements were great, including the abolition of slavery and serfdom, advances in science and technology, a rising standard of living in Western society, and the spread of democratic values. The individualism that accompanied the dominance of contractual relations in personal and institutional life inevitably led to a sensate culture in which the only reality was sensory experience. Its corollaries and consequences included belief in progress, materialism, the unchecked profiteering by captains of industry and corporations that led to the rise of socialism or totalitarianism, and eventually the collapse of the validity of contracts and their attendant obligations and values.

For the family, contractualism involved the change of marriage from an institutional, if not sacramental, basis to a contractual relationship. The continuing decline in the contractual society in the twentieth century was paralleled by "a progressive disintegration of the contractual family" (p. 187) with increasing divorce, desertion, and intergenerational conflict along with a loss of the family's religious, parenting, and socializing functions. The results included juvenile delinquency and antisocial characters without "moral integrity or spontaneous altruism" (pp. 190–191). Sorokin attributed the general "atrophy" of the family in size, functions, and significance to the excesses of the sensate culture of the West.

Sorokin (1941) concluded that "contractual society is rapidly crumbling" (p. 202) as a result of the excesses of the sensate culture. His forebodings came into reality in the 1980s with the extensive family disruption and the Reagan and Bush administrations' greed-and-gain ethic, reckless borrowing and spending, the savings and loan scandals, and widespread corruption and lying, along with the blaming of the family, scapegoating of the schools, and heartbreaking neglect of children's needs and problems. The only solution for the withering of values and meaning and the shrinking of human relationships was "a transformation of the forms of social relationship, by replacing the present compulsory and contractual relationships with purer and more Godly familistic relationships" (p. 320).

We can see that by the end of the 1930s, family scholars were in two opposing camps. In contrast to Zimmerman and Sorokin, the advocates of the companionate family saw it as an appropriate sociocultural advance. They recognized the fundamental problem—the family's responsibility for the children and their character formation—and agreed with Ogburn and Tibbitts's 1933 statement: "The chief concern over the family nowadays is not how strong it may be as an economic organization, but how well it performs services for the personalities of its members" (p. 661). But they were confident that the family was in a process of change, not disintegration, and that the bonds of affection and companionship would ensure its survival. The minority camp headed by Zimmerman and his colleagues saw the condition of the family and its well-being as inextricably linked to the stability and vitality of its society. In socializing the children and shaping their character, the family was determining the character of society and thus the future of the state. Excessive individualism could jeopardize the family and eventually have an unwholesome effect on the society.

The concerns about the changing family and its future persisted throughout the 1930s. Westermarck (1936), who had fiercely defended concepts of the evolution of the patriarchal and monogamous nuclear family, acknowledged that marriage and the family were in serious difficulty and that there was widespread unhappiness. He agreed that divorce was a "remedy for misfortune," but he doggedly insisted that home, family, and children were "too deeply rooted in human nature to fade away, and . . . [humans] can find adequate satisfaction only in some form of marriage and the family founded upon it" (p. 170).

WORLD WAR II

Concern about the status and future of the family was lessened by the improved economic situation after World War II. The often disastrous effects of war upon families were not studied intensively until the end of this conflict, which is surprising inasmuch as historians, dramatists, and novelists have long described the harrowing effects of war on the family. Classic accounts of the tragedies of war were described by Euripides (1952) in 415 B.C. in *The Trojan Women,* by Brecht (1961) in his apocalyptic *Mother Courage and Her Children,* and by numerous other accounts spanning the centuries between those two dramas. Burgess and Locke (1945) stated: "War is one of the major crises which the family has periodically experienced. Total war, as exemplified in World War II, drastically affected the family by mobilizing not only men but women for service in the Armed Forces, in home defense, in war industries, and in other essential activities" (p. 663).

Burgess and Locke (1945) discussed four major family problems produced by war. One was the dispersion of family members that interfered with communication and family unity. In March 1945, 12 million men were in the armed forces, and more than 15 million persons had migrated within the country to work in war industries or to live with families and friends in various parts of the country "for the duration" (p. 668). Rural areas and small towns lost population while the big cities, especially on the southern and western seaboards, experienced a great population increase.

The second was the increased marriage and birth rates, especially early in the war. Often, marriages were either hurried up or were hasty meet-and-marry unions. Some were postponed until after the war, but generally the wartime prosperity increased the marriage rate, as did decline in parental restraint, desire for personal security, and the contagious effects of romance and war.

The third major problem was family disorganization and reorganization. The war loosened sexual taboos and weakened social control, including the influence of the home and community. During the war, the divorce rate rose, and afterwards it skyrocketed. The disruptions caused by the entry of young men into the armed services and the flocking of women to war industries were associated with "reports from all over the country [that] indicated considerable neglect of small children, locked in the house, the apartment, or the trailer, during the hours the mother was employed" (p. 689). Also, juvenile delinquency rose 19% just from 1940 to 1942.

Fourth on the list was the envisioned mass of postwar problems. These included economic readjustments, housing shortages, marital conflicts and adjustments following separation and reunion, the changing status and roles for women, the instability of marriages and the high divorce rate (generally, wartime and immediate postwar marriages tended to be unstable), and the problems of children and youths. Burgess and Locke (1945) concluded that

> the basic effect of World War II, however, was the impetus it gave to further modification of the American conception of marriage which has been in process of accelerated change since the landing of the Pilgrims at Plymouth Rock. . . . The surface and immediate effect of war upon the family seems disruptive; the deeper and long-time effect is probably to increase the trend toward its companionship form. (pp. 702–703)

Reuben Hill (1949) reported on a detailed study of a random sample of 135 Iowa middle- and lower-middle-class families in order to examine family adjustment to the stress of separation during the war and reunion afterward. The most common type of successful adjustment pattern was a roller-coaster profile of disorganization succeeded by recovery and readjustment. Hill concluded that the families that were well adjusted and integrated before the war tended to meet the stresses of separation and reunion much better than others; that "family forms may vary but it is the content of family living which counts" (p. 333); and that families that succeed share decision making.

In 1960, Burgess and Locke discussed both the delayed and immediate effects of World War II on the family. One of the immediate impacts had been the increased number of marriages, especially an increase in hasty marriages by returning servicemen just after the war. Although the immediate effects of war upon the family appeared to be disruptive, the long-term effects were "increased freedom and higher status [for] women and youth [resulting from their] participation in the total war effort" (p. 639).

Many wartime marriages did not survive the return to peace and domesticity. The divorce rate had jumped 60% after World War I; after world War II, it jumped almost 70% from 2.01 per 1,000 population in 1940 to a drastic new high of 3.5 per 1,000 in 1945. It dropped to 2.6

per 1,000 in 1950 and reached a postwar low of 2.2 per 1,000 in 1960, but was still higher than before the war and was a persisting concern. It climbed again to 3.5 per 1,000 in 1970.

One explanation for the instability of postwar marriages is that although the persons might have known each other before or during the war, they were young when they married and had matured or changed attitudes during the wartime absence from each other. Another explanation was that there had been a rush of marriages after only brief acquaintance to "make up" for the missed war years. A third was the "disparity between the real and ideal husband" (Burgess & Locke, 1960, p. 485).

Problems for veterans and their families in the late 1940s included the difficulties of adjusting to civilian life, postwar recessions, housing shortages, marital adjustments, more women working outside the home, an increased number of births including illegitimacies, lack of paternal authority, and increased juvenile delinquency. Burgess and Locke (1960) emphasized that the veteran's readjustment could be difficult for him and his family because the army was authoritarian, subordinated its members' personalities, and repressed individual differences, whereas the family had democratic features, tended to develop personality, and valued individuality.

Burgess and Locke (1960) concluded, as they had earlier, that the basic effect of World War II on the family was the acceleration of change in the conception of marriage and family functions. The changes had been slow in the latter part of the nineteenth century, when women's status was barely rising, but World War I and the depression stimulated changes that World War II accelerated. Both wars "accentuated the trend toward equality of vocational opportunities and equality of pay" (p. 465) for women, and their increasing economic independence and greater social equality were conducive to the acceptance of the companionate family based on mutual affection (pp. 464–465).

THE POSTWAR FAMILY AND THE 1950s

Burgess and Locke (1945) asserted that the family was only in transition. Its problems and the indicators of disorganization were evidence of strains in the family, not in the wider society, that could be attributed to changing functions during the transformation from an institutional to a companionate family type. During this transition, traditional family folkways and mores were disappearing, new patterns of behavior were emerging, and family functions were changing. Burgess and Locke emphasized that "the family of today . . . is so different that Rip Van Winkle, if again resurrected, would hardly recognize many a present-day family" (p. 517). In the past, familial patterns "formed a 'cake of custom'" (p. 517) that prescribed behaviors, but older patterns of behavior were disintegrating, and there was family disorganization because current patterns contained a confused mixture of older and new behaviors. The authors contrasted the older and newer families:

> The institutional family was characterized by permanence of marriage, unplanned parenthood, and a sense of duty as the highest obligation of family members. The companionship family relies upon divorce as a means of rectifying a mistake in mate selection, upon planned parenthood, and upon happiness as the goal and *raison d'etre* for marriage and family living. This new type of family is coming into being on the American scene. (p. 518)

Burgess and Locke (1945) recognized that the companionate family was less stable than the institutional, but maintained that the instability was mainly transitional. In accord with Sorokin's views, they considered mobility to be the key factor producing family disorganization (p. 550). Family disorganization was not necessarily pathological, but rather part of the organization-disorganization-reorganization process. Family reorganization was dynamic, "being modified by forces within it and reaching to those impinging upon it" (p. 58). Analysis of the total process was needed, because such disorganizing features as divorce and delinquency had been publicized and "made-to-order reforms of family structure" proposed (p. 714).

One of those reforms was "the revival of the traditional family patterns" advocated by Zimmerman and Frampton (1935), who raised the question, "Is it necessary to reemphasize family life as an emergency to save our society from complete moral and social destruction?" (p. 357). Burgess and Locke (1945) maintained that Zimmerman and Frampton would have replied affirmatively, that "a 'strong family type' is required in the United States" (p. 715). Another reform would be a change to Sorokin's "reinstitutionalized family." Burgess and Locke (1945) stated that Sorokin "paints a black picture of the family and of present-day society [and] . . . ignores the fact that the same forces which found expression in family instability are creating a family unity based neither upon competition nor upon contract but upon the binding affection and loyalties growing out of intimate association in the companionship family" (p. 715). But Burgess and Locke were unwilling to let their companionate family develop to its logical conclusion. They rejected the legalization of companionate marriage for childless couples, although it had been proposed as early as 1906 by Elsie Parsons (in 1989, it was legalized in California as "domestic partnership").

Instead of advocating reform and reinstitutionalization of family functions and structure, Burgess and Locke (1945) asserted that the companionship-based family—with its emphasis on intimacy and affection, husband-wife equality, democratic decision-making, freedom of self-expression, personality development, and interpersonal associations—was "becoming so much a part of our culture that it is difficult to consider it objectively and critically" (p. 716). The forces that stimulated the development of the companionship family were "derived from crude beginnings in the pioneer and frontier situations" in the seventeenth and eighteenth centuries and their even earlier ideological foundation. Those pioneer situations included a breakdown of status and subsequent evaluations of family members according to "initiative, originality, independence, and, particularly, the contributions each could make to the family" (p. 717). Free land in the New World enabled young couples to build separate homes, and the women and children worked alongside the men on the farms. Second, the isolation of the pioneer allowed for "relaxation of rigid patterns of control of the traditional family" (p. 717) and for role flexibility; also, roles were defined by performance and not solely by custom. Third, the scarcity of women led to their having higher status and increasing equality. And fourth, democracy contributed to greater freedom for children and higher status for women.

The earlier ideological foundation to which Burgess and Locke alluded was the Anglo-Saxon individualism that had been a feature of life in England since the early Middle Ages. It was evidenced by the democratic heritage that began with the Magna Charta in 1215, by Wycliffe's 1380 translation of the Bible, and by the striving for ownership of land that accompanied the rise of capitalism as described by Marx. As discussed earlier, the nuclear family had been prominent in England since about the thirteenth century.

The post–Civil War industrialization and urbanization in the United States led to a diminution of some historic family functions and greater opportunities for the family to fulfill "its essential function, that of developing the personalities of its members through intimate association, affectional interdependence, and emotional security" (Burgess & Locke, 1945, p. 718). Burgess and Locke rhapsodized about the growth of industry early in this century and its potential to give women economic independence and higher status. Also, public education had increased intellectual and cultural activities for couples, and the authors praised the cinema for portraying the companionship marriage romantically. Their major theses were timely; the United States had just won a worldwide war with the atomic bomb at Hiroshima and Nagasaki. Victory was heralded as the triumph of American individualism and achievement. We were entering an era of optimism that, although it was shadowed by the spectre of communism, would mean "the good life" for many, especially the white middle class.

Despite the optimism of the times and their enthusiasm for the new companionate family, Burgess and Locke (1945) expressed concern about the family's lack of economic security: "The insecurity of the family in the modern world is a paradox" (p. 719). The United States had been successful in one of the great wars of history, but to obtain security the American family had four as yet unmet "chief wants": a minimum economic basis, decent working hours, good nutrition, and adequate medical care (pp. 714–715). Burgess and Locke's conclusions about the future of the family were that (a) it was in transition but still had some institutional characteristics; (b) it would survive; (c) increased disruption by divorce would continue into the postwar years; (d) the family would stabilize within 20 to 30 years as a result of the slowing down of population increase and immigration, "the transition of our economy from a risk to a security basis" (p. 750), and the expansion of family services and marriage counseling; (e) continued urbanization would involve a decline of familism and increased individualism of family members; (f) there would be a continuation of long-term trends—smaller family size, younger age of marriage, declining birthrate, increasing proportion of married persons, increasing proportion of women gainfully employed, and a decline in historic family functions; (g) new inventions (especially the automobile, cinema, and radio) would have a major influence on family life; (h) services to families would expand; (i) the family would make choices that determined its future; and (j) increased research was necessary (p. 750).

In contrast to Burgess and Locke's prediction of family stability by the 1960s and 1970s, Zimmerman (1947) expressed forebodings. His comprehensive historical and sociological study indicated that Western society, especially the United States, would "reach the final phases of a great family crisis between now and the last of this century" (p. 798). The crisis would be similar to that which occurred during the decline of Greece in the fourth century B.C. and of Rome in the third and fourth centuries A.D.

> Civilization grows out of familism; as it grows it loses its original connection with the basic spring which furnishes the essence of civilization. When this process has gone too far, the civilization soon exhausts its inventory of social "material." Then occurs a reaction or decay. The amount of reaction and the decay and the length of these "Dark Age" periods seem to depend

upon how quickly the culture finds it way back to the fundamental mother-source—familism. (p. 783)

From his cyclic view of history, Zimmerman associated the type, status, and stability of the family with particular stages in ancient Greece and Rome and in the United States in the middle decades of this century. His family typology consisted of the *trustee* family system, the *domestic* family system, and the *atomistic* family system; each varied in prominence throughout history relative to the power and vitality of the state. The trustee is the large extended family that controls family relationships and activities. It flourishes when central authority is weak and diffuse and clan law can prevail. It was the dominant type in early Greece of Homer's time, in Rome during its early years (the Twelve Tables epoch), and in Western society during the Dark Ages. It could be found in the mountainous regions of eastern Kentucky until World War II; vestiges were still apparent in 1950. Some of the Mafia families in the battered cities on the eastern seaboard are modern equivalents of the trustee family system.

The domestic family system succeeds the trustee as a result of the growth of the authority of the church and state, improvements in the standard of living, the excesses of the trustee family and its humanization, "and the desire of the domestic unit for more equitable treatment than that afforded by clan rule" (Zimmerman, 1947, p. 749). Thus, the change from the trustee to the domestic family system is caused by both external and internal forces. The domestic family is stable, integrated into society, and the dominant type when a society is in a healthy, vital stage and prizes the family as its essential unit. It was the dominant type in classical Greece during its height from about 650 B.C. to 400 B.C., in Rome during its great period from about 500 B.C. to A.D. 150, and in Western society from the sixteenth to the twentieth centuries.

In contrast, the atomistic family is usually small, often fragmented, and is not integrated into the community and the wider society. It was the dominant type in the decadent stages of ancient Greece, in Rome during its decline, and to some extent in Western society (especially the United States) in the latter part of the twentieth century. The change from the domestic to the atomistic family system is produced largely by external forces. Zimmerman (1947) explained: "The 'cause' of the rise of the atomistic family to dominance is the extension and elaboration of concepts, ideals, practices, and beliefs which made the domestic system take precedence over the trustee until, in due time, these beliefs (e.g., individualism, private property) and practices no longer permit the system of faith of the domestic family to be dominant" (p. 762). At that time in the civilization, the culture is integrated against familism. The family loses or gives up its institutional functions and emphasizes affection and personality. Eventually, Zimmerman theorized, "general cultural determinism takes over and the family system gradually loses its significance in the total social scheme" (p. 775).

Prominent characteristics of the atomistic family system are increased no-fault divorce, few children, lack of meaning of the marriage ceremony, antifamilism among the urbane and intellectual classes, "pessimistic doctrines about the early heroes" (e.g., questions about Columbus and the antihero), the belief that looser family forms will solve the problem, relaxation of inhibitions against adultery, revolt of youths against parents, increased juvenile delinquency, and acceptance of alternate lifestyles. These behaviors "become accepted as the things to do" (p. 777). Zimmerman asked: "What [do] these forms of behavior represent? What is lacking in the social system of which these forms are symptoms? What is the fundamental disease?" (p. 777).

He maintained that "atomism in family relations is not important because of its symptoms but primarily because of the decay of the basic components of social life. . . . Atomistic familism causes a dispersal of the infinite faith underlying the family system . . . [and] the breaking up of families" (p. 782). The atomistic family system and its alternative family forms become so amorphous that they do not provide sufficient structure to give meaning and coherence to everyday life. Eventually, "the negative spewing of antisocial doctrines into the social order" and/or the "inner decay" of a great civilization lead to a revival of familism (pp. 782–783). Thus, Zimmerman saw the strength or weakness of familism as a major cause of the rise and fall of civilizations; family change—along with favorable or adverse economic, military, and political events and processes—has been "the final decisive force" (p. 783).

On history's big screen, we can see that the trustee family system was associated with societies (e.g., Homeric Greece or western Europe between the sixth and eleventh centuries) that lacked unity and were limited by the power of groups, tribes, clans or extended families that demanded loyalty. The failure of the ninth-century Carolingian Renaissance to mature can be attributed to the prevailing factionalism, wars of succession, and the disunity in France, Germany, and Italy in the ninth and tenth centuries.

The domestic family system, in contrast, was in step with the development of societies because the equivalence between the domestic family and the wider society allowed for their interaction and was conducive to both family well-being and a stable social order. Zimmerman acknowledged that the individuality and loosening of bonds essential to the development of the atomistic family might be related to "the first flowering of a great civilization [and] seems necessary to its final culmination" (p. 783). But the atomistic family contains within it the seeds of its own destruction and the breakdown of the social order. Its negative (if not antisocial) biases and trends, along with its excesses, require reform, restitution, and the revival of basic faiths and rules.

Thus, as early as 1947, Zimmerman expressed grave concern about the future of the family. In many ways, the American family in the 1920–1947 era began to resemble that of Greece in its decline from about 400 B.C. to A.D. 100. About 360 B.C., Plato (1952) expressed doubts about the Athenian family in his last dialogue, *The Laws*. Let us recall that *The Laws* represented a change that had occurred in less than a century—in 451 B.C. Pericles could praise the Athenian family as the strength of the state. But from about 320 B.C. (when Aristotle committed suicide) to A.D. 90 (when Plutarch gave his moral lectures), the Greek family was in decline. "By the time of Plutarch, virtue, chastity, fidelity, having and rearing children, and even the loyalty of brother to brother had disappeared among all classes of Greece" (Zimmerman, 1947, p. 786). He documented existing orations and legal records that described the demands of funds for more public feasts, the farmers who wanted the "demoralized sensualism" of the city, the men who cared more for sex than their businesses, politicians with scandalous personal lives, unscrupulous lawyers, and women who limited having children so as not to interfere with pleasure (pp. 785–787). After about 440 B.C., the Greeks even developed two types of marital relations under one system of law: a private legally-based traditional marriage and family, and public relations with hetaerae. "Toward the end of the Hellenistic period in Greece, marriage and familism became simply a farce" (p. 792).

The cycle was repeated in Rome in A.D. 100 to 300. Zimmerman pointed out that a review of Roman laws and legal records showed evidence of extensive family decay, but the decay was slow because of the power and vastness of the Roman Empire and because of two countervailing forces. One was the steady influx of the "barbarians," with their ancient virtues of chastity and domesticity, who brought new blood and customs into the empire. The other was the profamily stand taken by the early fathers of Christianity. As noted in Chapter 2, the Romans also experimented with looser forms of marriage, developing types of legal marriages: *dignitas*, with the mixing of property, authority in the hands of the husband/father, procreation, and an emphasis on permanence; *concubinatus*, a less binding relationship with some husband-wife equality, no joining of estates, probably no children, and relatively easy divorce; and *in sine manu*, with the husband having no authority. Zimmerman stated that "toward the end of what the French call the *haute empire* period (c. A.D. 300) marriage and freedom in Roman society also became farcical—a grand vulgarization—with extremely devastating social consequence" (p. 792).

Zimmerman (1947) reiterated Sorokin's assertion that Western culture was breaking down, that "the family will continue to disintegrate.... Children will be separated earlier and earlier from parents.... The home will become a mere overnight parking place mainly for sex relationships" (p. 796). Thus, he was critical of many sociologists' rosy views of the future of the American family and their apparent disregard of history. He disputed "Burgess and Locke's opinion that the family [is] getting better and better all the time" (p. 797). Zimmerman concluded that "this process of atomization is hastened by the Pollyanna stories and pseudo-histories given by the family sociologists" (p. 797), and he made ten predictions about the family:

1. The United States and other Western nations "will reach the final phases of a great family crisis" (p. 798) by the end of the century.
2. Efforts to meet the crisis will be exaggerated.
3. There is little public knowledge of the crisis, and it is avoided or rationalized by intellectuals.
4. Each major change in the family system has been associated with a shift in power among the three vehicular systems (clan, religious institution, and state) "which mitigate between family and society" (p. 799). The great shift in Western society has been the increasing power of the state since the seventeenth century.
5. When the state has relinquished or lost control of families, devastating social changes have occurred.
6. Inasmuch as the state is not able to preserve the family system there will be a crisis, not just changes.
7. The state cannot maintain control of familism because the law has a "changing conception of the family" (p. 800).
8. Social work and other state agencies are not prepared to preserve familism, and drastic measures could make the crisis worse.
9. The state could obtain some help from the other vehicular agents, such as the clan or religious institutions.
10. Research is needed on family problems and means for rectifying them.

The solution that Zimmerman (1947) advanced was to make "familism and childbearing the primary social duties of the citizen. This will have to be voluntary—not compulsory. The solution will . . . be in the strong union of *proles-fides*—children and familism" (p. 810).

It has been necessary to look in depth at the opposing views about changes in the family at midcentury in order to bare the roots of the family crisis described in Chapter 1. Burgess and Locke tended to focus their analyses on family functions and, significantly, to regard the family as an almost independent unit when in reality it both produces and reflects what is happening in the wider society. In contrast, Zimmerman repeatedly linked either family well-being or instability throughout the ages with societal conditions and the vigor or decline of the state. Burgess and Locke and many of their colleagues used social indicator data to support their contentions that the family was not disintegrating but only in transition to an appropriate form in accord with the social change that was occurring. In contrast, Zimmerman relied largely on his immense grasp of history and the social sciences to declare unequivocally and unpopularly that the American family was in decline and was approaching a crisis. The most important point, one that Burgess and Locke and their colleagues tended to de-emphasize but was implicit in Zimmerman's views, is that the family determines its own and the society's fate by the way it socializes the young and shapes character, and that the society exerts reciprocal influences on the family.

The stress of the war years greatly increased demands on family agencies and clinics in Great Britain and the United States. After World War II, the family therapy movement developed from the shoots that had been planted by such pioneers as Flügel (1921) and Ackerman (1937) before the war. In the 1940s in London, H. V. Dicks (1967) began to use his "couples interview," and he and his colleagues developed family therapy programs, many of which were based on Melanie Klein's (1932) contributions and on the foundations that Bowlby (1965), Fairbairn (1954), and others built for object relations theory and therapy. In the United States, the increased family disruption and juvenile delinquency produced by World War II, along with the family problems of postwar adjustment and the high divorce rate in the 1940s, overloaded family agencies and mental health services. A generation of family researchers, theorists, and therapists rose to meet the many needs; *stress* was becoming a household term. Some of the leaders in this effort were T. Lidz, Fleck, Bateson, Bowen, Reuben Hill, and their colleagues. In the 1950s, family therapy was stimulated by advances in communications, cybernetics, and general systems theory.

Just as there had been such developments as the introduction of ego psychology after World War I, psychoanalytic theory underwent substantial change after World War II. The societal regressions—the distress of the Great Depression, and the horrors of the World War II era—were paralleled by increasing emphasis in psychoanalytic theory on regressive pre-Oedipal characteristics, including infantile rage, aggression, and dependency. Just as it is not mere coincidence that World War II brutalities were seen in pre-Oedipal terms, Fairbairn's (1954) object relations and Sullivan's (1953) theory of interpersonal relations became dominant themes in psychiatry and psychology in the 1950s. The continuing shrinkage of the family's institutional base and the reliance on affection to hold the family together required new supports, and the high divorce rate was a persisting concern. In the best American tradition, the public looked to experts for advice and assistance. Throughout the 1950s, an increasing number of therapies sprang into life to meet the immense demands of frustrated and disappointed women/men/husbands/wives for consolation, counsel, communication skills, and help with their interpersonal, family, and other "relationship problems."

During the 1950s functionalism, especially as represented by the work of Talcott Parsons (Parsons & Shils, 1951; Parsons & Bales, 1955), emerged as a major approach to family study. In sociological theory, functionalism is a "system-determined and system-maintaining activity" (Martindale, 1960, p. 445). The development of functionalism fit the prevailing zeitgeist; object relations theory had attained prominence in psychoanalysis, and Sullivan's theory of interpersonal relations dominated psychiatry and psychology.

Parsons and Bales (1955) emphasized theory to a greater degree than empiricism. They were especially concerned with the interrelationships of personality, culture, and the social structure as systems. Personality and social systems "are empirically inseparable from each other and from their culture.... They interpenetrate" (p. 31). Personalities, culture, and social systems can be understood only by referring to their interrelations; "sociology presupposes psychology, but equally, psychology presupposes sociology and both presuppose knowledge and analytical understanding of culture" (p. 33).

Parsons and Bales (1955) maintained that the nuclear family was "a differentiated subsystem of the society" (p. 356) and had a democratic structure as a result of continuing structural-functional differentiation and specialization that included a lessening of the importance of kinship units other than the family, a decline of some traditional family features, and the beginning "stabilization of a new type of family structure in a new relation to a general social structure" (p. 356). Characteristic features of the modern family were its isolation, living in a dwelling separate from other family members, and economic independence from kin.

According to Parsons (1970), the basic, irreducible functions of the family are the socialization of children "so that they can truly become members of the society" (p. 17) and the stabilization of the adults' personalities. He maintained that the modern isolated nuclear family with its four main role-types (adult, child, male, and female) "incorporates an intricate set of interactive mechanisms whereby these two essential functions for personality are interlocked and interwoven" (p. 21). The parents' role differentiation is important for the children's socialization, which occurs along two axes: one according to decision making or power, and the other along instrumental-expressive lines.

Parsons and Bales (1955) acknowledged that the family had been going through "a profound process of change" (p. 3) and that the change involved some degree of strain, but the latter "could be considered aspects of 'the disorganization of transition'" (p. 4). They expressed doubt that the disorganization would continue because the divorce rate had dropped during the 1950s, most divorces were of childless couples, a large proportion of the population was married, and the birth rate was stable. Also, the postwar boom in home construction indicated that the family was not breaking up.

Parsons and Bales (1955) did not see the changes in the family as being evidence of loss of functions, as did Ogburn, Burgess, and others. Instead, family members were carrying out the necessary functions "'as individuals' (in societal functions, e.g., parental participation in P.T.A.), not [just] in their roles as family member" (p. 16). The most important change was that the family was becoming highly differentiated (specialized), and its functions "in a highly differentiated society are not to be interpreted as functions directly on behalf of the society, but on behalf of personality. . . . It is because the human personality is not 'born' but must be 'made' through the socialization process that in the first instance families are necessary. They are 'factories' which produce human personalities" (p. 17). According to Parsons and Bales, this production would entail "the internalization of the culture of the society. . . . The most important part of this culture . . . consists in the patterns of value which in another aspect constitute the institutionalized patterns of society" (p. 17). "Underintegration" or lack of internalization of cultural norms resulted in the psychopathic personality, whereas an "overintegrated" personality type would resemble the compulsive personality type.

According to Parsons and Bales (1955), the isolation of the nuclear family had significance for character formation inasmuch as it sharpened the child's perception of "the difference in status" (p. 19) between family members and nonmembers. Also, the dominance of the nuclear family at the expense of intense kinship relationships reinforced the affective relationship between the parents and strengthened the emotional climate in the family in which the young child would invest all of his or her emotional resources, but later gradually become emancipated. The child's accepting the father's authority and values and relinquishing the affectively gratifying relationship with the mother provides the incentive to acquire "the skills, values, and other characteristics of the adult role" (Lasch, 1975, p. 115). Therefore, Parsons and Bales (1955) stated that "the family must be a differentiated subsystem of a society; not itself 'a little society' or anything too closely approaching it" (p. 30). They also insisted that the continuing differentiation was mainly a process of reorganization.

Parsons and Bales (1955) pointed out that strains in the family were being alleviated by mental health professionals and that increasing reliance upon them was in accord with the American tradition of turning to experts. But they acknowledged that the "vogue of psychiatry" indicated difficulty in personality and human relationships, and that "much of this strain relates to family and marriage" (p. 25).

Parsons and his colleagues attempted to supply a theory that related personality, culture, and society. Parsons tied elements of role theory to psychoanalytic concepts of personality development and fitted them into early systems theory. His efforts were ambitious and influential. Schools of personality development generally had given much more attention to the parents' affective influences on the child's personality development than on parental functions and roles and had largely avoided, if not overlooked, larger societal and cultural factors influencing the family and the children's personalities. Lasch (1975) stated that Parsons "grafted Freud onto Durkheim" (p. 113) and that his analysis of the family attempted to "show that the functional differentiation of instrumental and expressive roles, not the biological and the emotional connection between parents and children, provides the decisive element of socialization" (p. 120). The resolution of the Oedipal conflict, in Parsonian terms, allowed the child to outgrow dependence on the mother, acquire skills, and take a step toward becoming integrated into the family (and, later, into the larger society). But it has not yet been possible to test aspects of Parsonian theory empirically.

Lasch (1975) has been critical of the Parsonian family because "the transfer or loss of family functions included the father's withdrawal into the world of work which has not only deprived his sons of a 'role model' but has also deprived them of a superego or transformed the contents of the superego so that archaic, instinctual, death-seeking elements increasingly predominate" (p. 123). He pointed out that sons need to learn "more than techniques and roles" (p. 123) from their fathers. Often, during the 1950s, a common complaint from middle-class families was that the children and even adolescents did not know what Dad did all day. When the father is absent from the family or unavailable for limit setting, according to Lasch, "the child remains a slave to pre-Oedipal impulses and external stimuli with which he is bombarded by a culture devoted to consumption and immediate gratification. He resorts to violence in order to satisfy his desires or else represses his violence and anger at a high psychic cost" (p. 124). Also, Lasch was critical of Parsons for advocating that parents turn to professionals for help with child rearing, because their theories and practices varied in confusing, conflicting ways, and the parents' reluctance to exercise authority diluted child care and led to "the weakening of the psychic mechanism whereby the young internalize their parents" (p. 123).

In the 1950s, the height of optimism about the family was expressed by Ogburn and Nimkoff (1955), who began by obtaining a list of the "10 outstanding changes in the family in recent times" (p. 4) from 18 family scholars. All 18 agreed that there had been increasing divorce and changing attitudes toward divorce, but only 50% to 67% agreed on the remaining changes, which included a wider diffusion of birth control and/or declining family size; the declining authority of husbands and fathers; increasing extramarital sexual activity; increasing numbers of wives working for pay; and increasing individualism and freedom of family members (p. 7).

A major question was whether the more liberal attitudes toward sexual behavior reflected changes in mores. Some national polls showed that there was greater tolerance of women's premarital sexual behavior than in the previous generation. Although ten of the experts considered the reduction of family size to be significant, the decline was not as great as often believed. In 1790, the average number of persons per family was 5.8; in 1950, it was 3.5 (Ogburn & Nimkoff, 1955, p. 14). Smaller family size placed increased emphasis on the husband-wife relationship.

The husband/father's declining authority was accompanied by enhanced status for women and children (p. 10), as well as trends for wives to work outside the home and for husbands to do more of the household chores and child care. Ogburn and Nimkoff (1955) recognized that such changes were profound: "Authority over children has diminished . . . [and] obedience in children is not valued as highly as in times past . . . permissive attitudes . . . are encouraged" (p. 11). The increasing number of wives in the labor force reflected desires for a higher standard of living and, compared with the past, was associated with smaller families, greater economic security and equality for women, and more time at work, in automobiles, and other places than at home (p. 13).

Ogburn and Nimkoff (1955) viewed the changes as indicating a lessening of "dependence on the family for the satisfaction of our needs and wishes" (p. 15). Many family functions had been taken over by agencies, the community, or the state. Thus, the "business of the world" was being carried on apart from the home and more by individuals than by family groups: "The accent has shifted to the individual, so that the family is relatively less influential, the individual more so. The control of the family over its members is less" (p. 15). But Ogburn and Nimkoff maintained contradictorily that "the intrinsic role of the family is as significant as formerly, in shaping character, in inculcating morals, and in providing happiness" (p. 17).

The causes of the changes in family functions were seen as reaching back to the Industrial Revolution and were social, not biological, inasmuch as "a factor that does not change cannot be responsible for change" (p. 255). Some of the major causes were urbanization, with separation of residence from place of work; consuming becoming a major family function; the growth of the welfare state; birth control, with smaller family size; greater equality for women; and discoveries in the sciences that emphasized the social environment as a determinant of either well-being or pathology and also increased secularization. Ogburn and Nimkoff (1955) concluded that many of the changes could be attributed to the decrease in production as a family function and insisted "that the family has changed largely because of forces outside the family impinging on it" (pp. 263–264).

The final chapter was an overly optimistic statement of even the rosy views that pervaded American society in the mid-1950s. They foresaw a growth of transportation, an increase in family income, a dispersal of urban population or a "loosening up of congestion in cities" (p. 270), and a great increase in the number of mobile homes and/or prefabricated mass-constructed houses. Consumption would become an increasingly more important and time-consuming family function. Also, they predicted an increase in leisure time and more recreation, especially television. Outside influences would have major effects on the family inasmuch as the radio, telephone, and television brought the outside world into the home (p. 283).

Ogburn and Nimkoff's (1955) optimism became expansive when they pointed out that the increase in production in the 1950s and the continuing technological advances would increase family income: "The effect . . . will be to abolish poverty and to raise the income of working class families into those of the present middle class" (p. 286). Other changes would include a smaller percentage of rich families, a decrease in the size of the household (with fewer relatives and adult children in the home), and some diversification of family types. Furthermore, changes in communications and the distribution of income would tend to make families more alike than in the past. The major functions of the family of the future, aside from purchasing and consuming, would be its personality functions—affection, and companionship for the members.

We have described Ogburn and Nimkoff's views in detail because they represented the prevailing opinions and sentiments about the family and depicted the familism of the 1950s, the most familistic decade of the century. Seldom, however, have eminent scholars' opinions turned out to be so wrong. Such a judgment of their misperceptions and rose-tinted views is not just retrospective; it appears that they and many others simply did not see the "other America" that Michael Harrington (1963) would be writing about in a few years and the terrible racial segregation that was beginning to be the focus of protest and dissent. Blacks had been migrating from the South since World War II to tenements in such cities as Chicago, and ghettoization was taking place even in the 1950s. Ogburn and Nimkoff's mistaken opinions probably contributed to the complacency of the 1950s and to the short-lived glow of the pre-*Sputnik* era. Their failure to see inequities within the society, mainly poverty and both racial and sexual discrimination, were matched by their not foreseeing the major social forces that would convulse the United States in the 1960s and the shrinking of the middle class and growth of the underclass in the 1980s. Also, they did not anticipate the growth of the military-industrial complex that worried even Eisenhower, and they did not consider the sinister implications of the paranoid politics of the 1950s that dominated the American scene for decades. In the mid-1950s, the impending Vietnam War was feared, but its folly and devastation and the drug and crime culture that scarred the 1970s and 1980s were unimaginable.

In the second edition of *The Family: From Institution to Companionship,* Burgess and Locke (1960) documented the continuing changes in family functions. These included an increase in the percentage of married women working outside the home during the familistic 1950s (pp. 463–464); the reduction of the family responsibilities for the elderly as a result of social security programs; increasing educational and school activities (high school enrollment rose 523.7% from 1910 to 1950) (p. 467); more recreation outside the home (p. 468); and a waning of religious activities (pp. 469–470).

Burgess and Locke viewed these changes as being mainly in emphasis. The family was losing its institutional significance, and instead, "more and more the American family is becoming a union of husband and wife, parents and children, based on the sentiments of love, common interests, and companionship" (p. 470). A host of factors were contributing to changes in sexual attitudes and roles within the family. Puritanical attitudes were being swept away by women's entry into the workplace and higher status, advances in contraception, and urbanization. Also, the family was being influenced by "the emancipation of youth from parents that was accelerated by the automobile; the rise of the motion picture with its commercialization of sex appeal and its presentation of passionate patterns of love-making; the rise of a radical school of young writers in revolt against the tyranny of morals and convention . . . [and] the dissemination of the Freudian theory of suppressed desires" (pp. 470–471). And roles within the family were changing as a result of mothers working outside the home, adolescents earning relatively high wages, fathers commuting to work or traveling a great deal, and a decline in the husband's authority over the wife and of parents' authority over children.

The changes in the family had been accompanied by an increasing divorce rate. Between 1887 and 1891, the divorce-marriage ratio was 1:17; in 1950 it was 1:4.3, an almost ninefold increase (p. 474). The children involved in divorce rose 15%, from 6.3 per 1,000 in 1950 to 7.2 per 1,000 in 1960. Burgess and Locke reiterated that "the companionship family relies upon divorce as a means of rectifying a mistake in mate selection" (p. 479), but paradoxically stated that "the American home [was] the most transient of any in the world" (p. 505). They attributed the lack of permanence to four overarching social processes: urbanization, secularization, individualism, and especially, mobility.

Burgess and Locke (1960) stated that there was a need for caution when drawing conclusions about the future of the family; the companionship family had lost many of its traditional functions but retained its institutional functions "as a social group in society" (p. 684). They predicted that the family would survive not only because of its long history of adaptability but also because its functions of giving and receiving of affection and of personality development contributed to personal satisfaction. The increased family disruption evidenced by the high divorce rate would continue at an accelerated pace for a few years, but certain factors already apparent in 1960 would help stabilize the family in 20 to 30 years. These included a slowing down of the increase of population, the stopping of immigration, the transition of the economy to a security basis, and the expansion of family services. Urbanization, they predicted, would continue and would be associated with a decline of familism and greater individualism.

The 1960 predictions by Burgess and Locke were almost the same as their 1945 forecasts. In the intervening years, the divorce rate had declined after its postwar jump, and there had been an expansion of family services and of social security and similar programs. Some of Burgess and Locke's predicted longer-term trends had continued, especially the younger age at marriage and the increasing number of women gainfully employed outside the home. But other trends had not followed their predictions; the birthrate had risen sharply in the late 1940s and the 1950s.

Burgess and Locke seem to have overlooked the manifestations of family distress and social pathologies that were appearing as well as couples' and families' skyrocketing demands for mental health services. Novelists and social scientists were raising disturbing questions about identity and values, for example, in Wilson's (1955) *Man in the Grey Flannel Suit* and about the pressures for conformity and status in Whyte's (1956) *Organization Man*. Even though television glorified "typical" family life and parodied fathers' ineptness, the increasing juvenile delinquency and gang warfare in the cities were predictors of institutional flabbiness, if not decadence, and of social disorder as well as family disorganization.

By 1960, a generation that viewed happiness as the goal of marriage was coming of age. The emphasis on marriage as a companionate relationship, based on affection but not institutionalized, was accompanied by major developments in social science research. Kinsey and his colleagues' studies of male and female sexuality catalyzed interest in marital relations (Kinsey, Pomeroy, & Martin, 1948; Kinsey, Pomeroy, Martin, & Gebhard, 1953).

Anxiety about nuclear war affected the family during the decade. Many families drained their financial resources and strained their energies to build bomb shelters. "Duck and cover" drills in schools and televised news about even more destructive weapons led to the realization that power was out of control. The proliferation of nuclear weapons and the paranoid politics that culminated in the Cuban missile crisis in 1962 made it Auden's "Age of Anxiety."

The Korean conflict, McCarthyism at home, and international politics, along with anxiety about "the bomb," sparked interest in such classics as Toynbee's (1934) *Study of History* and Spengler's (1929) *Decline of the West*. Sartre's novels and dramas expressed the pessimism and malaise of Western society. Existentialism gained recognition as a meaningful philosophy in the 1950s, and there is little doubt that the nihilism intrinsic to the belief that God was dead spread to the younger generation. In *Existence*, May, Angel, and Ellenberger (1958) described the applicability of existential concepts to the psychotherapies. In psychoanalysis, the emphasis on object relations brought into focus Marx's prescient insight—labor had become a commodity, and relations between people would assume the same fragmented character as their relations to objects on assembly lines where workers handled only bits and pieces, not the completed products, and where continuing interactions with parts limited wholesome thoughts and feelings.

Optimism about the well-being of the American family peaked; the divorce rate declined from 2.6 per 1,000 in 1950 to a postwar low of 2.2 in 1960, and the median age of first marriage fell in 1955 to the lowest figure of the century (22.6 years for men and 20.2 for women). Even though the marriage rate dropped from 11.1 per 1,000 in 1950 to 8.5 per 1,000 in 1960 (the low for the century), the birthrate climbed to 23.7 per 1,000 population in 1955 (16.2 in 1989). The average family size rose from 3.54 in 1950 to 3.67 in 1967, peaked at 3.70 in 1970, and then started falling to a twentieth-century low of 3.16 in 1989. The declining divorce rate during the 1950s and the low age of first marriage were strong indicators of familism.

Unfortunately, major historical developments that would alter family life were under way. City life became ghettoized as upwardly mobile middle-class families moved to the suburbs; in 1957, *West Side Story* depicted the gang wars that had grown from the hazards of the slums. For middle-class adults who had grown up during the 1930s and had gone to war in the 1940s, the 1950s was to be the decade of the family—a "haven in a heartless world" (Lasch, 1975).

Despite the prevailing optimism about the future of the new companionate family and its members' well-being, a few critics were concerned about the long-term consequences of the changes in the family that were occurring, especially those affecting personality development and character formation. Iago Galdston (1958) stated flatly that the American family was in crisis. Any concerns about mental health and illness, he averred, should include questions about the health of the community and about how the community contributes to the health and illness of its members. He insisted that scrutiny should be focused on the family, "the social integer of society" (p. 229), which was abandoning traditional patriarchal patterns, values, and mores and was in transition to becoming *matriarchoid*. The features of a matriarchive society were not yet discernible, but its pathologies—juvenile delinquency, divorce, alcohol, and drugs—were appearing. Galdston maintained that they could be attributed, in part, to the defective character formation resulting from impairment of superego development because of the absence of the father.

Riesman et al. (1950) described the American character as changing from the inner-directed type, with its internalized controls, to the other-directed type, which was attuned to group mores and behaviors. But Parsons doggedly argued that, historically, American culture had valued instrumental activity, individualism, and achievement and that by specializing in the "production of personality" and by giving the child independence, the family was preparing him or her to face the unpredictability of the modern world. Even as late as 1961, in *Character and Society*, Parsons maintained that the family had emerged from crisis and was beginning to be stabilized. The following year, he asserted that parents were "firmly committed to a policy of training serious independence in their children" (Parsons, 1962, p. 115). Thus, he rationalized that parents were not abdicating responsibility but were being realistic, inasmuch as social change was moving too fast for them to anticipate and to prepare their children for the future (Lasch, 1975, pp. 127–128).

THE SEARING SIXTIES

The family sociologists' glowing and sometimes expansive views of the family in the 1950s and of its future were dimmed by the events of the 1960s and relegated to historical obscurity in the 1970s. The early indicators of family distress were the disaffection of white middle-class youths and the newly developing youth culture of the late 1950s, along with increasing gang violence in the slums. In retrospect, we can see that a host of factors combined to produce the problems, if not the alienation, of the young that progressed during the 1960s to rebellion against society and its values. Demographically, for example, there was a disproportionately large number of children and adolescents. Traditionally, a large number of children has been associated with familism and strong family units, but throughout this century, a disproportionate number of adolescents has been linked with turmoil and an increase in the suicide rate in the young. As Friedenberg (1964) explained, large numbers of young persons are frightening to adults, who sense that their beliefs and values will be challenged. Consequently, adults tend to maintain a defensive distance from the young. Salinger's (1951) *Catcher in the Rye*, which described the void between the generations in the 1950s, became a testament of youth.

In *The Vanishing Adolescent,* Friedenberg (1964) foresaw many of the problems that would soon erupt, particularly the unease and alienation of middle-class youths and the delinquency and antisocial activity in the lower class and among gangs. The large number of young people heightened competition for jobs, athletic achievements, and educational opportunities. Steady pressures were placed on them by the extended training and preparation needed in order to participate in the increasingly bureaucratic and technological society, with its impersonal interpersonal relationships and sometimes obsessive depersonalization. Friedenberg was critical of adults, many of whom "treat adolescents more like things than people . . . [and of] how impersonal the high school environment had become" (pp. x–xiii). But his greatest indictment was of American society in the late 1950s: "The whole society is worse than I thought; and it is bad for more fundamental reasons and reasons that are merely the obverse of its most highly prized values. . . . Our problem is not conformity. . . . The difficulty is that *we have only norms to conform to, rather than standards*" (pp. xiv–xv; italics added). He added that the young "rightly distrust from the depth of their hearts the jolly establishment" (p. xvii). In the schools, "the youngsters crouched in the corridor like see-no-evil monkeys during compulsory Civil Defense drills [and heard] the blatting jocularity and pompous patriotism that [came] . . . over the public address system into every corner" (p. xii). He asked, "What does Don Quixote do when the windmills become atomic piles and go underground?" (p. 142).

Friedenberg (1964) feared that adolescence as a distinct life stage with its particular development process was becoming obsolete. Traditional adolescent high school years were being eroded by the precocious maturity of the 10- to 15-year-olds, whose extensive exposure to TV and peer influences made them worldly-wise at a young age. Young people were having difficulty defining themselves because the culture was frustrating the emotional processes necessary for healthy development, and they were reacting by playing it cool. The young, according to Friedenberg, were struggling against the timidity, corruption, and brute Orwellian power of the adult world. He deplored their "having no concept of fixed stars, [as well as] . . . no gift for navigation" (p. xvi). They were "rebels without a cause" in an increasingly technological world that was becoming a bureaucratic maze until the blacks, with purpose and integrity, launched their battles for desegregation and obtained some support from a few brave young whites who joined their struggle.

The major problem for the young and eventually for our society was that, in Friedenberg's (1964) words, "homo sapiens is undergoing a fundamental model change [that] . . . involves great alteration in the processes of personality development. A different kind of adult is being produced. . . . The change . . . [is] a weakening in the relationship between maturity on one hand, and stability of identity on the other" (pp. 133–134). He concluded that the young person's efforts to define the self, build a sense of integrity, and respect both self and others could be helped only by strengthening our cultural roots and institutions.

Many of Friedenberg's views supported Galdston's contentions about an increase in character pathology resulting from instability of the family and the ascendance of the "consumer culture." Also, his focusing concern about personal identity and integrity foreshadowed the mass of identity problems that became so prominent in the 1960s and 1970s and would be succeeded by the even more grievous problem of integrity and commitment in the 1980s. In the 1970s and 1980s, many of our patients presented these problems, which sometimes appeared clinically as multiple personality disorder or, more often, as borderline personality disorder.

In his introduction, Riesman described *The Vanishing Adolescent* (Friedenberg, 1964) as a profound and imaginative diagnosis of our time. He added that the young were alienated because society was amorphous and asked little of them other than to oppose communism at home with the aid of Joseph McCarthy and abroad with weapons when necessary. In 1950, Riesman and his colleagues defined character as "the more or less permanent and socially conditioned organization of an individual's drives and satisfactions—the kind of 'set' with which he approaches the world and people. . . . 'Social character' is that part of 'character' which is shared among significant social groups and . . . is the product of the experience of these groups" (p. 18).

The linkage between society and character is age-old. Hippocrates (1952) wrote about it in the first treatise on ecological medicine, *Airs, Waters, and Places*, and the classical Greeks emphasized it, as evidenced by Lycurgus's laws for training Spartan children, by the attention given to it by Plato (1952) in *The Republic* (character formation was too precious to be entrusted to the parents' variability and, instead, needed to be under the control of the guardian-philosophers of the state), and by Heracleitus' assertion that "character is fate." Freud and his colleagues offered the first systematic formulation of personality development and character formation. This stimulated cultural anthropologists and others to study the relationships between family structure, child-rearing practices, and personality and character in various societies. Riesman (1950) noted that Erikson's study of the social character of the Yurok Indians showed that "systems of child training . . . [created] the configuration of attitudes" that would be optimum under the tribe's "natural conditions and economic-historic necessities" (p. 19). Also, Riesman cited Erich Fromm's opinion that character formation requires the children's desiring "what objectively is necessary for them to do. . . . Outer force [therefore] is replaced by inner compulsions, and by the particular kind of human energy which is channeled into character traits" (pp. 19–20). Freud had described such processes in the development of the ego-ideal and the superego, and Parsons and his colleagues emphasized the ways in which roles were the articulations between the individual and society.

Riesman et al. (1950) described two revolutions that influenced social character. The first was the increasing separation of the person from his or her family that had been begun with the Renaissance and the Reformation, and the other was the "shift from an age of production to an age of consumption" (pp. 20–21) that had begun early in this century. From an organic-cyclic historical perspective, Riesman conceptualized three societal stages and associated each with its particular character type. The first, that of high growth potential (with an explosive increase of population), was associated with the tradition-directed character; the child was intensively socialized in accord with cultural traditions and regulations that were reinforced throughout life by established customs, etiquette, and the institutions. Familism and a relatively slow rate of social change were prominent features. Tradition-directed societies were common in the Far East and in the West until the decline of feudalism in the fourteenth and fifteenth centuries.

The second stage, that of transitional growth (slowly declining birth and death rates and a relatively stable population curve), has been associated with the inner-directed character type. The strict external controls of tradition and custom are replaced by an internalized control mechanism—a "psychological gyroscope" that is implanted and "set" by parents and other authorities early in the child's life to keep him or her "on course," to ensure behavioral conformity and a "consonant self-consciousness and individuality" (Riesman et al. 1950, pp. 31–32). Prominent features of the inner-directed society are mobility, expansion, production, a future orientation, and a goal orientation. Eventually, the individualism that has been a distinctive force in the life of the inner-directed person is accompanied by a decline in familism, and increasingly the person is linked directly to the state and society. Familism wanes, and the family loses its influence on its members. The government and society become centralized and bureaucratic, and other people become "The Problem" (pp. 33–34).

The third stage, that of incipient population decline, is associated with the emerging other-directed character type. Riesman et al. (1950) insisted that their other-directed character was a contemporary product of capitalism, industrialization, and urbanization:

> What is common to all the other-directed people is that their contemporaries are the source of direction for the individual—either those known to him or those with whom he is indirectly acquainted through friends and through the mass media. . . . This source is "internalized." . . . The goals toward which the other-directed person strives shift with that guid-

ance.... [Only] the process of striving itself and the process of paying close attention to the signals from others ... remain unaltered throughout life. (p. 37)

Thus, the tradition-oriented person was controlled externally by firmly established precepts and customs, and the inner-directed individual by a psychological gyroscope. In contrast, the other-directed person has to rely on radar for guidance and control. Also, each of the character types has its own internalized emotional controls. For the tradition directed, it is shame; for the inner directed it is guilt; and, for the other directed it is diffuse anxiety.

When Riesman et al. (1950) were writing, the other-directed individuals were mainly young persons who lived in the big cities and were in the upper-income groups. They foresaw that prominent features of the developing other-directed society would be a rise of "white collar and service trades ... an increased corruption of words and images from the new mass media ... [and] many 'socialized' behaviors both for success and for more marital and personal adaptation" (pp. 36–37). Such changes would be accompanied by "chips in the family and child-rearing practices" (p. 37). Already "the latency period in childhood was getting shorter and shorter and as a result adult males try to create or retain artificial latency periods" (Riesman et al., 1950, p. 321). As families became smaller in the 1960s and 1970s and urban life dominated the American scene, family instability increased, parental and school discipline tended to relax, and our society was labeled permissive. The peer group with its cult of popularity became increasingly important, and by the 1980s, the other-directed population were the children and adults with the herd instinct who engaged in fads, joined the crowd, and followed the popular (and usually self-serving) social and political groups. Some even became cultists.

The other-directed character type was observable in Athens, Rome, and Alexandria during their decline: "Fashion not only ruled as a substitute for mores and customs, but it was a rapidly changing fashion that held sway" (Riesman et al., 1950, p. 38). The "insatiable force" (p. 38) of the other-directed character's need for approval, however, was a distinctive American feature. For the other-directed society, the product in demand "is a personality." Inasmuch as the culture does not emphasize established values and does not have clear-cut goals, parents have doubts about child rearing and turn to friends, the media, and often to so-called experts for advice. Parents pass on to the child "their own contagious, highly diffused anxiety ... by giving the child approval ... [which] becomes almost the only unequivocal good in this situation" (p. 66). The consciousness of the self becomes heightened awareness of the self, especially in relation to others. The child has both to make good and to define "what making good means" (pp. 64–66).

The family of the other-directed character type, according to Riesman et al. (1950), is "merely part of a wider social environment to which he (or she) early becomes attentive. . . . The other-directed person is, in a sense, at home everywhere and nowhere, capable of a rapid if sometimes superficial intimacy with and response to everyone" (p. 41). Riesman et al. (1950) noted the concern about disintegration of the family; the relatively high divorce rate was indicative of the new demands people were making on their mates and their marriages. They stated that a new model of marriage needed to be developed, one that "finds its opportunity precisely in the choices that a free-divorce leisure society opens up. Because women are less privatized than they have traditionally been, marriage offers more for millions of people than ever before in its long history" (p. 320).

Although Riesman's discussion of the different character types (and particularly the development of the other-directed type) was both incisive and ahead of his time, it is difficult to understand what his concept of a new model of marriage and the choices to which he alluded would mean for the family. The artificial latency periods in young adulthood and the other-directed orientation tend to increase dependency, lead to instability in relationships, and impair family cohesion and vitality. The now-accepted serial monogamy and millions of children of divorce seem to have been logical outcomes of the other-directed character and the society.

Despite the problems for society and for the family that were surfacing, especially the rebellion of youth and the early development of the counterculture, Parsons (1962) described youth as being "less rebellious" (p. 116), somewhat apathetic politically, and "better integrated in the general culture" (pp. 113–119). Some youthful dissatisfaction was a sign of commitment and high standards that society could not meet. Parsons (1962) concluded that "American society in a sense appears to be running a scheduled course. . . . [The] strain demonstrated by youth . . . may be considered normal for this (type of society) and . . . the patterns of reaction on the part of American youth also seem well within normal limits" (p. 122).

In contrast to his opinions about youth in the early 1960s, which were appallingly wide of the mark, Parsons (1962) saw accurately that youth groups were occupying an increasingly differentiated position in society. They were under special conditions of strain, particularly in education, because of the impact of social change and developing anomie (which he did not see). Also, youth was caught in the conflict between the societal conservatism of the Eisenhower era and the burgeoning social activism of the 1960s.

Lasch (1975) declared that "Parsonian theory has been overtaken by events [and Parsons had] . . . hardly anticipated the emergence of a youth culture that condemned American society in the most sweeping terms, repudiated the desirability of growing up in the usual way, and sometimes appeared to repudiate the desirability of growing up at all" (p. 129). Also, American youth of the 1960s saw society as having betrayed its ideals and "sold out"; society could be accepted only with guilt. "Youth culture itself has made the family a prime target—not just something to 'rebel' against but a corrupt and decadent institution to be overthrown. . . . Hostility to the family has survived the demise of the political radicalism of the 1960s and flourishes amid the conservatism of the 1970s" (Lasch, 1975, pp. 129–130).

During the 1950s and 1960s, the parenting by adults who had endured the hardships of the Great Depression tended to be benign, if not permissive and at times indulgent. In the dominant white middle class, many of those adults were experiencing upward mobility and achieving status. Inasmuch as they had lived in two cultures (economic strain and affluence), they displayed a mixture of values to their children. Youth responded with an efflorescence of identity problems that in the 1970s would be supplanted by the problem of "commitment" in personal relationships.

A number of developments in the early 1960s coalesced to change American political and social history and to contribute to the forthcoming family crisis. They included the high level of anxiety about nuclear weapons, the beginning of the Vietnam War, the discovery of "the pill" and the loosening of sexual strictures, the cultural acceptance of the credit card and its promise of immediate "buy now, pay later" gratification, and the technological triumphs in space, air travel, computers, and television. Change in mores and values penetrated the family. Youth revolted, at first "without cause" but later with the counterculture's disdain of parental norms and precepts and still later with defiance and "dropping out." The divorce rate climbed enormously within just a few years during the mid-1960s. The courageous battles of blacks (aided by young white allies) for their constitutional rights, which began in the 1950s, intensified during the 1960s. Also, the women's movement stirred after the familistic 1950s, when millions of well-educated women did their best to fit the model of the typical suburban mother/housewife.

Jules Henry (1963), in *Culture Against Man*, maintained that there was a disequilibrium between the production of material goods and the unlimited desires of our society; the demands for goods and consuming were continuously stimulated by advertising and had no natural ceiling. "Ours is a driven culture. It is driven on by its achievement, competitive, profit, and mobility drives, and by the drives for security and a higher standard of living" (p. 13). Anxiety stemmed from the "race between consumers and products. . . . At present there is no visible middle ground between the needs of the caveman and the cravings of space-man" (pp. 17, 21).

In our "Era of Consumption," according to Henry, the first commandment is to Create More Desire and the second is to consume. "Advertising helps sustain the culture and is an expression of an irrational economy that has depended for survival on a fantastically high standard of living incorporated into the American mind as a moral imperative" (Henry, 1963, p. 45). Advertising was directed toward the family as the basic unit of consumption. Americans were undergoing a psychic revolution, of which the first phase was the deliberate creation of needs and the second an "unhinging of the old impulse controls" (p. 26). Optimistically, the eventual third phase would be a restoration of balance and a new level of integration. In the meantime, "a high-rising standard of living has become a moral ideal. . . . Only a people who have learned to decontrol their impulses can consume as we do" (p. 44).

An internalization of "the drive toward a higher standard of living" is now a part of the cultural configuration (Henry, 1963, p. 25). To compensate for personality impoverishment, the worker substitutes the goal of a higher standard of living and security for the inner self. Restlessness, frequent job changes, and the search for the perfect job, however, become ways of life in which individuals can hide their narcissistic wounds while they live and work with a great deal of fear. Lack of involvement in work results from the specialization of tasks and the declining loyalty between employee and employer; work is "an emotionless connection" and is desocializing. Consequently, workers turn to family or friends for meaning and involvement, for love and feelings, for life without competition, and for a sense of humanness (p. 128).

Henry (1963) was particularly concerned about the effects of the culture on the young. His poll of teenagers' "personal problems" showed that they were preoccupied with acceptance, appeal, and conformity, which he attributed to "the great population flux . . . that makes the personal community so uncertain from day to day that people must use every possible device to guarantee that they will not be alone" (p. 189). Also, "relationships are never guaranteed but must be won, [and the result is] anxiety in inter-personal relationships . . . [and] the hunger for popularity among teenagers" (p. 180).

With the declining age of marriage in the 1950s and changed attitudes toward sexuality, Henry (1963) found that young girls were becoming more sexually aggressive and that there was increased competition for boys:

> It is no exaggeration to say that the teenage American girl lives on a razor-edge of sexual competition. . . . Courtship and friendship, presumably two of the greatest joys of life—are discussed with considerable anxiety. And this is a central paradox of the age—that its pleasures are often negated by a concomitant anxiety so that love itself, one of the dearest values of our culture, becomes a drive—the courtship drive. (pp. 180–182)

In Henry's description of teenagers' problems, we can sense many of the features of the other-directed character type Riesman described only a dozen years earlier. Thus, many aspects of our culture in the early 1960s were combining to stress the family. The technological developments, rapid change, and new freedoms, compounded by consumerism and depersonalization in the workplace, produced stimuli and demands that threatened to exceed family members' coping abilities. The results were the continuing barrage of relationship problems that Henry saw in their early stages, the fantastic rise in the divorce rate in the late 1960s, and the rapidly increasing demands for mental health services.

H. V. Dicks (1967) expressed confidence in the future of the family as he summarized his 16 years of experience in marital study and therapy at the Tavistock Clinic in England. After World War II, he noted, the caseload "swelled into a flood as one symptom of social change and dislocation in the wake of this cataclysm" (p. 1). Demands for help for families came from many sources. The magnitude of the problem of marital instability led to the establishment of the Royal Commission on Divorce in 1951 and its 1956 pronouncement that there was a "disquieting social epidemic" (p. 3). The crude divorce rate in England and Wales rose from 0.02 per 1,000 in 1910 to 0.67 per 1,000 in 1953, a figure still tremendously lower than in the United States. "Had this fabulous increase of 3,350 percent been recorded for tuberculosis or dysentery—what a panic would have been caused, and what an outcry for most drastic measures of research and prevention" (p. 4). Dicks also pointed out that there had been no such increase in the incidence of mental illness, juvenile delinquency, or crime, and asked whether many tensions and discontents were being "worked out in this intimate field of marital relations, thereby saving other manifestations of stress? Perhaps marital strife was a kind of substitute psychiatric illness, or at least a symptom of disordered biosocial adaptation following the war?" (p. 4). Dicks expressed special concern about divorce depriving children of healthful home conditions, of security, and also of "subtler, less objectively measurable factors, of the essential elements of love, security, and understanding discipline which are the nutrients of personality growth and mental health" (p. 4). He voiced fears that the increasing number of broken and disturbed homes would have adverse long-term effects on the young, who eventually would be the adult members of the society.

In evaluating the social setting for marriage and the family in England in the early 1960s, Dicks (1967) emphasized the unprecedented "technological transformation of society" (p. 26) following the two great wars of the century. The rapid erosion of the old order and the social changes were responsible in part for marital conflict, because they produced a "constriction and atomization of the modern family" (p. 26) that increased each spouse's dependence upon the other and requirements for satisfaction and security that previously had been met by a "more diversified and structured family milieu buttressed by social and religious sanctions" (p. 26). Consequently, the modern trend toward autonomy and independence would meet resistance both from within the person and from society, because the resistance would spring from "the older, more familiar and secure order, handed down by the culture lag of generations" (p. 26). According to Dicks, some persons would not be able to adapt to the demands of the more complex marital roles and to the social conflict. Also, there were changed public attitudes toward broken marriages, adultery, and abuse in the family; in the past, marital breakdown and family disruptions were concealed or dealt with by members of the extended family and were not as public as in postwar society.

In addition, Dicks insisted that marriage is a system of interpersonal relations that includes the interactions of three interrelated subsystems. The first, and most public, is that of sociocultural values and norms that involve homogamy. The second is that of the ego, which operates at the level of personal values, conscious judgments, and expectations developed from childhood. Mature dependence, with its flexibility and tolerance of ambivalence in oneself and one's partner, is necessary if this second subsystem is to function well. The third consists of the unconscious forces that form the positive and negative bonds between spouses and determine many of their interactions. According to Dicks, this conceptual framework could be a basis for assessing the contributions of each subsystem either to spousal conflict or to integration.

Dicks (1967) emphasized the parallels between the family and society; in both, there were "contradictions, between respect for individual growth into equality and the archaic defensive postures of dominance and possessiveness. . . . [Contemporary] *nuclear families are the microcosmic reflections of what goes on in the larger society*" (p. 27; italics added). He concluded that there was an evolutionary trend in marital relations and the family toward "greater integrity" and "spontaneous goodness" (p. 319); regression and disruption could be the beginning that led toward a new integration. He reminded us that women's rights were historically "quite new," as were concepts of personality development and the right to happiness. It might take a hundred years to establish new social norms because "we live on the unconscious of our grandparents' generation which our parents transmitted as our cultural heritage" (p. 319). He expressed hope that the new norms and their social system would be more flexible than those of the past and would recognize "the instability of biological and social equilibria in growth processes" (p. 320). Psychiatry and the behavioral sciences could assist the striving toward growth.

Dick's insights add to our understanding of the modern family. He saw that the social system and the family system were in step and that the stresses in one were also appearing in the other; thus, the widespread societal turmoil and family conflicts in the 1960s were counterparts. His discussion of the contradictions between the past and the present produced by rapid social change have direct clinical applicability in, for example, the use of the three-generation genogram in family therapy.

In the United States, the events of the 1960s—desegregation, the revolt of youth and the development of the counterculture, women's protests, and especially the folly of the Vietnam War—battered the family and shook the wider society. Generational differences stunned many parents, some of whom trembled with disbelief at what was happening, while others began "to do their own thing" and still others grimly resisted change.

THE 1970s AND THE LOOMING CRISIS

The bewildering array of events that threatened the social order stimulated interest in their influences on families and also in the concepts of generational differences. Why the presumably advantaged children of the 1960s were so dissatisfied with the American way of life and societal institutions was a pressing question for which there seemed to be no adequate answers. As R. Hill (1970), Goode (1964), Elder (1974), and Hareven (1977) showed, historical time influences family life. For example, Hill (1970) maintained that "each generation is bounded in its career choices by its peculiar biography. . . . To determine why certain options are preferred over others we need to consider the historically bounded childhood experience and socialization of each cohort" (p.

285). Hill found differences in family attitudes about consuming among the grandparents born in 1907, the parents born in 1931, and the third generation born in 1953 that could be linked to differences in the historical context of their marriages, secularism, and the trends toward greater prosperity and a planned economy. The grandparents' generation was characterized by caution and modest goals, and that of the parents by prudence, especially in regard to family planning and acquisitions; but those married in 1953 were forward planners in that they bought houses early in their marriages and usually relied upon credit to obtain automobiles, furniture, and the like.

Interest in the concepts of generational differences in marriages and family life climbed during the 1970s and has continued. Why such interest developed when it did is intriguing inasmuch as major studies of the family since World War II, except for Sorokin's and Zimmerman's, have been remarkably unhistorical. It is possible that the severe family problems of the late 1960s have been so baffling that historical studies are needed in order to place them in perspective. Another possibility is demographic, in that the longer life span has led to a great increase in the number of elderly persons and three- and four-generation families, and thus to interest in generational differences. Still another is that as the century was drawing to a close, it was only natural that there would be interest in its events and sociopolitical processes.

Elder (1974) analyzed data gathered from 1934 to 1964 in the longitudinal Oakland Growth Study initiated by Jones and Stolz in 1932. The subjects were 167 Caucasian children from working- and middle-class families who were born in 1920–21 and had experienced the Great Depression during their early pubertal years and adolescence. His objectives were to determine how economic deprivation had affected the subjects' adult lives and was associated with generational changes. He conceptualized family adaptation as the primary link between economic hardship and the individual's behavior, personality, and life course.

Financial loss (of one third or more of annual income) affected families by producing changes in the division of labor, changes in relationships, and social strains. The division of labor in the family following the father's unemployment, and often the family's downward social mobility, made it necessary for all family members to help meet the needs for maintenance. The changes in family relationships were mainly a diminution of the father's social prestige and emotional significance and an increase in the power of the mother, who became the decision maker and emotional resource. "Roles in the deprived household and the matricentric family joined forces in structuring a conducive environment for traditional sex roles and an accelerated movement toward adulthood" (p. 279). The social strains included marital tensions, a sense of inferiority, and uncertainty about status and identity stemming from changes in family income: "They believed that they were held in lower esteem [by their peers] than was actually the case" (Elder, 1974, p. 280). These perceptions led to recognition striving, achievement motivation, and an orientation toward the future. As they grew older, those from such ambiguous social situations reported self-consciousness, emotional sensitivity, and emotionality that prompted relatively early marriages.

The depression had three enduring effects over the life course to adulthood. One involved the paths through which the young achieved adult status. For men, family deprivation made achievement dependent on effort, whereas women often neutralized their educational handicaps by marriage. The second, adult health, was negatively related to economic hardship, mainly among those from working-class homes. The third was values. As Elder (1974) asserted, "The one common value across men and women is the centrality of the family and the importance of children in marriage" (p. 282). Others included a premium on job and security, the importance of work over family and leisure time, and a heightened belief in "the power of money" (p. 283). In Elder's opinion, those values contributed significantly to the "familistic aura of the postwar years" (p. 282). Also, parents who viewed the future in terms of the depression pushed their young to find secure jobs more appropriate to the 1930s than to the prosperity of the 1950s (p. 276).

Thus, the Great Depression contributed to the "baby boom" of the late 1940s and 1950s and to an increasing emphasis on consumption and education. The offspring of deprived families tended to be conservative and to hold traditional values; having children was a higher priority than marital understanding or companionship. Largely from "intuition and self-reflection," the depression became linked to "an extraordinary work commitment, a self-conscious desire for security and an inability to partake of pleasure or leisure without guilt feelings" (p. 277). Elder (1974) quoted Hoar: "We search for affluence with neurotic intensity so that our children will not have to go through what we went through" (p. 277).

For the children and teenagers of the Oakland subjects, the prosperity since World War II, increased population, and educational upgrading had led to an extension of the dependency years and an "increasing segregation of the young from the routine experiences of adults" (Elder, 1974, p. 292). In the consumer-oriented "society of abundance," the young did not need to be productive, were a surplus group, and were experiencing problems in the 1960s and early 1970s. The 1970 White House Conference on Children emphasized the issue of age segregation and the necessity to "bring adults back into the lives of children and children back into the lives of adults" (p. 293). Parents of the Great Depression were uneasy about the "beneficent life that required so little from their children" (Elder, 1974, p. 293).

The Great Depression and World War II were collective experiences that fostered sentiments of self-sacrifice and of earned success and inspired action in the national interest (Elder, 1974, p. 295). Between 1929 and 1946, Americans experienced hardships that increased the value of material goods and the desire for children. The economic upswing after the war allowed those dreams to materialize. "In one lifespan, Americans had moved from scarcity to abundance, from sacrifice to the freedoms made possible by prosperity" (p. 296). Parents who grew up in the 1930s tended to give a much greater priority to finances and possessions than would their adult offspring. In the late 1960s and early 1970s, many young persons took a comfortable standard of living for granted. A job that offered a chance for personal growth and achievement and to contribute something unique was as important or more so than one that offered just security.

Elder saw the depression as conducive to the increasing endorsement of "the companionship form of the family" (p. 286) described by Burgess and his colleagues. According to Elder, the companionship model of marriage, with its emphasis on equality, was rejected by those who reached marital age in the first decade of this century, accepted by those who reached marital age in the early 1930s, and endorsed by those who reached marital age in the 1950s.

Later, Elder was able to obtain data from the Berkeley Guidance Study on a cohort of 214 middle-class Caucasian children born in 1928–29 and also on their parents and grandparents. Thus, he could compare the effects of the Great Depression on the young Berkeley children with the effects on the Oakland adolescents, study the effects of historical events and processes across three generations, and conduct both cohort (referring to a group sharing a demographic characteristic, e.g., year of birth) and generational (referring to family as well as to time) analyses. In the Berkeley cohort, Elder and Rockwell (1979) found that during the depression, the 8- to 10-year-old children from deprived families had more positive feelings toward their mothers than their fathers:

> The principal result of economic deprivation for parent-child relationships was a weaker tie between fathers and sons and much stronger ties between mothers and daughters. "This female bond stands out as the strongest intergenerational tie among families in the Great Depression." . . . It represents a general pattern in situations where male support is precarious or absent. (p. 47)

In adolescence, the Berkeley girls from deprived families were more adequate and goal oriented than the nondeprived. Also, their mothers' taking jobs outside the home provided them with a model that "broadened their ideas about women's options" (Elder & Rockwell, 1979, p. 49) and laid a foundation for the women's movement of the 1960s. The deprived boys were more ambitious, resourceful, and sensitive to others' needs than the nondeprived but were also more vulnerable to their peers' judgments. Those in the middle class tended to have a view of the world as meaningless (p. 48).

Elder and Rockwell (1979) concluded from their Oakland-Berkeley cohort comparisons that the children had been affected differently because the two groups of families had endured the depression at different periods in their lives; also, the children had been affected by the quality of the parents' marriage. Similarities between the deprived in the Oakland and Berkeley groups were that both experienced hardships and difficulties during their developmental years and had limited educations, but their work had provided compensations, and they saw life as becoming "more satisfying since adolescence" (p. 301). Among the differences were that the younger Berkeley children were exposed to deprivation over a longer period of their early life and sustained more adverse outcomes than the Oakland subjects. "It is among the Berkeley offspring of deprived families that we can see the greatest discontinuity between childhood and adult experience, and their significant [deleterious] contributions to psychological well-being in middle age. The legacy of family deprivation remains a problem at mid-life even among the most successful men" (p. 301). Studying the life course showed that favorable adult experiences could lessen, if not overcome, much of the adversity that had been the legacy of the Great Depression.

In view of the "limits of growth" that our society began to feel in the mid-1970s, Elder (1974) speculated that the inequalities in income and wealth prominent in the 1920s would again become apparent. The "image of limited resources has much in common with the realities of Depression life in the 1930s, with the problem of 'making the best of what we have.' . . . For children of the Depression generation and especially for their children, some disciplines practiced in the 30s—frugality, conservation, and so forth—were likely to become imperatives in the years ahead" (p. 297).

We have devoted significant space to Elder's work because the data base enabled him to look at one of our interests that is important for family studies: the influence of sociopolitical events on childhood socialization and the American family over two to three generations. Also, much that Elder described is within the senior author's personal experience.

Zimmerman (1972a) pointed out that in each century in modern history, both the family and its social system have undergone major changes. In the United States in the twentieth century, the marriage vows, especially "till death do us part" (p. 323), had lost much of their meaning. The outstanding feature had been the movement away from familism toward individualism. The atomistic family type that described the American family in the 1970s referred to the loss of family rights that had been transferred to individuals. Also, the family had much more social responsibility and less power than in the past; the resulting disequilibrium was responsible for much of the family crisis (pp. 323–324). In the middle class, despite the earlier age of puberty, children and youths were dependent for a longer period of time than ever before in history. Preparation for an occupation had moved during the century from about age 14 to age 24.

According to Zimmerman (1972a), the problem was, "Can the family continue to exist?" (p. 324). He noted that Aldous Huxley in *Brave New World* and George Orwell in *1984* had answered negatively. Zimmerman asked: "But what will its ceasing to exist mean for society? Will we continue in the same direction until we eliminate mother-love, paternal-obligation, and spousal loyalty?" (p. 324). He emphasized the basic nature of the family, noting first that it is "a unit in the web of the total sociological structure" (e.g., all great religions are familistic). It has functions, rights, and purpose, and in contrast to Parsons's views, "It gives the [family] members 'roles'" (p. 324). Second, the family "has as many fields of action as are necessary to life" (p. 327). Zimmerman's "triple field theory" about the family was that it must (a) satisfy the individual members; (b) participate in the moral structure; and (c) have societal rights and obligations. Third, one member can color, discolor, or stain the family.

As a consequence of these three principles, "when the ideological structure of the family system loses its virility and strength, the social system generally gets into trouble" (p. 325). And when both are in trouble, then the "casual nexus" reverses direction, and the family recreates the society. But before that breakdown, "the agents of the big society work against the family because . . . individuals do not ordinarily like restrictions—such as against divorce and sex freedom—or duties and responsibilities such as unlimited family support" (pp. 325–326).

The modern family, according to Zimmerman (1972a), still had its biological basis—its fundamental mammalian characteristics that are constant. But it also is a "legal structure" in the greater society and is part of the moral structure, and those two fundamental aspects of the family are cyclic, not constant. At present, "we seem to be in one of those extreme periods verging on anarchy in family-controlled social relations" (p. 326). Zimmerman noted that in the late 1960s, "young boys and girls fornicate nakedly and openly in the middle of crowds in broad daylight" (p. 327). Except in military combat or periods of revolutionary demoralization, this "type of reversion" had not been seen since the twelfth century.

The breakdown of the educational system, as evidenced by the assaults on college campuses, mob action, the students' forceful occupation of administrators' offices, students' and teachers' strikes, and the lack of use of the libraries, was a special concern. To Zimmerman, it would have long-term consequences, but he insisted that family behavior "tends to move in cycles" (p. 330). Such movement, however, is slow; it might take generations for extreme behavior to be at a maximum, but then a counter-revolutionary process begins in the next generation. An example is the antifamilism in the USSR after 1917, with either marriage or divorce (factual familism) being simply a matter of sending a postcard to the government so that one or the other would be officially registered. By the mid-1930s, the adolescents roaming Moscow's streets were "the wolves." Family codes were officially "remoralized" in 1936; in 1945 the gangs' activities had diminished markedly (Zimmerman, 1972b).

Zimmerman (1972a) saw our family system as having become "a very extreme type" and our institutions as being assailed. Churches were being pushed to give in and make radical changes quickly, and schools had lost the authority to discipline children. The public welfare system had to provide for millions of children abandoned by their fathers. "A society which permits men to breed carelessly and then go off casually with other women should not be surprised if it becomes the mode among the proletariat, leaving the demoralized woman with the total burden" (p. 331).

According to Zimmerman (1972a), a struggle between the antifamilistic and the profamily groups cannot endure more than two or three generations. The first is the generation in which "the trouble becomes evident and violent" (p. 332). The second is the one that is in the battle between the opposing forces, and the third sees the emergence of a new social order and of another type of family. He maintained that the third generation "might be here before the end of the century" (p. 332). Zimmerman stated that he knew his conclusions were often unorthodox, but that "insofar as they have been predictive, they have been proven to be fairly accurate" (p. 332).

Zimmerman (1972b) asserted that "the family has to reestablish itself by the end of the century or it will be too late" (p. 1). The domestic anarchy of the 1960s had weakened the family system. With his superb grasp of historical processes, Zimmerman was able to explain that several factors had coalesced to produce the youth rebellion. They included the raising of the age of consent and the lengthening of nonage for the young, which eventuated in an "overbalance of rights without obligations [that] gets out of hand" (p. 1) in a high civilization; adolescents' earlier physiological maturation also was contributory. The main result of these developments was anarchy directed toward the culture. Major problems in the early 1970s were (a) confusion about the moral and legal aspects of sexual relations, which in the past had been largely family controlled; (b) the anarchic youth movement; (c) the "overburdening of the public" (p. 5) to take care of families and the bankruptcy of our cities by relief expenditures; and (d) the disruption of the educational system.

Zimmerman (1972b) concluded that the question before our society was whether the middle class was sufficiently organized and motivated and the culture conducive to furnishing needed new direction and leadership. The answer would be in the affirmative; the "issue will be settled by the end of this century" (p. 9), and the family would be stabilized.

Veroff, Douban, and Kulka (1981) compared the results of their 1976 nationwide mental health survey with those of the 1957 survey conducted by Gurin, Veroff, and Feld (1960) to describe the problems that would become critical in the 1980s. In many ways there had been stability over the 20 years, but there also had been some generational and cohort changes in subjective mental health. One major generational change was that in 1976, young respondents reported more common symptoms of anxiety and a greater frequency of worry than their counterparts did in 1957. They attributed the emotional distress to uncertainty about the future, the job market, and especially about family roles that were in transition. Veroff and his colleagues (1981) stated: "Commitments to family and work are harder for young people to make than they once were. The culture at large is probably more uncertain about these issues" (p. 529).

Another major change was "the movement from social to personal integration of well-being" (Veroff et al., 1981, p. 529) which involved a shift toward individualism. It was supported by three changes that had occurred since 1957: (a) a diminution of the use of role standards to define adjustment and well-being, as reflected by reports of some ambivalence about parenthood, acknowledgement of the negative aspects of marriage, and increasing approval by young persons of decisions not to marry; (b) an increased emphasis on self-expressiveness that included concerns about individuality at work and women's commitments to work outside the home; and (c) a dramatic shift from "social organizational integration to interpersonal intimacy" (p. 529), as evidenced by a decline in the use of prayer, more turning to one's spouse or friends for emotional support than in the past, and a heavy emphasis on affiliative relationships and intimacy. These three changes "illustrate the general theme of a shift from the comfort of society and social integration to personal growth as a way of defining well-being" (p. 531). Also, in 1976, both men and women were thinking about themselves more in psychological terms and tended more often to seek professional help for problems than in 1957.

The uncertainty about the future included more reports in 1976 than in 1957 of parents' worrying about their children and their jobs. Also, parents in 1976 recognized that the dominant forces in their children's world were their peers and television. Overall, there was a significant tendency for people to be less optimistic about the future in 1976 than in 1957.

Thus, many findings indicated that people were becoming increasingly more oriented toward the self, self-fulfillment, and individualization, but Veroff and his colleagues (1981) expressed hesitation about whether there was increased narcissism. "There is an inevitable refocusing on the self. We do not see it as a disintegration of values, but as an adaptation that people have made to a complexity of choice in a heterogeneous society" (p. 535). The reports of self-sufficiency were considered to be adaptive in view of the likelihood of divorce, the many years most women spent as widows, and the increasing number of single persons; however, these could contribute to incompatibility in interpersonal relationships. Finding that there were more reports of marital satisfaction and happiness in 1976 than in 1957 was surprising, but the high divorce rate probably indicated that many persons were unwilling to live in a less than happy marriage.

In 1976, interpersonal difficulties were reported to be a major source of problems and symptoms; in 1957, however, such external events as the illness or death of a loved one or financial difficulties were more likely to be considered the cause. Veroff and his colleagues (1981) expressed concern about interpersonal intimacy becoming "a self-conscious arena for achievement rather than an automatic social activity.... More people now 'work at' intimacy rather than experience it as a spontaneous reaction to their relationships with others" (p. 538). Also, the concomitant decline of ritualized experiences and participation in organizations meant that persons were losing certain social guarantees of self-affirmation; not participating in organizations and in the community deprives persons of a sense of social stability and comfort in troubled times (p. 538).

Most of the changes that had occurred from 1957 to 1976 were seen as evidence of a cultural shift rather than as cohort changes. Cohort changes did include the younger subjects turning toward more formal help seeking, their more negative orientation toward parenthood, their acceptance that a woman might not marry, and the strong commitments younger women were making to their work. According to Veroff and his colleagues (1981), those cohort effects were reflecting "either expressive styles or value commitments made in late adolescence or early adulthood as part of young people's consolidation of values. This early commitment may be impervious to further social change" (p. 541).

A surprising finding was that there was no increase in reports of performing marital roles inadequately, even though there had been a large increase in reports of problems in marriage. Veroff and his colleagues (1981) asked insightfully:

> Could it be that the new vision of marital role difficulties as a system of interpersonal communication problems rather than as one in which one spouse or the other is at fault, reduces the guilt that men and women feel about marital difficulties? Perhaps the increased interpersonal focus on life problems reduces the responsibility of illness or incompetence.... Perhaps difficulties can be thought of as *system* problems, rather than personal flaws. (p. 543; italics added)

Veroff and his colleagues (1981) concluded that we were a happy society overall, but we were worried about the future. The emphasis on satisfying and fulfilling interpersonal relationships would mean that those who could not make the necessary interpersonal adjustments "would find living in our society a very isolated and detached experience" (p. 545). Also, there was some dwindling of optimism about the future, although many seemed to be confident about their own efficacy. Finally, the dominant mode of adapting to worries or unhappiness was by talking about troubles to other people. "Turning to friends has increased . . . at the same time that marriage and participation in formal organizations have become less common" (p. 549).

The Inner American (Veroff et al., 1981) provided a valuable and timely assessment of our society and of the family that revealed the diminished optimism following the Vietnam and Cambodian tragedies and the Watergate disgrace. The declining confidence in the government was paralleled by increasing family disruption, a strong trend toward individualism at the expense of family and community, and a definite weakening of familism. The data and the trends revealed by Veroff and his colleagues complemented Christopher Lasch's incisive 1975 social analysis of the modern family, *Haven in a Heartless World.*

As we have seen, ego psychology and group therapy began after

World War I, and the theory of interpersonal relations and object relations theory dominated psychiatry and other mental health disciplines in the 1950s and 1960s. Such changes were responses to the needs of individuals and the society; pre–World War I libido theory simply was not relevant to the complexities of life in the 1920s and 1930s, and the numerous problems of marriage and the family in the late 1940s and 1950s following World War II necessitated theories and therapies that were aimed toward salving or solving people's problems with each other. Individualism triumphed over familism; the turbulence of America in the 1960s, the Vietnam tragedy, and the disillusionments of the 1970s, coupled with divorce, distress, family disorder, and the high rates of mental illness (especially epidemic depression in the young), led to a search for survival.

For the individual, self-concept and self-esteem became topics of concern, as well as buzz words at a time when America's self-esteem was deflated by the defeat in Vietnam. Putting faith and trust into either the society or the family seemed to be as risky as it was unwise; well-being depended on the self, not others. Psychoanalytic theory was modified by the development of self-theory, which was touted as new but in fact was largely borrowed from the work of George Herbert Mead, Charles H. Cooley, and their colleagues in the 1910–1930 era. In psychiatry and psychology, as well as psychoanalysis, self-theories and therapies were developed, and there was an efflorescence of both popular and scientific therapies, including EST, assertiveness training, and groups aimed toward improving the self-concept and maintaining a requisite level of self-esteem. Self-interest changed from being a leitmotif to becoming a dominant theme as American society tumbled pessimistically into the 1980s and the rising antifamilism was increased by narcissism and divorce.

By the late 1970s, the family crisis that Zimmerman (1972a,b) had predicted was at hand. As described by Lasch (1975), among the fundamentals was, first, that the crisis had been developing since the late nineteenth century. Second, social control over individual and family activities, especially as exerted by the state, had been increasing for about four centuries. Third, private life increasingly was being guided and supervised by such experts as doctors, teachers, and authorities on child rearing; as a consequence, the socialization of production was now followed by the socialization of reproduction Marx (1952) had described. Fourth, most family studies had not asked why family life was now so painful, marriages so shaky, and parent-child relationships so hostile. Fifth, almost all the family studies assumed that the nuclear family was "isolated" from the kinship network, the world of work, and the wider society.

Lasch's (1975) *Haven in a Heartless World* began with the question, "Do the very storms out of which the need for such a haven arises threaten to engulf the family as well?" (p. xiii). As Henry (1963) had also pointed out, family life for decades had been expected to compensate for the routinization of work life, but "increasingly the same forces that have impoverished work and civic life invade the private realm and its last stronghold, the family" (Lasch, 1975, p. xvii). In the past, tensions and some distance between the family and society had protected the growing child from the competition and conflict that pervaded the outside world. But it was doubtful whether the family was now able to shelter its members, and the results were a concomitant weakening of family loyalty and the emergence of the narcissist, with the "ethic of survival and immediate gratification" (p. xviii) as the dominant personality type.

The concept of the family as a haven of refuge developed in the nineteenth century, according to Lasch, not because the family had become "warmer and more attractive . . . but because the outside world came to be seen as more forbidding" (p. 168). Also, as Harvey Cox (1969) explained, the puritanical work ethic of capitalism combined with "the forces of organized virtue" to eliminate many holidays and festivals that had enriched community life; neighborhoods and communities became arid. A damning condemnation of early nineteenth-century capitalistic Christian society and its exploitations and hypocrisy is that in the United States, even Christmas did not become a holiday until 1837; in England, Scrooge's allowing Bob Cratchit to be off from work on Christmas Day (albeit begrudgingly) was not an accepted practice. Lasch emphasized that "the glorification of domestic life simultaneously condemned the social order of which the family allegedly served as the foundation. In urging a retreat to private satisfactions, the custodians of domestic virtue implicitly acknowledged capitalism's devastation of all forms of collective life . . . [but] defended [it] as the price that had to be paid for material and moral improvement" (p. 169).

Lasch (1975) attributed much of the weakness of the American family in recent decades to parents' increasing reliance on psychiatrists, pediatricians, educators, and other authorities. Permissive child rearing led to the peer group's becoming the director of attitudes and the regulator of behaviors; consequently, "relations within the family have come to resemble relations in the rest of society" (p. 174). Inasmuch as standards have been replaced by norms and the other-directed personality type looks to peers for approval, the excessive dependency exhibited by so many young adults may be a result of their self-esteem level being dependent upon their peers' approval or disapproval. Such dynamics may explain, in part, the high prevalence of depression in children and adolescents and the high rates of suicide in the young.

Lasch (1975) discussed major factors that had led to the crisis of the American family. They consisted, first, of the changing relationships between parents and children and the problems exemplified by the youth revolt of the 1960s. Popular culture—comic strips, novels, and movies—depicted parents as amusing figures, as ineffectual, and/or increasingly as absent from their children's lives. He expressed particular concern about the loss of the father's authority as a result of his being separated from the family by work, travel, or divorce. Consequently, children were unable to internalize authority and instead projected their hidden impulses onto the external world, which then becomes a "nightmare" (p. 178).

Second, there had been a "normalization of the abnormal" (Lasch, 1975, p. 179). Inasmuch as modern parents often are shadowy creatures, their remoteness allows free play for the child's aggressive fantasies; as a result, fear, guilt, and rage become pervasive features of the young person's emotional life. "The counterculture's quest for emotional detachment, put forward as a program of emotional liberation, reflects a deeply held belief, rooted in the psychodynamics of the contemporary family and much more pervasive than the counterculture itself, that strong feelings lead to self-destruction" (pp. 182–183). He saw the widespread acceptance of oral sex, masturbation, and homosexuality as evidence of fear of heterosexual passion. Contemporary sexuality implies a repudiation of all but primitive forms of sensuality; analogously, the extreme interest in personal relations "conceals a thoroughgoing disenchantment with personal relations. . . . A narcissistic withdrawal of interest from the external world underlies both the demand for immediate gratification—resoundingly endorsed by advertising, mass promotion, and the health industry—and the intolerable anxiety that continually frustrates this demand" (p. 183).

The third was "corruption as a form of social control" (p. 183). Lasch maintained that authority has been devalued. Officials abused the authority and trust given to them, as evidenced by Watergate in the mid-1970s, and were not identifying with the institutions they served. Lasch was perspicacious; Reagan forcefully campaigned against Washington in the 1980 presidential election and did it successfully again in 1984, even though he had multiplied the powers of the presidency by fantastic expenditures of borrowed money.

As a result of the corruption, Lasch (1975) pointed out, social control became a matter of the half-truth or even the official lie or of manipulation of individuals and groups by the media and by institutions. He cited Friedenberg's students' belief that the law is "an indispensable technique for controlling behavior" (p. 187). Just as the rapid increase in mental health professionals in the past 25 years reflected the increasing needs for their services, the call for law and order was evidence of a collapse of moral standards and of the resulting need for external restraints and deterrents (p. 187). Lasch expressed fear that the "rip-off" had been legitimatized in our society at a time when the public was displaying cynical indifference about government and even expected lies and corruption at high levels, such as the Iran–Contra deception that surfaced in the late 1980s.

The remoteness, corruption, and manipulation that were such prominent features of the Watergate years mirrored the disorganization of the family that was occurring. In the late 1960s, the divorce rate climbed to reach 3.5 per 1,000 population (a rate seen before only in 1945) and then rocketed to the unbelievable high of 5.0 per 1,000 in 1976. Of the almost 56 million families in the United States in 1975, more than 7 million (13%) were headed by women with no husband present; those fatherless families contained more than 9 million children under the age of 18 (*Information Please Almanac,* 1990, p. 785). Lasch (1975) cited Rogow's thesis that the superstate is the only alternative to the superego (p. 189).

The socialization of children, Lasch (1975) feared, had in many ways been taken over by society. The conditions of life were seen as dangerous and unpredictable even by middle-class youths and young adults who were adopting strategies for survival similar to those used by ghetto children. Other middle-class strategies included a search for nonbinding commitments and a pseudotoughness that concealed dependency. Lasch stated that "middle-class 'Momism,' a muted version of black 'matriarchy,' can be understood as a product of the general deterioration of the social environment" (p. 165).

CONCLUDING REMARKS

As we look back, we can see that in the early 1960s, Parsons and others had maintained that the family had been only changing, not losing vitality. They clung to their opinions even though the objective indicators of instability and distress—the increasing divorce rate, the growing number of single parents caring for children, the many demands for marital and family therapy and the efflorescence of family therapies, and the multiplication of family forms and living arrangements—pointed toward family atomism and social anomie. Zimmerman's predictions, repeated from 1935 to 1972, about the coming crisis had been accurate. Also, he had stated that the societal and family instability could not continue indefinitely. According to the three-generation struggle he described, the first featured disruption was instigated by the youth of the 1960s. The second, the battle and the turning point, would involve the young who came of age in the mid-1970s and the 1980s. The third generation, those who matured in the 1990s, would have the task of consolidating the newly emergent family system or systems depending on the outcome of their predecessors' battles. Zimmerman was optimistic about the outcome, mainly because the family throughout history had undergone cyclic changes and regained its vigor.

Lawrence Stone pointed out in 1990, however, that there was no precedent in Western history for what had happened to the American family beginning in the 1960s. Even Zimmerman (1972a,b) focused mainly on the dissent of youth and the social unrest of the 1960s and gave relatively little attention to the dire national and international corruptions and to the conflicts that were denervating American society. Such disasters as Vietnam and Watergate were coldly calculated—neither spontaneous nor accidental. They reflected the self-deceptions and miscalculations of a nation that had been led "off the track" by its leaders and the military-industrial complex. Moreover, the Vietnam tragedy was chronic, and persisted despite warnings for at least 10 years that it was a malignant failure. As the 1970s drew to a close, internal and external disintegrative forces adversely influenced the nation, its social system, the nuclear family, and the American character. The individual had not been exempted from the changes, influences, and manipulations that battered America in the 1970s and were reflected by family turmoil. The historic first resignation of a United States president paralleled the divorces and desertions that were disrupting families. The adjective *narcissistic* began to be applied, widely and pejoratively, to the rising tide of self-interest that would be manifested in the 1980s by the open proclamation that "greed is good."

As we look back at the end of the 1970s, we can see that in the "century of concern" the patterns of family life changed in accord with inventions, industrialization, urbanization, and social movements such as women's and blacks' struggles for rights and equality. The fundamentals, however, are the circular influences of society and social change, family and personality development, and the American character.

CHAPTER 4

Family Research

> What we call the beginning is often the end
> And to make an end is to make a beginning
> —T. S. Eliot (1971, p. 144)

Systematic family research has had a relatively slow development in Western Society. It started only in the nineteenth century after the American and French Revolutions and after industrialization and urbanization changed the structure of society. Also, family research could not be more than individual scholars' efforts until the social sciences evolved as distinctive fields of study that could address the problems of society and its institutions, including the family. Their development has allowed for the multidisciplinary approaches needed for family research. Unfortunately, family study was impeded by concern about invading the privacy of the oldest institution. In this chapter, we look at early studies of the family as an economic unit, adjustment to and satisfaction with marriage, family functioning, and especially, at the immensely increasing number of studies of the family and mental disorder.

THE PIONEER RESEARCHERS

Social Research

The Beginning: Le Play (1850–1860)

Concern about the stability of Western society after the French Revolution and the political unrest of the first part of the nineteenth century was largely responsible for the first systematic research on the family in Western society. It was carried out in the 1850s and 1860s by Frederic Le Play, a French mining engineer who later became the leader of a conservative political science school in Paris. In his travels throughout Europe as a consulting engineer, Le Play developed empirical methods for studying families by combining the quantitative data he gathered with his qualitative field observations. His immediate objective was to evaluate the relationships between workers' employment, their family types, their family members' well-being, and the vitality and stability of the societies in which they lived. He studied about 300 families in western Europe and Russia; according to Silver (1982), this was "the first time in which the largely silent and the illiterate masses of Europe were studied in a scientifically intelligible way, with methods that essentially resemble modern-day sociological and anthropological procedures" (p. 6). His approach consisted mainly of obtaining detailed accounts of family income and expenditures and essential sociodemographic data, which he compiled into family monographs and used to develop typologies of societies, families, and workers.

The monographs consisted of three sections. The first contained a description of the physical and social characteristics of the family environment, the type of work done by the head of the family, each member's contribution to the household economy, the family lifestyle and history, and its "moral habits." The heart of the monograph was the second section, which included budget information about all sources of revenue from each member's type of work and the number of days at each job, as well as five sections on expenditures: "food, dwelling, clothes, moral needs [e.g., health and recreation], and financial expenses" (Silver, 1982, p. 69). The third section contained qualitative information, mainly short descriptions of the history, laws, economy, and vitality of the community (p. 73).

Le Play used the family budgets and monographs to develop a family typology. The first of the three types was the large patriarchal or traditional family, consisting of the male head, his wife, all of the unmarried children, and the married sons' families. Often they lived under the same roof, or the married sons lived only a short distance away. Ultimate authority belonged to the father. These families were common in eastern Europe where the societies were family-based and families were the only significant social organization. The second was the stem family, consisting of the parents, their unmarried children, and the married son who had been chosen by the father to continue his work and to inherit the family property. The stem family maximized the interests of both the individuals and the group; the father had freedom of testation and could assure continuity of the family line. Le Play maintained that it was the major type in stable societies in which private property was prized and that it met both the moral and economic needs of its members more completely than other family types. He attributed the success of the English and the American societies to the predominance of the stem family, with its combination of paternal authority and individual freedom.

The third type was the unstable family: "It establishes itself by the union of two free adults, grows with the birth of children, shrinks with the successive departure of the members of the new generation, and dissolves finally, without leaving a trace, with the early death of the abandoned parents" (Silver, 1982, p. 80). Paternal authority was eroded because the father could not provide for the members. Thus, the children were left to fend for themselves and eventually the family property was divided among them and dispersed. Unstable families were found most often in Western industrialized urban centers.

Le Play also distinguished between types of workers. Of the 36 monographs published in 1877, 15 were devoted to so-called provident workers, who saved to buy necessities and acquire additional property or a business, and 19 to the improvident, who were reckless or were not required to save. Many of the improvident were passive, unable to engage in long-term relationships, and lacking in religious feelings. Le Play linked success and stability to religious beliefs, a firm family structure, parental authority, good worker-employer relationships, and the worker's having institutional affiliations. Also, he praised working-class women for their moral leadership in the family and their domestic activities that bettered the family's chances of improving its social condition.

Le Play's research was an auspicious beginning for family studies. The development of the family budget as a research tool and of the monograph method have served family scholars in this century. According to Silver (1982), "Nisbet considers Le Play the first researcher to carry out the truly scientific study of communities and the first to use the comparative method as a way to understand the concrete processes of change rather than as a way to promote general theories of societal development or 'progress'" (pp. 9, 195-269). Zimmerman (1959) stated that Le Play's chief contribution "was the discovery of the important relations between family type and the rest of society" (p. 957). Le Play's theory of cyclical changes in society associated with changes in family mores was unpopular because it was in opposition to the prevailing ideas of progress held by Comte, Spencer, Durkheim, and other nineteenth-century social scientists.

Despite Le Play's paving the way, family research developed slowly. The fruitless search for the origins of the family, which began in 1861 and continued into the first few decades of the twentieth century, drained energy and resources that could have been used to develop methods for studies of the many family problems that were beginning to appear. By the turn of the century, industrialization and rapid social change were transforming Western society, and urbanization and mobility were affecting the family. Developments in ocean travel facilitated massive immigration, mainly from southern and eastern Europe to the mines and factories of the United States that needed cheap labor.

Booth and Rowntree

The horrible conditions of families in the industrialized centers began to be studied late in the nineteenth century. In 1890, Charles Booth's (1982) survey of lower-class districts in London found that 30.7% were in dire poverty. In 1899, Rowntree (1903) surveyed all of the households in York (with its population of almost 75,000 persons) by a "house-to-house visitation [to find families] living in . . . obvious want and squalor" (p. 297) and, following in Le Play's footsteps, to ascertain income and expenditures. The number of persons in poverty—lacking the basic necessities and not in a state of "merely physical efficiency"— was 29,302, or 27.8% of the total population (p. 296). Of these, about one third, or 10% of the population, were in "primary poverty" (i.e., earnings would not provide the necessities), and two thirds in "secondary poverty" (i.e., earnings would have provided the necessities if monies were not used for other purposes or wasted; p. 296).

> That, in this land of abounding wealth, during a time of perhaps unexampled prosperity, probably more than one-fourth of the population are living in poverty, is a fact which may well cause great searchings of the heart. There is surely need for a greater concentration of thought by the nation upon the well-being of its own people, for no civilization can be sound or stable which has as its base this mass of stunted human life. (p. 304)

In the United States, Byington's 1910 study of 90 families in a small community with a new steel mill showed that the long hours of work adversely influenced family life by shrinking time and energy for family interaction. Bahr, Wang, and Zhang (1991) stated: "Her study provided a case example of how industrialization weakens family solidarity" (p. 5). In the 1960s, the industrialization of the small cities of the Southeast was associated with increased psychosomatic disorders, especially a high incidence of coronary artery disease, and Bruhn's study of Rosita, Pennsylvania, presented an illustrative analysis of the detrimental and deleterious effects of industrialization on community life and health. In 1913,

More studied 200 New York City families' incomes and expenditures. Basic necessities required about 80% of the average family's income (Bahr et al., 1990, p. 7). The results of More's study are much like those Rowntree obtained in York only a decade earlier.

Although there were no specific studies of the family and mental illness early in this century, research showed that the family was being stressed, if not battered, by the increasing industrialization and urbanization. At the turn of the century, three developments stimulated interest in the study of the family. One was the influence of Darwinian concepts of evolution that spurred the study of the origin of social institutions, including the family. Another was the acceptance of early principles of genetics and a fascination with pedigree studies, especially those related to mental disorders. The third was Freud's introduction of psychoanalysis.

Darwinian Concepts (1859)

Darwinian concepts kindled scientific interest in the age-old observation that heredity influenced mental health or illness. In 1877, Dugdale (1910) described the Jukes, a mentally retarded kin group in New York State that could be traced back to a prostitute who died in 1740. Many members of the family were mental retardates, alcoholics, prostitutes, criminals, or psychiatrically ill. In 1912, Goddard (1973) presented the classic study of the notorious Kallikak family. He traced the ancestry of Deborah Kallikak, who was then a 22-year-old inmate at the Training School for Backward and Feeble-Minded Children at Vineland, New Jersey, through ten generations. In the early 1700s, Caspar Kallikak came from England and fathered a "family of good stock" that had a reputation "for honor and respectability" for four generations (p. 50). But during the Revolutionary War, Martin Kallikak, one of Washington's soldiers, tarried for a few hours at a New Jersey tavern and met a young woman who was known to be "defective." After being wounded in the war, he "married a woman of quality" and became a respected businessman. Nine months after the chance meeting at the tavern, however, the young woman had a baby and thus became the ancestress of a long line of "defectives," mentally ill, alcoholics, and/or criminals. Martin Kallikak's descendants through his wife, the other family line, were normal. Goddard stated, "We thus have two series from two different mothers but the same father [that] extend for six generations [and] . . . live in the same region and in the same environment" (p. 50). Of the 480 descendants of the woman at the tavern, 143 "were or are feeble-minded," 46 were normal, and there were no infirmities in the others (p. 18). Goddard (1973) called the study a natural experiment: "The biologist could hardly plan and carry out a more rigid experiment or one from which the conclusions would follow more inevitably" (p. 69).

Pedigree Studies

The emergence of the new science of genetics about 1900 prompted psychiatrists to undertake early case-control studies of their patients' blood relatives. Even before the principles of Mendelian genetics were brought to light, Kraepelin's associates in the 1890s launched genealogical studies of the ancestors and other relatives of mentally ill patients to ascertain hereditary patterns (Koller, 1950). By 1916, the Rüdin School in Munich had developed stringent methods for family studies. After studying almost 1,000 schizophrenic patients' family members, Rüdin (1961) reported that the rate of schizophrenia for siblings of an index case ranged from 4.5% to 23.0% and that it varied according to the parents' psychiatric diagnoses. The results of such early studies provided a slowly enlarging base of knowledge about family patterns of mental illness that was increased considerably by work in psychiatric genetics following World War II.

During the past two decades, such family studies as Winokur, Tsuang, and Crowe's (1982) Iowa Five Hundred, Egeland and Hostetter's (1983) continuing study of the Old Order Amish, and the studies led by Gershon (Gershon et al., 1982; Gershon & Guroff, 1984; Gershon, Hamovit, Guroff, & Nurnberger, 1987) provided data on risk for mental disorders in the family members of a mentally ill person. When one parent has mental illness, the risk for a child is 36.5%, and when both parents have mental illness, it is 75.1% (Merikangas, 1982, pp. 1173–1180). Data from those studies are being used to strengthen diagnostic criteria for specific mental disorder entities. And Egeland and her colleagues' (1987) research on affective disorders in the Old Order Amish and the work of some other investigators include blood and tissue studies directed toward the identification of genes that might be involved.

Anthropological Studies

In the first few decades of this century, cultural anthropologists were stimulated by the psychoanalytic theory of personality development to look for relationships among culture, family structure, and personality in various groups. Malinowski (1927) found that a variation of the Oedipal complex existed among the Trobriand islanders, with their matrilocal family system in which the mother's brother was the parenting father. The biological father, who merely visited his wife, parented his sisters' children. The children showed features of the Oedipal conflict that were directed toward the parenting father, not the biological father.

Later, Franz Boas's students, especially Margaret Mead and Ruth Benedict, studied South Seas islanders and Indian tribes in North America. Mead's classic studies in Samoa and New Guinea in the 1920s and 1930s revealed various cultures' methods of conditioning their adolescents. Her continued interest in the vicissitudes of childhood and adolescence (Mead, 1970) is a haunting remonstrance to the conscience of our era. Ruth Benedict's (1934) study of North American Indian groups was an ambitious attempt to relate various societies' values, customs, and child-rearing principles and methods to the psychological characteristics typical of the group; for example, the Pueblo Indians were socialized to be Apollonian—restrained, ritualistic, and group-oriented.

Psychoanalytic Contributions

Freudian Theory

The third stimulus to family research was the development of psychoanalytic theory. The Freudian theory of psychosexual development was based on clinical work with middle- and upper-class nuclear families in pre–World War I Vienna. Children's emotions of love, lust, fear, rage, and jealousy were seen as reactions to their socialization within the family early in life. Introjection led to the development of inner representations of the parental figures. Later, the superego developed through the process of identification with the parents and, still later, with peers, authority figures, and institutions. Case studies described trauma in childhood that had been produced by parental attitudes toward children, rules and constraints, or the births of siblings.

Psychoanalytic theory, as promulgated by Freud, often appears to have underemphasized family factors. But, in his 1923 classic *General Psychopathology*, Karl Jaspers (1963) stated that

> the way the family structure molds its members has been recognized by the psycho-analysts. . . . "The unconscious of the parents affects the children without their being aware of it. The family-psyche-body connections are like communicating wires." For example, "The life which parents would have liked to have lived, but which they were too timid or too weak to do, is now passed on as a task for the children to perform." (p. 718)

Also, Bell and Spiegel (1966) noted that Freud "frequently gave the impression that the disposition to neurosis could be laid at the door of the environment—whether pictured in terms of the family, the community, or the culture" (p. 117). Family relationships were central features of his famous case studies. Little Hans was a 4-year old whose phobia stemmed from fears of his father, and Dora was a young woman whose family consisted of a mother with a "housewife's" psychosis, a father who was an intermittently depressed philanderer, a hypochondriacal aunt, and her father's mistress's husband, whose sexual advances contributed to Dora's neurosis (p. 117).

According to psychoanalytic theory, the family was responsible for psychosexual development and also could be the cause of neurosis. The Oedipus complex signified the combination of possessive love for the parent of the opposite sex and of jealous death wishes for the parent of the same sex—feelings that crystallized into complex emotional attitudes during childhood and, if unresolved, would be at the core of neurosis later in life. Fenichel (1945) asserted that "in this sense, the Oedipus complex is undoubtedly a product of family influence. . . . Not only do the personalities of the parents make a lot of difference, but also the conceptions of love and death vary from child to child" (pp. 91, 97).

We should not forget that psychoanalytic theory and its clinical concepts and precepts were based on extensive work with patients. Long before there were scientific case-control and other family studies, psychoanalysts described the often adverse influences of parental conflicts, divorce, and separation on children and their potential for distorting personality development. Fenichel (1945) explained that when children were the subjects of, or were brought into, parental arguments, the Oedipus complex would be intensified "because of the exaggerated interest in the children and the consequent narcissism" (pp. 97–98). Psychoanalytic theory also held that such parental behaviors as either extreme sexual repression or an unusual degree of sexual freedom could be harmful to the child.

Fleck (1980) pointed out that Freud tended to concentrate upon the individual, but that the core of his work involved "family-related unconscious processes, such as his rediscoveries of Oedipus and Electra, of the family romance and incest" (p. 213). Also, in psychoanalysis, the patient relives and reworks childhood experiences in the transference with the therapist. Although psychoanalysis has been charged as being narrow, biased, and having neglected the family in favor of the individual, Fenichel (1945) dispelled some of those accusations with his family emphasis:

> Neurotic parents bring up neurotic children, and the children's Oedipus complex reflects the parents' unsolved Oedipus complex. Very often the

mother loves the son and the father loves the daughter. The parents' unconscious sexual love for their children is greater when their real sexual satisfaction, due to external circumstances or their own neuroses, is insufficient. (p. 93)

Abraham, Adler, Flügel

In 1912, Karl Abraham (1968) presented the first psychoanalytic study of manic-depressive illness. From patients' recollections, he concluded that lack of gratification by the mother led to the child's developing an unusually strong oral drive and dependency that was often frustrated. During adolescence, relationships with parents and others tended to become increasingly ambivalent. As a result of their early childhood experiences, potential manic-depressives were unduly vulnerable to rejection later in life. Disappointments could trigger regressive modes of relating to others and to conflict. Such basic concepts derived from early psychoanalytic studies have been observed repeatedly and complement the newer information being provided by pedigree, genetic, and clinical studies of bipolar illness.

Alfred Adler (1964), who formulated the concept of lifestyle, emphasized that during development a child selects events from experiences, especially interactions within the family, and consolidates them into attitudes and behaviors. Social feeling develops in the growing child mainly as a byproduct of the relationship with the mother. Adler saw neurosis as being derived from various childhood experiences—overindulgence and overprotection, neglect, or an inconsistent mixture of love and protection. As a result of negative experiences, the child could develop a negative self-image characterized by helplessness and a view of the social environment as hostile and dangerous. Self-centeredness and exaggerated feelings of insecurity led to excessive attempts at self-protection or neurotic strivings for superiority.

In his neglected book *The Psycho-Analytic Study of the Family*, J. C. Flügel (1921) extended psychoanalytic concepts and the insights from his clinical work with individuals to the family. He expressed disappointment because the psychoanalytic literature emphasized the relations between parents and children and between siblings, whereas "those between husband and wife which probably will be regarded as equally fundamental to any consideration of the psychology of the family are but lightly touched upon" (p. v).

He emphasized the importance of the family, especially a healthful psychological atmosphere" in the home, for the child's development. But, too often, parents used their children to work out their own neurotic conflicts. He credited Breuer and Freud's 1895 *Studies on Hysteria*

(1957) as being the first scientific work that described the influence of strong emotional forces in the home and the continuing significance of a child's early emotional experiences on his or her relationships later in life. The origin of psychic conflict lay in the family environment where, during the course of personality development, the child's instinctual drives were inhibited by the socialization process.

Flügel's 1921 views seem amazingly up-to-date. Many of his statements about healthful parent-child relations, and his emphasis on the importance of the parents' happy marital relationship for them and their children, have been confirmed by such current studies as those of Beavers and Hampson (1990), Beavers and Voeller (1983), Lewis, Beavers, Gossett, & Phillips (1976), Lewis (1989), and Westley and Epstein (1969). Also, Flügel's work can be looked upon as an early clinically based study of the family life cycle. As the children mature, parents needed to loosen their ties to them and make their own readjustments by developing outside interests and hobbies. Flügel (1921) concluded that the adult children's care of their elderly parents was culturally desirable, although of necessity it would have some limitations. The family was biologically and socially necessary: "On the psychological side, the thoughts, feelings and impulses that centre round the family belong to the most intimate and fundamental part of Man's spiritual nature" (pp. 241–242).

Obstacles to Family Studies

In 1915, Goodsell pointed out that there were obstacles to family studies, even though the family should be "the basis and starting point of social research" (p. 1). Reasons for the opposition were that the family was the institution "closest to men's and women's hearts" (p. 2), that it involved sexual relations and intimacy, and that family studies had to look at the problems of prostitution and venereal disease. Also, researchers deemed it unethical to invade the privacy and sanctity of the marriage relationship by investigating it. In 1945, Komarovsky and Waller asserted that "the worker in this field is shackled by taboos and ancestral superstitions, which he has the more trouble in combating because they are in his mind as well as in the environment" (p. 433). Nimkoff (1948) attributed the short history and lack of development of family research to the "relative stability of the family in Western society for some 2,000 years during the period of the agricultural economy preceding the Industrial Revolution" (p. 477). Hill (1958) contended that resistance to the study of families was reinforced by religious and political pressures.

Family Studies

Ackerman's Family Studies (1937–1984)

Despite the obstacles, in 1937, Nathan Ackerman (1957) began his pioneering efforts to adapt psychoanalytic formulations to the study of family life. His long-range objective was to develop a typology of families in health and illness that would have clinical significance. In 1941, he started an ongoing study of 50 families in which at least two of the members had received psychotherapy. He developed criteria for evaluating the family's psychosocial functioning and mental health, assessing each member's effectiveness in carrying out his or her family role, and determining each member's ability to meet the requirements of multiple roles. The evaluations identified the relatively healthful and unhealthful areas of family functioning, the balance between them, and trends in family relationships.

Ackerman (1957) insisted that mental illness must be considered at three levels: (a) the intrapsychic; (b) the interactions between the individual and the human environment; and (c) the distortions in the environment. Thus, mental illness was a process that takes place both inside and outside the individual, but "the matrix of human relationships, whether healthy or sick, is the family" (p. 203). For the individual, problems arose when he or she had to meet the often conflicting requirements of multiple family roles. Problems included disabling conflict within the family that surfaced as the need for psychiatric treatment. Also, conflict influenced the fate of symptoms or contributed to the development of new ones. Family problems could be circular because members' conflicts and deviant emotional development are reinforcing. Traditionally, a family member is seen as "sick" and identified as the patient.

Spiegel and Bell (1959) criticized Ackerman for being too narrow and mainly theoretical and procedural. Psychoanalytic formulations had not been correlated with sociological and anthropological theory, and procedural observations had been confined to the nuclear family. Also, he had neglected the horizontally extended networks to the community and the vertically extended networks to other generations. But Ackerman had recognized that psychoanalytic concepts could not simply be extended from the individual to the family and to the community without a primary bridging concept.

In accord with role theory, the popularity of functionalism in the 1950s, and Parsons's emphasis on roles as the articulations between the personality and the social systems, Ackerman then conceptualized the individual's "social self" as the link between the individual and society.

"Social role [was] . . . the operation of the integrational aspect of the total personality (the social self) that was configured by the individual's goals and values" (Bell & Spiegel, 1966, p. 138). Also, he developed typologies of marital interactions according to role dominance and of family groups according to the quality of their internal and external integration (Ackerman & Behrens, 1956, p. 66).

As Ackerman's work proceeded, he modified his earlier methods. The diagnosis of family psychopathology came to involve assessing the internal organization of the family, its external adaption, parental roles and child-rearing practices, and how those roles and policies were integrated during the child's development. According to Bell and Spiegel (1966), with Ackerman's reformulation of family assessment, it was no longer necessary to "phrase the diagnosis in terms of the child's inner processes or the mother-child relationship" (p. 138), and it was essential to treat the individual as a member of the family. Thus, Ackerman's work could alter the nature of diagnostic and treatment procedures.

Ackerman and Behrens (1974) emphasized the need for a model for family diagnosis that would include an ecological perspective and account for the "contagious and communicable nature of pathogenic emotion in family group process" (p. 38). Their guide for family diagnosis included (a) identifying the "destructive levels of conflict, the contagious flow of anxiety, and the family relationships within which conflict and anxiety are trapped" (p. 43); (b) identifying role relationships and patterns of complementarity in regard to self-esteem, need satisfaction, a shared search for solution to conflict, the buttressing of defenses against anxiety, and support of growth; and (c) assessing the family's capacity to fulfill its multiple functions—survival and security, affection, the balance between dependency and autonomous development, social and sexual training, and growth and creative development (p. 44).

Ackerman and Behrens noted that a theory of family dynamics had not yet been developed. The biopsychoanalytic model of the family was inadequate because it was based too completely on the medical model of mental illness. The systems model was ecologically oriented and had a rich potential, but systems theory was abstract and lacked methodology. What was needed was a psychosocial model that focused on the family's internal dynamics. But Ackerman and Behrens (1974) recognized that it was difficult to develop such a model and whimsically quoted Einstein: "Insofar as the laws of mathematics refer to reality, they are not certain; insofar as they are certain, they do not refer to reality" (p. 42).

Ackerman died in 1971, before the comprehensive family diagnostic system on which he had worked for years was completed. Nevertheless, he made substantial contributions that included his conceptualizations of the problems and the goals of family studies, the development and testing of research methods, the consistent linkage of the family to its social environment, and the many advances in family therapy. The Ackerman Institute for Family Therapy in New York is a center for training that provides therapy to many persons from all social classes and is an enduring testimony to his achievements.

Systems Theory

In the 1950s, the development of general systems theory gave a needed impetus to family research. General systems theory grew out of the changes that took place in the intellectual climate, especially in mathematics and the physical sciences, during the early part of the twentieth century. In 1905, Einstein enunciated the theory of relativity, which was confirmed in 1919. In 1927, Nils Bohr described the uncertainty principle and showed that, even in the exact sciences, simple linear models of causation were inadequate. The way was open for a new paradigm for science—general systems theory—as well as for an altered view of external reality. Relativity and uncertainty fit the new view of the world that included the Freudian unconscious, Joyce's stream-of-consciousness writing, Schoenberg's and Stravinsky's musical dissonances, and in painting, the work of the surrealists, futurists, and postexpressionists.

General systems theory developed from its roots in gestalt psychology, with its emphasis on the whole rather than isolated elements, and Kurt Lewin's (1951) field theory. Field theory provided a basis for the integration of etiological principles needed for comprehensive concepts of health and illness, especially for the family. Advances in communication theory further enriched general systems theory, as elaborated by von Bertalanffy (1966). He defined a system as a "complex of component parts that are in mutual interaction" (pp. 1–21). Instead of viewing each part or element in a field or situation as isolated, and instead of simply adding the parts to arrive at a whole, general systems theory emphasizes the relationships between the parts. To understand how the whole works, it is necessary to assess the transactional process taking place between the components of the system (von Bertalanffy, 1966, pp. 705–721).

During the past 30 years, general systems theory has been enlarged significantly by James Grier Miller's (1978) elaboration of "General Living Systems."

> General systems theory holds that the universe is composed of a hierarchy of concrete systems, defined as accumulations of matter and energy orga-

nized into co-acting, interrelated subsystems or components and existing in a common space-time continuum. . . . It provides a conceptual framework within which the content of biological and social sciences can be logically integrated with that of physical sciences. (p. 75)

A system was defined by Miller as "a set of interacting units with relationships among them" (p. 16). Systems exist at levels of ascending complexity, such as cells, organs, organisms, groups, societies, and even planets and/or galaxies. Each living system's suprasystem is the next higher system; for example, the suprasystem of the cell is the organ in which it is located, and that of the organ is the individual of whom it is a part.

Every system consists of components, structures, and 19 subsystems that process matter-energy and information. For example, the ingestor subsystem processes or brings matter-energy into the system; the distributor subsystem carries inputs to the outputs, and the extruder subsystem eliminates or discharges the matter-energy. Subsystems that process information are, for example, the input transducer that brings markers bearing information into the system and the memory subsystem that stores information. The decider is an executive subsystem. The boundary subsystem at the perimeter processes both matter-energy and information. The reproducer subsystem gives rise to other systems similar to those to which it belongs.

Conceptually, general living systems theory provides for "an integration of biological and social approaches to the nature of man" (Miller, 1978, p. 75), resolves the age-old mind-body dichotomy, and contributes to the development of personality theory. Karl Menninger (1963) described normal personality functions and psychopathology in terms of general living systems theory, and Engel (1977) used it as the theoretical basis for his biopsychosocial model of health and illness.

In Miller and Miller's (1980) discussion of general living systems and the family, they cited as an example the inadequacy of the ingestor subsystem: If the family is receiving too little food, clothing, and medicine, it suffers from deprivation. Another common family difficulty that can become pathological is conflict about family decisions resulting from problems with the decider subsystem that processes information. Still another example of family subsystem pathology is impermeability of the boundary subsystem, which can be associated with excessively rigid family rules that either stultify personality development or, as happens frequently, lead to a teenager's rebellious reaction. Also, rigid family boundaries can be associated with the development of depressive symptomatology because of lack of external stimulation and variety in everyday life. Conversely, when the boundary is extremely permeable, the family may not have a sense of family identity or cohesion, and adolescents may develop characterological disturbances.

Family researchers hailed general systems theory. By the late 1950s, a systems approach to family study and therapy was being established on the groundwork laid by Köhler and other gestalt psychologists, Kurt Lewin's field theory, von Bertalanffy's introduction of general systems theory, and the pioneering studies of interpersonal communication and of families by Bateson, Ruesch, Jackson, Haley, Bowen, Wynne, and others. Goldenberg and Goldenberg (1980) declared that

> in contrast to psychoanalysis, with its psychopathological orientation, general systems theory views man as a complex being operating within a system where concepts such as "sick" or "well" are irrelevant; a symptom developing in one person merely means that the system [e.g., the family] must be studied because it has become dysfunctional. . . . The patient is not reduced, mechanistically, to Id/Ego/Superego struggles of an intrapsychic nature but rather the emphasis is on multiple causality at various levels. (p. 85)

According to Epstein, Bishop, and Baldwin (1984), basic aspects of a systems orientation are that (a) the parts of the family are interrelated; (b) one part cannot be understood in isolation from the rest of the system; (c) family functioning cannot be fully understood by simply understanding each of the parts; (d) a family's structure and organization are determinants of the members' behavior; and (e) the transactional patterns of the family system shape family members' behavior. The fundamental family therapy orientation is a view of the family as a system (p. 77).

The use of the term *systems approach* spread in almost epidemic fashion. It has been widely acclaimed with fervor by family scholars and expert clinicians but also sometimes by clinically inexperienced marriage and family counselors. Too often, it has not been defined or has been so vaguely defined that the concept is stripped of its significance.

DEVELOPMENTS DURING THE 1950s AND 1960s

Interest in the family and mental illness in the 1950s was not paralleled by advances in studies of family functioning and mental disorder. There was agreement that the field had been handicapped by its late start and the complexities of such research. Spiegel and Bell (1959) stated that "up to the present time, the area of the psychiatric patient and his family has shown more promise and less achievement than almost any other segment of psychiatric work" (p. 141). Comprehensive guides for family diagnosis and treatment had not yet been developed, and there was no coherent theory of family mental health and illness. Also, if studying the individual in isolation from the family was artificial, then was it not equally artificial to isolate the family from the community? Such gaps could not be neglected.

Although there was concern about the lack of progress in family research in the early 1960s, promising developments included the work of the Group for the Advancement of Psychiatry (GAP) Committee on the Family, Spiegel and Kluckhohn's (1971) transactional approach, Bowen's ongoing efforts to formulate family theory that had clinical significance, and family sociologists' attention to the need for theory. GAP was the first major national organization to look at family research. In 1950, William C. Menninger recommended that it form a committee for family study; John Spiegel was the first chairman of the committee, which included Bowen, Wynne, and other illustrious family scholars. Their first report (GAP Committee on the Family, 1954) emphasized the importance of the family's lateral and vertical extensions and that "the structure of the family was inextricably associated with the structure of the society of which it is a part" (p. 927). Variations in the structure and functions of the family were related to "the variations in values of a culture and subcultures" (p. 928). The family was seen as an organized system that bridges the social system and its needs and the individual and his or her needs (p. 943).

The report presented Spiegel and Kluckhohn's (1971) value orientations (the family reflects basic cultural variations in terms of the human being's temporal orientation, relationships with other persons, etc.). Middle-class families' problems included those associated with adjustments to an "action-oriented, future-time minded society" (p. 278), such as the father's frequent absence from the home, the mother's anxiety about conflicts between her maternal and housewife roles, and the adolescent's family-versus-peer group strains. Lower-class families' problems reflected different value orientations: a present-time ("live for today") orientation and powerlessness in relation to "the system." The report concluded that there were some successful integrations "within family patterns, and among the family, the social system, and the system of value-orientations. . . . The typical roles within the middle-class family structure appear . . . to be fitted to the functions of the family within the larger social system" (p. 979). Thus, it reflected the familism and optimism of the 1950s.

Bowen considered the next GAP Committee on the Family report (1970) to be the best survey of the field up to that time. The committee sent questionnaires to social workers, psychologists, psychiatrists, and others who practiced family therapy, and ranked the 297 responses on a scale from A (concentrating on individual psychopathology and the therapist-patient relationship, and practicing mainly individual psychotherapy) to Z (thinking in terms of family systems, relationships, and breakdowns in communication, and practicing family therapy). The report emphasized that "the most striking characteristic of family therapy at this time is the tendency of therapists to cluster into two groups—those who view the family as a complicating factor in any individual member's psychic struggles and those who view the transactions of the family as determining, in a dynamic way, the responses and attitudes of its members" (p. 604). It deplored the polarization and suggested strongly that it would be advantageous to therapists (as well as to their patients) for the two extremes to learn from each other and to meld their approaches. Research was necessary because of the relative absence of theory.

Family problems were seen in an optimistic perspective. They involved struggles about sharing power and responsibilities that also are the root of many intergenerational, interracial, and international problems. "Although this is a long-range hope, it may be that what can be learned about restoring or creating equilibrium within the family can be extrapolated to larger system levels—to the university, the city, the society of a nation, and the community of nations" (GAP Committee on the Family, 1970, p. 607).

The Transactional Approach: Spiegel and Associates

Spiegel and Bell (1959) praised the emerging family-centered approaches to the study of the family. They noted that those approaches had been developed from psychoanalytic theory and credited Ackerman's pioneering studies. During the 1950s, Spiegel and Florence Kluckhohn (1971) developed their transactional approach to the study of the family, which was based on field theory.

> The events involving the sick individual with his family occur within a total system of interdependent subsystems, any one of which—for example, the individual, the family, the community, the value system—may become temporarily, a focus of observation. The "world" being observed must include the observer and his active observing . . . [and thus, concepts of causality change from] "What in the family causes pathology in the individual" to "What processes occurring between the individual and the family are associated with the behaviors which are called pathology?" (p. 139)

The transactional approach specified sources of strain at three interlocking levels—the culture, the family, and the individual. At the cultural level, strain in the family occurs, for example, when a family's original value orientations differ greatly from those of the dominant society (e.g., recent immigrants) or when the older generation holds to its original orientations while the younger generation is adopting a newer set. At the family level, interpersonal strains occur in regard to social role and role-conflict resolution. Both the sick and well families studied by Spiegel and Kluckhohn (1971) showed evidence of role and value conflicts; however, the sick families had been attempting to change a broader spectrum of values and at a more rapid pace than the well families. The rapid changes resulted in intrapsychic conflict for individual family members, as well as interpersonal problems. No sharp dichotomy existed between sick and well families inasmuch as all families were involved in both neurotic and healthy interactions. At the level of the individual, strain was viewed according to psychoanalytic concepts of intrapsychic conflict and object relations. Treatment needed to be directed toward "the interplay of the homeostatic mechanisms which have gone astray. It involves the restoration of homeostatic controls of cross-cultural, social, psychological, and somatic boundaries" (Spiegel & Kluckhohn, 1971, p. 141).

Spiegel and Kluckhohn's transactional approach was a significant addition to family research and treatment because it had a meaningful theoretical base, included reciprocally influential community-family-individual interactions, and placed an emphasis on values, a relatively neglected topic in family research. Their approach is applicable to families in our highly mobile, pluralistic society, and its utility increases with increased immigration and the variety of values and ways of life displayed by television. Unfortunately, it has not received the attention it merits.

Bowen's Family Systems Theory

Kerr and Bowen (1988) presented an excellent summary of Bowen's family systems theory, which he developed over almost five decades. We shall pinpoint a few of his key concepts that we think are especially important. Bowen emphasized the distinction "between the *family relationship system* and the *family emotional system*" (p. 11). The emotional system provides a "behavioral *link* between the human and other animals" (p. 27) analogous to Darwin's physical link, and the emotional system drives and regulates behavior (p. 28). In addition, family systems theory conceptualizes the feeling system (e.g., guilt, anxiety, ecstasy) and the intellectual system (or the "thinking brain").

A key postulate is the interplay between the counterbalancing forces—individuality and togetherness—that influence behavior. Individuality is a "biologically rooted life force" (p. 64). The growing child differentiates the self from the family of origin, but differentiation is counterbalanced by togetherness, and early attachments are never fully resolved. When there is a low level of differentiation of the self, "emotionality and subjectivity have a strong influence on family relationships" (p. 96). Kerr and Bowen (1988) described the scale of differentiation as the degree to which people are able to distinguish "between the feeling process and the intellectual process" (p. 97).

Togetherness also is a biologically rooted life force "that propels an organism to follow the directives of others, to be dependent, to be connected, an indistinct entity" (p. 65). Thus, in human relationships, the balance between individuality and togetherness will be variable. Relationships exist on a continuum ranging from a great deal being tied up in the relationships to only a small amount being "bound." When a great deal is bound, the relationship is undifferentiated or fused. The amount of energy bound up in the relationship is a function of the individual's level of differentiation; the lower the level of differentiation of the self, the greater the amount of energy that will be tied up in a relationship (p. 68):

> "As differentiation decreases, individual functioning and well-being become more dependent on the relationship and . . . [the person involved becomes] threatened by perceived threats to its balance. . . . The emotional boundaries between people become progressively blurred. As boundaries dissolve, anxiety becomes an increasingly infectious agent." (pp. 76–77)

Adaptations can absorb some of the anxiety; for example, gaining emotional distance or doing one's utmost to maintain harmony can reduce anxiety. But "when conflict prevails, *it is the relationship that is symptomatic*" (p. 83).

Another basic concept is that of *triangling*. Relationships between two people generate anxiety that leads to their becoming involved with other people through predictable triangular patterns, and "through the process of triangles, a relationship may absorb anxiety from other relationships" (p. 88). Examples of triangling involved with symptom formation are a wife's becoming distressed and involving a friend in her marital problems, or the birth of a second child that leads to a mother-children triangle in which the mother becomes anxious about meeting the children's emotional needs and ends up radiating tensions while the children engage in sibling rivalry (pp. 148–149). Detriangling is "probably the most important technique in family systems therapy" (p. 150), but loosening the emotional connections linking a triangle requires objectivity and emotional neutrality.

Levels of differentiation are both basic and functional. "It is the basic level of differentiation that is largely determined by the degree of emotional separation the person achieves from his family of origin" (Kerr & Bowen, 1988, p. 98). Basic differentiation is not dependent on "the relationship process," whereas functional differentiation is. Kerr and Bowen (1988) emphasized that differentiation is handicapped by

> societal reinforcement of a togetherness and feeling orientation [that is transmitted through the media, novels, sermons, and gossip]. . . . Blame is irresponsibly affixed for most issues about which society is anxious. We are implored to have more feeling for one another, all the while being bombarded by feeling-laden communications that stir up still more of the feelings we are supposed to lack. (p. 132)

Differentiation involves defining the self, which in turn requires awareness of the influence of anxiety and emotional reactivity. The level of functioning is explained by two inversely related variables: differentiation of the self and chronic anxiety. Anxiety can spread through the family and change imagined problems into real ones. Increasing anxiety leads to greater need for closeness; eventually, chronic anxiety leads to regression.

Symptom development is influenced by the basic level of differentiation of the self and the level of chronic anxiety. The level of the differentiation of the self determines the type of adaptation (symptom), and the level of anxiety quantifies the degree of disturbance. "Symptoms are rooted in the undifferentiated or togetherness aspect of human functioning. . . . The more the members of a relationship system function *in* reaction to one another, the more likely someone in the system will get into a position emotionally that interferes with his or her functioning" (Kerr & Bowen, 1988, p. 256). Whether and in whom a symptom develops are determined mainly by the pattern of and balance in the emotional functioning of the family system. For example, when parents project their anxieties into the relationship, the result is marital conflict; but when patterns of emotional functioning include the child, the anxiety can lead to the child's developing symptoms.

Symptoms can be those of either physical or emotional illness; however, Kerr and Bowen (1988) prefer not to think in dichotomous terms, and instead conceptualize all clinical dysfunctions as being associated with disturbances in the "basic patterns of emotional functioning in the nuclear family" (p. 164). Thus, in a systems model, "many factors or processes interact to produce a particular clinical syndrome. . . . Sickness is not the result of the presence of any one or of all the factors, but develops due to a disturbance in the balance of the relationship system between them" (p. 258).

One of Bowen's most significant contributions has been that of the "multigenerational emotional process" (Kerr & Bowen, 1988, p. 221). All types of major clinical dysfunctions are seen as products of a multigenerational emotional process that is "rooted in the instinctual nature of man" (p. 253). Thus, family dysfunction inevitably is linked to dysfunctional trends in previous generations. Even in a three-generation family, it is possible to observe discrepancies in functioning (e.g., mild dysfunction in the oldest generation, chronic dysphoria and conflict in the next, and definite pathology in the third). It may take five to ten generations for schizophrenia to develop.

The multigenerational emotional process is characterized by its predictability because nuclear families have only a limited number of patterns of emotional functioning. A family is influenced by the functioning and problems of its families of origin, and that functioning and the problems are repeated, sometimes with only minor variations, from one generation to the next. Grasping the multigenerational process can be therapeutic. Kerr and Bowen (1988) emphasized that "if a person can look at a four or five generation diagram of his own family and really see it as a living organism, a multigenerational emotional unit that changes gradually over time in accordance with precise principles, he is beyond blaming self or others" (p. 255).

Family Evaluation (Kerr & Bowen, (1988) contains the important epilogue "An Odyssey Toward Science," in which Bowen describes his research and the formulation of his concepts over the years. In many ways, this personal anecdote summarizes the development of family theory and therapy in the latter part of this century and is a valuable historical reminiscence. He concludes optimistically: "When the human believes he can do something, it will be done. It leads me to believe human behavior will become a science by the middle of the next century. The human will be richer if the favorable trend continues" (Bowen, 1988, p. 386).

Bowen's work over more than 40 years has significantly advanced the field of family theory and therapy. His contributions are the products of extensive family research and clinical practice, and they are sound. Murray Bowen stands as one of the giants of "the family movement" in this century.

Conceptual Frameworks in Family Sociology

Hill and Hansen (1960) noted that there had been an increase in family studies during the 1950s, but that little attention had been paid to theory. They identified major family study areas and described five approaches, including the interactional approach that had developed mainly out of sociology and social psychology and was exemplified by the work of Angell and Burgess; the structure-function approach, developed out of sociology and social anthropology and exemplified by the work of Goode and Parsons; and the developmental approach that arose out of sociology, child psychology, and human development and was exemplified by the work of Farris, Sussman, and Hill.

Christensen (1964) described five emerging sociological theoretical approaches to family study. They were (a) the institutional approach that had focused on the origin and evolution of the family as an institution and was being used in cross-cultural designs; (b) the structural-functional approach that viewed the family as a social system and focused attention on both its internal workings and the relationships between it and other social systems; (c) the interactional approach, based on the work of Mead and Burgess, that looked at the family in terms of role-playing, status, communication problems, decision making, stress, and so forth; (d) the situational approach that viewed the family "as a social situation affecting behavior" (p. 22) and that Christensen considered to be too individualistic; and (e) the developmental approach that focused specifically on the stages of development as the family moved through the life cycle.

In family sociology, the realities of the almost cataclysmic events of the 1960s dwarfed the repeated pronouncements about changing family functions—the family obviously was changing, if not disintegrating. In the 1960s and 1970s, major efforts were directed toward the development of theory and, later, toward studying family functioning. As the reader will see, by the 1980s the foremost family researchers were devoting their efforts to studies of generational differences and the family life cycle; assessing family functioning, family competence, and stress and the family; and, to an increasing extent, the study of the family and mental illness (at first mainly schizophrenia, then depression, and more recently the identification of genes responsible for mental illness). Holman and Burr (1980) emphasized that during the 1970s, family theories had proliferated and the field had moved beyond the five conceptual frameworks described by Hill and Hansen (1960). Broderick (1971) added three conceptual approaches: balance theory, game theory, and exchange theory.

Holman and Burr (1980) placed the conceptual approaches to family studies in three categories: the major theoretical approaches, the minor theories, and those peripheral to the field. The major theoretical approaches were symbolic interaction, exchange theory, and systems theory. Symbolic interaction had been used frequently during the 1970s and had been expanded to encompass role attribution and self-processes. Exchange theory focused on the rewards and costs in relationships and increased the understanding of "precarious human relationships, such as courtship processes and . . . [marriages in which] the relationship has deteriorated and the positive and rewarding aspects are few" (p. 36). Holman and Burr noted that exchange theory lacked utility when it encompassed such nonrational factors as love and jealousy, but Nye (1988) praised it in his Burgess Award address. Systems theory continued to develop during the 1970s; Kantor and Lehr (1975) described how it could provide a clinically useful understanding of family relationships. Satir also emphasized the clinical applicability of systems theory, but Holman and Burr (1980) stated that although it was widely accepted, in many ways it was only descriptive.

The second major category consisted of the five minor theories: conflict theory and the developmental, behavioral, ecological, and phenomenological approaches. Conflict theory had expanded during the 1970s but had not been used extensively. In contrast, the developmental approach had been used effectively, for example, by Elder (1974), and its use had stimulated interest in the family life cycle. Holman and Burr (1980) considered the behavioral approach controversial and the ecological approach to be a modification of the household economics–home management approach. The phenomenological approach had been used mainly in family therapy. The third major category, peripheral approaches, included structural-functional concepts, psychoanalytic theory, learning theories, and game theory.

According to Holman and Burr (1980), in 1945, Merton urged social scientists to develop small, modest theories that could be tested and revised, but such middle-range theories had developed unevenly. They concluded that there was no overarching general theory of the family, but that the field was still young and more research was needed before such a theory could be devised. It was necessary to begin with discrete approaches and to improve the methodology for family studies. Holman and Burr insisted that family research was more sophisticated in 1980 than in the past and that researchers were demanding scientific theory building.

Comment

It appears that theory and study of the family in sociology during the 1960s and 1970s did not keep pace with changes in either the family or the society, even though the groundwork had been laid down in the 1920–1950 era by the achievements of such leaders as Ogburn, Burgess, Terman, Angell, and Koos and their colleagues. The arguments about the functioning of classic theories and schools of thought may have drained energies that might have been used more productively in attempts to evaluate the reciprocal influences of the societal and historical processes on the family. Also, the disregard of history in favor of the emphasis on functionalism, as exemplified by Parson's domination of the new field of social relations (no long sociology) at Harvard and the downgrading of Sorokin and Zimmerman, probably contributed to what seems to be a lack of vitality at a critical time in the history of the family in this century. An overview of family research from 1937 to 1987 (see pp. 183–187), however, reveals that family sociology may be entering a Renaissance era.

Although there was concern about the seemingly slow development of family research, there were some outstanding studies. Koos's (1946) study of New York City tenement families, discussed in Chapter 2, supplied a model for future research on family function and competence. Koos found associations between the degree and type of family organization-disorganization on one hand and both the occurrence of troubles and their effects on the family and its members on the other. Studies of family function and the formulation of models of family function by Olson et al. (1983), Epstein, Bishop, and Baldwin (1984), Lewis, Beavers, Gossett, and Phillips (1976), Beavers, Hampson, and Hulges (1985), and their colleagues are in many ways derivatives of Koos's too-little recognized work.

Studies of family stress and coping also owe a debt to Koos that Reuben Hill (1949) acknowledged in his important study of family adaptation to the stress of World War II separations and postwar reunions in Iowa families. In the 1930s, Hans Selye (1956) had developed concepts of stress in laboratory work with animals that later were applied clinically to humans, especially patients with psychosomatic conditions. Grinker and Spiegel's (1945) *Men Under Stress* became a well-known documentary on wartime stress that reported the efficacy of psychiatric treatments for stress-related conditions and enhanced the popularity of psychiatry and psychology in the postwar era. Reuben Hill's (1949) ABC-X Family Crisis Model (p. 84) was used by Olson and his colleagues (1983) in their large and highly publicized but methodologically limited and conceptually flawed *Families: What Makes Them Work*. Hill's contributions extended to generational and family life cycle studies; his *Family Development in Three Generations* (1970) supplied a background for Elder's continuing studies of the effects of the Great Depression on samples of Oakland and Berkeley, California, children during their adult lives (Elder, 1974; Elder & Rockwell, 1979; see Chapter 3).

The major underresearched area was that of poverty and the family, even though such families have a host of health, marital, child care, abuse, and other problems. With few exceptions, only demographic data about the poor and their families are available despite the growing presence of a large underclass in the United States. Koos's (1946) *Families in Trouble* was an exception and another was Minuchin, Montalvo, Guerney, Rosman, and Schumer's (1967) penetrating study *Families of the Slums*.

Minuchin's *Families of the Slums*

Minuchin and his colleagues studied an experimental group of 12 disadvantaged families with two or more delinquent children at the Wiltwick School for such children and 10 disadvantaged control families with no delinquent children that were obtained from agencies in New York City. All the families were characterized by "a striking absence of fathers or father-figures living at home, a plethora of children, ethnic minority status, low educational achievement of mothers, and dependence on public financial assistance.... [Except for having no delinquents] the control group, in living styles and in home arrangements, was generally similar to the experimental group" (Minuchin et al., 1967, p. 20).

The investigators' goals were to "shed light on the dynamics of disadvantaged, 'hard-core' families which had produced more than one acting-out child (juvenile delinquent) . . . [and to] explore and to report on the efficacy of a specially developed technique of family treatment which employed a team of therapists working with family members as a group and in various subgroups" (p. 7). Key concepts were the absent or unstable father-figure, the need for "executive guidance" by the mother, her problems with nurturance and control, and the allocation of authority to "parental children" (p. 11). Major variables were aggression, cooperative responses, expression of positive or negative feelings, acceptance of responsibility, disruptive behavior, and leadership (p. 12).

The family therapy consisted of 30 weekly 1½ hour sessions with all family members over age 6. The sessions consisted of three stages; first, the entire family met with two therapists to explicate problems; second, the parents and the children met with the therapists as separate subgroups; and third, the whole family and the therapists met again to discuss approaches to the problems (pp. 14–15). Among the disadvantaged families, inadequate communication, family interactions, crowding, and noise produced a "developmental delay" for the children, who showed an "action and excitement orientation" (p. 30) and tended to relate to others physically and with aggression. The investigators emphasized that "poverty and pathology are decidedly associated with each other" (p. 34).

Of the 12 families in the experimental group, 7 were therapy "successes": They showed an increased capacity to cope, and parental roles and spousal subsystems had been strengthened (Minuchin et al., 1967, pp. 349–350). At the end of the study, the investigators' reconceptualizations included a recognition of the "paucity of roles," rigidity within the family, problems stemming from the absence of a stable male figure, and of families with grandmothers that did not function in "a three generational manner" (p. 351). They saw the families as less static than beforehand, and also that the training of the children curtailed their ability to "judge accurately the impact and implications of their behavior on others and themselves. . . . The family culture which organizes the child's dominant style of coping . . . clashes with the differently defined rules and boundaries within the larger sectors of the extrafamilial world" (pp. 351–352).

Minuchin and his colleagues (1967) developed *profiles* of disorganized and disadvantaged families. The *disengaged* family was an "atomistic field" in which the members' actions did not produce repercussions, the members moved in "isolated orbits," and the family grouping was characterized by delayed responses, lack of contact, and apathy. The *enmeshed* family was characterized by interlocked stasis, immediate reactivity of one member to another, and many complicated power struggles. The family with *peripheral males* was a more complex unit than either the disengaged or the enmeshed families; its prominent characteristics were lack of parental communication as equals, the mother's centrality, and exclusion of the male by the mother-children subsystems, who saw him as "responsible for the family unhappiness" (Minuchin et al., 1967, p. 361). The family with *nonevolved parents* contained a grandmother who was the executive while the mother and children functioned "as one vaguely differential subgroup. The mother . . . [was] an older sibling" (p. 364). In the family with *juvenile parents,* all members avoided adult roles and remained frozen at a preadolescent stage of development. The mother was a "fickle girl" who rejected maternal functions, and the male, who often nurtured the children, was dependent on her. The children suffered from "divided loyalties and frequently confused sex-role identity" (p. 366).

Minuchin and his colleagues' (1967) work with these difficult and usually neglected families deserves more attention. They saw the overlooked diversity of disadvantaged families and the need for a variety of therapeutic strategies. A larger study, built on the start supplied by them, could identify subgroups of families and predictors of response to various therapies and thus make significant contributions to American society at the end of the twentieth century. We should heed Minuchin and his colleagues' optimistic concluding words: "So striking is the variety of family forms through which personality comes forth unimpaired, that when such experiments fail, the event cannot be considered less than tragic" (p. 378).

RECENT FAMILY SOCIOLOGICAL RESEARCH

In 1987, The *Journal of Marriage and the Family (JMF)* celebrated its 50th anniversary by presenting overviews of topics by outstanding family scholars. Nye (1988) attributed the new "freedom in marriage" since the 1940s (praised by Burgess, 1945, and Locke, 1960) to the emergence from the Great Depression and the availability of jobs, the increasing use of effective methods of birth control, appliances that reduced women's chores and facilitated their employment, and the social security system. Also, the social climate had been favorable; Roosevelt's New Deal freed persons from institutional pressures, and their goals often became individual well-being and marital happiness.

Nye's (1988) review of five major sociological journals at 10-year intervals from 1937 to 1987 revealed that the major relationship topics studied were marital happiness, unhappiness, and conflict. In 1987, there was an increase in the number of articles devoted to family and individual problems, especially family violence, and also greater interest in such topics as sex roles, employment, achievement, and (to a lesser extent) global happiness and self-concept. There had been an increasing number of historical studies since 1977; time usually was the dependent variable. Over the 50 years, there was a "decline in the use of primary data and an increase in the use of secondary data—mainly large national surveys" (Nye, 1988, p. 310). The number of articles stating hypotheses increased from about 26% in 1957 to about 48% in 1987. But Nye stated that "less than 25% of the research reports in 1987 included a theoretical statement" (p. 313).

According to Nye (1988), continuing study needed to be centered on the dominant problem—concern about relationships and why almost three in five marriages end in divorce or are unsatisfactory. Also, studies of sex and family roles were promising avenues for research, and there was a growing interest in studying family violence and sexual aggression.

Nye concluded that much had been done, "but as we look at current family conflict, divorce and disillusion, family stress, violence, and unmet personal and relationship needs, *it appears that family problems are multiplying considerably faster than research and therapy can address them*" (p. 316, italics added).

Bert Adams (1988) noted that *JMF* had increased in size from 96 pages in 1941 to 910 pages in 1986, and the percentage of articles containing statistics grew from 6 in 1951 to 92 in 1986. It was difficult to characterize the overall content of the journal in the 1940s and 1950s, but under the influence of Reuben Hill, the 1960s were the "decade of conceptual frameworks" and the 1970s "the decade of path model theories" (p. 7). The decade of the 1980s, Adams felt, might end up being called "the decade of policy debates and concern for varieties of families."

Adams (1988) reported that the five major topics studied since 1941 were children and youth, sexuality, marital adjustment, divorce and remarriage, and violence. Children and youth topics were (a) "parent categories" and child outcome, in which the deficit model indicated that "the absence of a parent has adverse effects on children and youth"; (b) parental behavior, attitudes and characteristics, and offspring outcomes; the major conclusion was that the family's culture or behavior "is more important to adolescent achievement than is the presence or absence of one parent"; (c) relationships between parents and their offspring; and (d) "*attitudinal and perceptual similarities and differences between parents and offspring.*" Acock and Bengtson had reported in 1980 that parents have a "generational stake" in emphasizing "the similarities between themselves and their offspring whereas the offspring's stake is in emphasizing the differences" (Adams, 1988, p. 8). Adams also cited Sebald's study, which noted that adolescents' relationship to their parents had been curvilinear over the years—closer in the 1940s and 1950s and again in the 1980s than in the 1960s or 1970s, especially for boys.

In the study of sexuality, Adams reported there were four landmarks: Freud's theory of psychosexual development early in the century, Kinsey's reports on sexual behavior in the late 1940s and early 1950s, Masters and Johnson's studies of human sexual response in the mid-1960s, and I. Reiss's 1986 *Journey Into Sexuality*. Adams (1988) pointed out that Freud considered the human male as sexual and the female as being more of "a receptacle than an active sexual partner" (p. 8). The Kinsey reports (Kinsey, Pomeroy, & Martin, 1948; Kinsey, Pomeroy, Martin, & Gebhard, 1953) revealed the extent and variety of sexual activity and sparked numerous controversies. In 1966, Masters and Johnson's *Human Sexual Response* was "no less earth-shaking than the

Kinsey Reports had been 15 years earlier" (Adams, 1988, p. 8). And Reiss, who looked at the "traditional-romantic" and the "modern-naturalistic" views of sexuality, emphasized that sexuality is "more important cross-culturally for pleasure and self-disclosure than for reproduction" (Adams, 1988, p.8) and is linked to jealousy, gender role power, and beliefs about normality. Singh's (1980) evaluation of the National Opinion Research Center's surveys indicated that persons in each generation had been entering adulthood with more liberal views of premarital sex than those of the preceding generation.

Marital adjustment, according to Adams (1988), was the popular topic for study during the preceding 50 years. The terms *adjustment, satisfaction,* and *happiness* had been used almost synonymously, but such current research as Spanier's was emphasizing "quality" (p. 9). Adams pointed out difficulties with the concept of marital adjustment: Does a well-adjusted marriage mean mainly that the partners are two conventional persons? Another question was whether marital adjustments changed during a marriage, inasmuch as marital satisfaction generally declined over the first 20 to 30 years of marriage and then, at least until recently, increased in later years. Thus, there are problems with the study of marital adjustment, including the possibility that the topic is "male-biased" and possibly "a static concept." Also, it is possible that a marriage either is adjusted or is not.

Studies of divorce and remarriage included research on the causes and the consequences of divorce, the most apparent of which are postdivorce depressions, economic hardships for women, and loneliness for men. Studies also looked at adjustment to divorce, such as Bohannon's (1970) description of six states of divorce. Adams (1988), however, maintained that the most timely recent advance consisted of such studies of remarriage and step-relationships as Furstenberg and Spanier's (1984) *Recycling the Family* (p. 10). Also, Kinnaird and Gerrard (1986) reported that young daughters from intact families had much more positive views toward marriage and less sexual experience than daughters from families of divorce (p. 10).

Although there were no articles on family violence in the *JMF* until 1969, their number had increased steadily since then. Adams (1988) categorized violence in terms of the victim, with information appearing about spouses, children, siblings, dating partners, and elders, in that order of frequency. He cited Strauss and Gelles's (1986) finding that there had been a 47% decline in child abuse and a 27% decline in spouse abuse from 1975 to 1985. The changes were attributed to a rise in the age of the first marriage and a rise in the age of the parents at the time of the first birth; however, the major differences in the methodology used in the 1975 and 1985 surveys are most likely responsible for the reported declines. Researchers have emphasized the "cycle of violence" (p. 11); in violent homes, violence begets violence and there is an intergenerational transmission of violence. Possible causes of violence include low self-esteem, economic dependency, and having been abused as a child.

The five areas discussed by Adams (1988) covered different classes of topics inasmuch as studies of children is a group category, whereas "divorce and violence are events, sexuality is a behavior, and adjustment or quality is a condition" (p. 11). Therefore, it is necessary to identify topics as precisely as possible and to use the appropriate methodology for each. Analyses of events focus on rates, causes, and consequences, but the "line between events and behaviors is unclear" (p. 11). There are measurement difficulties with the studies of such conditions as satisfaction or quality, because they are "soft" variables.

Even though there has been considerable progress in family research during the past 50 years, Adams (1988) advanced three reasons why the field is still "relatively low in status" (p. 12). First, many of the variables are "soft;" second, family study is "value laden"; and third, the family may not really be a dependent variable, and studying it as such "lowers its status among the subfields of social science" (pp. 12–13). Studies of marital quality need to recognize that it may be culturally specific and should begin with the individual's definitions of high and low quality. Methodological issues burden family research; for example, just the analyses of family data are beset by complexities. Also, Adams agreed with the feminists' critiques of the male orientation of family studies.

Adams concluded that it is important to "cross boundaries." It is necessary to cross temporal boundaries, for example, to obtain greater historical understanding of the family, such as that provided by Elder and his colleagues, Hareven, and others. Also, cultural boundaries needed to be crossed. Research boundaries that needed crossing included the theoretical, the disciplinary, and the institutional. Adams (1988) also argued that the entire area of relationships between the family and other institutions and of the "family-in-society" needed further development. Although researchers had become "sophisticated chroniclers" of family life, most family research was still "value pervaded." Adams proposed the following questions for study: "Is cohabitation increasingly becoming a non-marriage rather than just a premarriage? ... What is the new 'glue' for marriage? ... In 50 years of research we have only begun the task of understanding family life" (Adams, 1988, p. 15).

The editor of the *JMF*, Berardo (1990), emphasized the concern during the 1980s "that our marriage and family institutions were being severely weakened and threatened under the press of accelerated and pervasive social change. Much of that change has been taking place within the context of altering attitudes and values; in particular, the long-recognized *shifting of emphasis away from familism toward individualism*" (p. 809; italics added). In family studies in the 1980s, he noted there had been four major themes. One was the role of economic variables in family life; history had shown that changing economic conditions have been intimately related to the state of family health and welfare (p. 817). Another was the increasing number of wives and mothers entering the labor force; they changed employment patterns, challenged traditional sex -and gender role definitions, and gave an impetus to negotiations and struggles about the division of labor within the family. The third was the "growing recognition and acceptance of the diversity of American families and their lifestyles" (p. 817). Researchers were shifting from a view of many families as being pathological, disorganized, or culturally deviant to looking at models of minority families that included their adaptive capabilities. The fourth was that "contemporary families function within the context of an increasingly complex milieu—one that exposes them to considerable conflict and stress" (p. 817). Berardo asserted that it was imperative for scholars and practitioners to "sensitize the public and policy makers to family needs" (p. 817).

FAMILY STUDIES OF SCHIZOPHRENIA

Soon after World War II, the introduction of general systems theory, with its emphasis on communication, stimulated research on the possible etiologic role of the family in schizophrenia. Fromm-Reichmann (1958) described "schizophrenogenic mothers" as hostile, cold, rejecting, and overprotective women who were not able to give themselves to their children even though they tried. Arieti (1959) stated that the mother of a schizophrenic young person was either extremely rejecting or extremely anxious during the patient's "tender years" (p. 469).

Even before the war, Theodore Lidz, Fleck, and Cornelison (1965), and R. Lidz and T. Lidz (1949) had begun longitudinal studies of schizophrenic children and their parents, especially the mothers. Their continued research after World War II focused on the formation of the child's identity and on the quality of family relationships in the child's early years. In schizophrenic patients' families, the parents had problems and their roles were unclear; instead of complementing and trusting each other, they undermined each other, threatened separation, and each enlisted the child's support against the other. Usually, both partners were disillusioned; the husband viewed the wife as defiant, and the wife was disappointed because the husband was passive. The fathers often were insecure, had a shaky sense of self-esteem, and exhibited demoralized, paranoid behavior.

Lidz and his colleagues (1974) emphasized that the "marital schism" in some schizophrenic families could split the family and that the children would be thrown into conflict by being compelled to take sides. In other families, they observed "marital skew" which was characterized by the severe psychopathology of one parent who was so dominant that other family members accepted it.

Lidz et al. (1974) described family disturbances that affected the children. A faulty parental coalition led to difficulties; sometimes a child was scapegoated or had to assume the role of a villain in order to mask parental discord or shift the blame. Conflicts arose in the family between the parents when, for example, fulfilling a social role interfered with fulfilling a spousal role. A family environment filled with conflict and anxiety thwarted the child's psychological development; the family operated in destructive fashion, and parental attitudes were transmitted directly to the child. Lidz and his colleagues concluded that a family member's schizophrenic breakdown occurred in a pathological family system and that the psychopathology was nurtured by the disturbed communication patterns in the system.

In a later discussion of schizophrenic patients' families, Lidz (1980) backed away from his earlier concepts of schizophrenogenic parenting. "It became apparent that the patient's nurturance had often been impaired during the first few months of life because of maternal depression; such findings did not explain the etiology of schizophrenic disorders for similar difficulties are found in other psychiatric and psychosomatic conditions" (p. 47).

In Finland in the 1950s, Alanen (1980) began a series of longitudinal studies of families with schizophrenic, neurotic, or normal children that merits serious attention. There were differences between the schizophrenic, neurotic, and normal children and their families during adolescence. Mothers of the schizophrenic children tended not to understand their children's needs and feelings, were overpossessive and hostile toward the children, and kept them closely tied by inimical bonds. Often those mothers were unable to be emotionally or physically close to their children. Alanen suggested that such mothers usually treated their children as they themselves had once been treated.

Schizophrenia developed as a multiphasic process; it began with a weakness in early individuation that increased the child's vulnerability during transitional stages. The vulnerability was heightened by adverse parental influences, especially parental "narcissistic self-expansion." Also, many of the parents had either narcissistic personality disorders or latent psychoses. Some of Alanen's results supported the view advanced by Lidz and his colleagues in the mid-1950s that parents can transmit their cognitive disorders to their offspring as a "transmission of irrationality" (Alanen, 1980, pp. 303–305).

Bateson, Jackson, Haley, and Weaklend (1956) postulated that a defect in communication—the "double bind"—was a specific cause of schizophrenia. It consists of two conflicting communications sent from one person to another, usually from a mother to a child; generally, one message is verbal and the other nonverbal. An example is a mother exhorting her adolescent son at lunch to "grow up and act your age" while cutting the meat on his plate into small pieces and hovering over him as if he had an eating problem. The concept of the double bind sparked interest in the role of communication in the family and the development of schizophrenia. Research in the 1960s (Rabkin, 1976), however, showed that the double bind could be found in families in which various types of psychopathology developed and that it was not specific for schizophrenia.

Some of Jackson's (1957) major contributions were his explication of the family as a system, his emphasis on communication, and his concepts of family homeostasis and of the "identified patient," usually an adolescent in a disturbed family system. Jackson argued that a system could be understood only in its entirety; it was its own cause. Feedback was necessary in order to maintain homeostasis in the system, and deviant individual behavior was a manifestation of the functioning of a disturbed family system.

Jackson (1957) cited clinical evidence showing that the lessening of a family member's symptomatology by individual treatment was sometimes followed by the appearance of pathology in one or more previously "healthy" family members. Family members had become so accustomed to dealing with each other in terms of illness that symptom relief in one upset the precarious balance and allowed other problems to surface. Also, Jackson theorized that often it was necessary for a family to have a "patient" to maintain a semblance of family life. The family could focus attention on the identified patient, whose symptoms masked or inhibited marital or other problems. Eggers (1989) has appropriately termed the identified patient a "pseudo-stabilizer."

In the late 1940s, Bowen and his colleagues at the Menninger Clinic began studies of schizophrenic patients and their families that they continued at the National Institute for Mental Health (NIMH), where patients and their families could be hospitalized for intensive study. Bowen conceptualized the mental disorders as being on a continuum, with normality at the healthy end, the neuroses in the middle, and schizophrenia at the pathological end. A family member's schizophrenia was a symptom of a faulty family system. Bowen viewed schizophrenia as a developing process that occurs in families over a number of generations—often as many as seven, but at least three. For example, it could be supposed that a grandmother ruled the family roost and her daughter, the mother of the future schizophrenic patient, was immature and adopted her own mother's domineering manner. Characteristics of the mothering thus would be conducive to the development of schizophrenia in the third-generation child. Such views are in accord with some current concepts of schizophrenia being only the tip of an iceberg, the bulk of which comprises several generations of family members' eccentricities and/or schizoid, schizophreniform, or paranoid disorders (Kerr & Bowen, 1988). Some of Bowen's observations about his multigenerational schizophrenia hypothesis have been supported by Alanen's (1980) findings.

Lyman Wynne (1984), who worked with Bowen at the NIMH, later developed a family schizophrenic research program at Rochester, New York. He and his colleagues, notably Margaret Singer (1958, 1963, 1965), looked for psychodynamic processes in schizophrenic patients and their families that involved the social organization of the family as a whole. They described patients' formal psychological disturbances, such as identity diffusion and disturbed communication, as resulting from the internalization of pathological aspects of family life. Wynne and Singer (1965) reported that at least one of the parents of a schizophrenic patient had a communication disturbance that was amorphous or fragmented. Also, they emphasized the importance of links between individuals and their cultures; thus, they had a more social psychological orientation than many other family researchers.

Wynne and Singer's research engendered a great deal of enthusiasm when Singer (1975) differentiated schizophrenic patients and their family members' Rorschach protocols from those of patients with other disorders and normal controls. The schizophrenic patients and their family members' protocols revealed a disturbance or disorganization of their thought processes and, even when family members were not clinically ill, there were similarities between the schizophrenics' and other members' protocols. The background for such work was established by Manfred Bleuler in the 1920s. In his doctoral thesis, he had reported similarities between schizophrenic patients' and their family members' (especially siblings') Rorschach protocols (Bleuler, 1983, personal communication).

Wynne and his colleagues (1958) formulated the concept of "pseudomutuality"—of family members becoming so tightly enmeshed in an effort to maintain harmony that they sacrificed individual identity and autonomy and thus had difficulty carrying out their roles. A breakdown in pseudomutuality could precipitate overt schizophrenic symptomatology. A schizophrenic family member was prima facie evidence of pathology in the entire family system, which usually was demonstrated by the family members' interactions. Families with a schizophrenic member had a more limited number of roles than those without a schizophrenic member; also, roles were more constricted, if not rigid, in the families that were more concrete and "sicker" than other families. Neither genuine autonomy nor genuine mutuality can exist in a family with a schizophrenic member.

Wynne, Singer, Bartko, and Toohey (1976) developed the concept of communication deviance (CD) from studies of schizophrenic patients' and their families' responses to the Rorschach and the Thematic Apperceptive Test (TAT). Wynne described four patterns of communication: functional, amorphous, guarded, and fragmented (Lewis, 1989, pp. 24–25). The patient's inability to maintain a shared focus of attention with the tester while being tested is scored as high, intermediate, or low CD; high CD is associated with schizophrenia or schizophrenia-spectrum disorders (Singer, Wynne, & Toohey, 1978).

By the end of the 1960s, family studies of the mental disorders were influenced by three major developments. The first was that, regardless of their brilliance, few of the findings were specific for schizophrenia. Second, there was increasing recognition of the scientific difficulty in distinguishing "between deviant parental behaviors which were a *response* to the child's psychosis and deviant parental behaviors which might have created and/or shaped the psychotic reaction" Goldstein et al., 1968, p. 233). The third was the early results of the study of schizophrenia in adoptees in Denmark by Kety, Rosenthal, Wender, and Schulsinger (1968). These authors matched 33 schizophrenic patients with a control group of adoptees who neither were listed in the psychiatric register nor showed evidence of mental illness, and then compared the two groups' biological and adoptive relatives' mental illness rates. The biological relatives of the schizophrenic index cases had the "highest concentration of schizophrenic spectrum disorders" (Rosenthal, 1973, p. 231), supporting the hypothesis that genetic factors are influential in the etiology of schizophrenia.

As a result of these developments, family studies of schizophrenia during the past 20 years have focused mainly on pedigree, twin, adoptee, and other genetic investigations. For example, Kendler et al.

(1992) have been carrying out large-scale pedigree studies in Ireland, and Sherrington and his colleagues (1988) reported presumptive evidence of an abnormality involving chromosome 5 in patients and pedigrees studied in Iceland and England. The chromosome 5 abnormality, however, has not been replicated.

Deinstitutionalization has produced serious problems for families of schizophrenics. With public hospitals no longer serving as asylums, many young, chronically mentally ill patients have become the responsibility of their families, who often are unprepared for the staggering burden of a family member's chronic mental illness. These families can become demoralized, and the untreated mentally ill persons (many of whom end up homeless) are a tragic public spectacle. Fortunately, families of the mentally ill have formed effective advocacy groups—such as the National Alliance for the Mentally Ill (NAMI)— and are mounting political pressure to gain improved care for the mentally ill. They maintain that they did not produce schizophrenia in their offspring and, like most investigators and clinicians, reject the concept of the schizophrenogenic mother. They insist that schizophrenia is a disease that requires more medical care and intensive research.

Disillusionment about the role of family factors in the etiology of schizophrenia can readily be seen in psychiatry. The space allotted to family studies of schizophrenia since 1966 in the successive editions of the *Comprehensive Textbook of Psychiatry* (Kaplan, Freedman, & Saddock, 1980) has been diminishing. Falloon, Boyd, and McGill (1984), Hogarty et al. (1986), and others' psychoeducational programs for schizophrenic patients' families have been significant contributions to the care of patients and helpful to their families.

Even the influence of family factors on relapse in schizophrenia is controversial. In England, Leff and Vaughn (1980) reported that high levels of expressed emotion (EE) in the family were associated with the schizophrenic member's relapses. But Kanter, Lamb, and Loeper (1987) disputed the reliability of that association and its possible cause-and-effect implications, citing studies that reported a "chicken-egg" relationship between high EE and the patient's disturbed behavior. Also, EE is not a pure construct; it contains three components—criticism, hostility, and emotional overinvolvement. Kanter and his colleagues feared that emphasis on EE "conceal[s] subjective judgments of families behind the objective veneer of a complex scientific methodology" (p. 379). They urged clinicians to concentrate on "establishing a livable home situation for all family members" (p. 379) and advocated studying the interactions of patient and family variables, as recommended by G. W. Brown and Harris (1978). These are cogent criticisms of EE research and valuable recommendations, but efforts to make sure that patients' families are not blamed for causing schizophrenia should not result in blaming the patient for the illness. The work of Doane, West, Goldstein, Rodnick, and Jones (1981) indicates that a benign affective style (AS) in the family is conducive to better mental health than a negative AS.

Goldstein (1985) reported the results of a 15-year prospective study of parental communication style, affectivity in the home environment, EE, and the development of schizophrenia and schizophrenia-spectrum disorders in teenagers. Schizophrenia-spectrum disorders were associated with the high parental CD described by Wynne (1984), the negative AS described by Doane and his colleagues (1981), and the high EE described by Vaughn and Leff (1976). Goldstein (1985) stated that "parental CD was a significant marker of the potential for subsequent offspring schizophrenia or schizophrenia-spectrum disorders" (p. 16) and that there were deleterious interactions between high CD, negative AS, and high EE. He concluded that the findings "strongly suggest that disturbed patterns of intrafamilial communication and affective expression antedate the onset of schizophrenia-spectrum disorders and are not reactions to psychotic behaviors in already schizophrenic offspring" (p. 7). But he recognized the limitations of the research: "Possibly, all we can say at the present time is that living in a high CD, high EE, negative AS family environment, to use an analogy with cigarette smoking, is not good for your mental health" (p. 17).

Scientists at the UCLA Clinical Research Center for the Study of Schizophrenia have proposed a vulnerability-stress model for schizophrenia. Two mediating factors—information processing and autonomic abnormalities—influence the interactions between stressors and protective environmental factors. In accord with evidence of genetic factors, disturbances of attention and information processing can be heritable and can increase vulnerability to family tensions, stressful life events (SLE), and adverse circumstances. Also, "the electrodermal arousal of schizophrenic patients may be sensitive to stressful events such as the presence of a high expressed emotion relative or the interaction of independent life events with the presence of a key relative. . . . [Thus] an autonomic hyperarousal state may serve as a mediating factor in exacerbating an already deteriorating environment and . . . in the development of psychotic symptoms" (Neuchterlein, Goldstein, Ventura, Dawson, & Doane, 1989, pp. 88–89).

The repeated finding that family psychoeducational programs reduce relapse rates is evidence of family influences, either salutary or deleterious, on the course of schizophrenia. In psychiatry, the current "biologism" is accompanied by a rather wholesale "the family has no part in it" thesis; however, it is wise to recall that dogmatic opinions eventually give way to evidence (e.g., *folie à deux* is an established verity). Although the early family studies of schizophrenia are out of favor, they focused attention on the topic of the family and mental illness and led to the development of such concepts as Lidz's marital schism or skew, Bowen's emotional divorce, Wynne's pseudomutuality, and Jackson's family homeostasis, which have clinical utility even if they have little or no specific etiological significance. Also, these studies emphasized the importance of the early home environment on children who later became mentally ill. The results of family studies (e.g., Alanen, 1980) do not preclude the possibility of genetic influences or the transmission of negative parental attitudes and behaviors toward children from one generation to the next. The schizophrenic phenotype may be produced by genetic factors in combination with other biological factors, as well as such life experiences as disturbed parenting during critical developmental periods.

FAMILY STUDIES OF DEPRESSION

Theories of Depressive Illness

Interest in schizophrenia dominated family research for two decades after World War II, and there was little systematic research on the family and depression. Since the early 1970s, however, there has been epidemic interest in depression aroused by rapid social change, rising suicide rates in the young, and such findings as those from our Florida Health Study, which revealed that respondents in the 16–20 age group had much higher scores on a depression scale than reported previously (Schwab, Warheit, & Holzer, 1973).

There are a number of major theories of depressive illness, including genetic and biological, psychoanalytic, behavioral, cognitive and attributional, and social stress models. It is surprising that until recently there has been a relative paucity of scientific work on depression and the family, because risk factors in the family combine to increase vulnerability to depression, often to precipitate it, and to affect its course and outcome. Family risk factors cover a spectrum that includes assortative mating, genetic factors, the child's psychosexual development, learning in the family setting, cognitions and attributions, interactions between spouses, family living, social stress, and multigenerational influences. Even before marriage, family influences are evident inasmuch as the nonrandom selection of a potential mate places wives of affectively ill husbands at increased risk (Merikangas, 1982).

Evidence from pedigree and twin studies indicates that heredity is a major etiological factor. The work of Winokur, Tsuang, and Crowe (1982) in Iowa and of Egeland and Hostetter (1983) on the Old Order Amish shows that depression runs in families. Gershon and his colleagues' (1982) pedigree study reported that the lifetime prevalence of major affective disorders in the relatives of index cases was 24.8% for bipolar I, 25% for bipolar II, and 20% for unipolar, in contrast to 7% for controls. For the offspring of one affectively ill parent, the morbidity risk was 27%; for two ill parents, it was 74%. Twin studies show that monozygotic concordance may be 74%, whereas dizygotic concordance is only about 20%.

In the family setting, psychological as well as genetic factors predispose to depression. Karl Abraham's (1968) classic 1912 paper revealed that prominent family factors during the childhood of adult manic-depressives were conformity to rigid rules, emotional withdrawal by the mother (who often was the dominant figure), and high expectations of the child that led to ego deficits and an inability to withstand disappointments later in life. Repeated clinical findings point to the importance of the family setting for unipolar depression as well. Parents of depressives tend not to express positive feelings directly, to be rigidly perfectionistic and relatively unaware of their own needs, and to be critical of the child (especially of his or her performance). The child internalizes such parental attitudes, develops a harsh superego, hinges assessment of the self on parental criticisms, becomes guilt-prone and self-punitive, and is dependent on external supports for maintaining self-esteem. Because aggressive behavior is not tolerated, the child controls anger or directs it toward the self and becomes repressive and ambivalent. Often, his or her life becomes a grim, unrewarding pursuit of goals such as unambivalent love from others and total success, neither of which can be attained this side of paradise. These attitudes and behaviors are transmitted to children in future generations and thus abet the intergenerational continuity of depression.

Clinical studies support the psychodynamic, if not contributory, significance of the child's home environment for depression. Parker's (1983) case-control studies of depressed young adults and of their parents (biological and adoptive) showed that "affectionless control" (lack of positive affection combined with overprotection) of the growing child, especially by the mother, was a measurable risk factor for depression.

Effects of Depression on the Family

Persons with depression tend to marry much more often than those with other serious mental illnesses. Consequently, the effect of a depressed person on the family has been a great concern. Fenichel (1945) pointed out that depressed patients "try to influence the persons around them to return their lost self-esteem by demonstrating their misery and by enforcing and even blackmailing their objects for affection. . . . The depressed patient, who seemingly is so extremely submissive, is actually often successful in dominating his entire environment" (pp. 391–392).

The most profound effects are on the children. Weissman, Paykel, and Klerman (1972) reported that 58% of 109 children of depressed mothers showed evidence of disturbed functioning. Depressed mothers found it difficult to provide emotional support to their children, experienced a great deal of discord with them, and had problems of guilt and resentment with the children, who often were exposed to the mothers for a significant part of each day. Also, Coyne (1990) reported that children of depressed patients "are at risk for a full range of psychological problems, academic difficulties, and even physical health problems. . . . As many as 40-50% of the children of a depressed parent have diagnosable psychiatric disturbance" (p. 43). Keitner (1990) found that the children of a depressed parent continued to function poorly even after the parent's condition improved.

Keitner (1990) reported that there was impairment of family functioning in 75% of families of depressed patients during acute episodes, in contrast to smaller percentages of families of schizophrenic patients or of those dependent on alcohol (p. 5). Such findings support the results of the important 1989 Medical Outcome Study; the impairments of depression were more severe than those of such chronic medical diseases as hypertension and diabetes mellitus and were equal to those of severe coronary artery disease (Wells, Stewart, Hays, et al., 1989).

In a study of 43 depressed inpatients and their families and a control group, Keitner (1990) found that the depressed had significant difficulties with communication, problem solving, and affective expression (p. 6). In another study, 64% of the families with a depressed family member reported that they had a host of everyday problems, emotional upsets, family role issues, and difficulties showing love or affection to each other. Although the disturbances in family functioning lessened during remission, even then the patients' families reported significantly poorer functioning than controls.

In a study of 38 unipolar depressed inpatients and their families, Keitner (1990) reported that the Family Assessment Device (FAD) showed that positive changes in family functioning were associated with shorter recovery times, and also that improved functioning lessened the likelihood of relapse. Family functioning was better in families of male than female patients. The investigators emphasized that many studies using various methodologies "agree that significant disturbances are experienced by families through all stages of the depressive illness" (p. 20). Their studies could not shed much light on etiology; probably there was an interactive (not a linear) relationship between family dysfunction and depression (p. 19).

Keitner (1990) categorized depressed patients and their families into four types: (a) those whose depressive symptoms remitted rapidly after family issues were treated; (b) those in whom there was little family pathology during the illness; (c) those in whom there was a wide spectrum of family pathology that improved when the patient was treated effectively and the family received family therapy; and (d) those with severe depressive symptomatology who entered therapy reluctantly, but when they were treated and their symptoms diminished, severe underlying character pathology or dysthymia emerged.

Weissman (1990) stated "that there is overwhelming evidence from clinical, family, epidemiologic, and pedigree studies that depression is a family affair. . . . The familial nature of depression and its serious impact on family functioning are sturdy findings" (pp. 187–188). But an exclusive family systems view of depression is inadequate because depression runs in bloodlines even when the biological relatives are not in direct contact or have no social impact on each other or the patient.

Our Pilot Longitudinal Family Study

Thus, depression has adverse effects on family members; however, studies of families in which a person is already depressed and studies at only one point in time can reveal only associations between depression and family life that may or may not have etiological significance. Only prospective studies can untangle the sequential relationships among disturbances of family functioning, the impact of SLEs, the quality of the home environment, disturbed interactions, and the development of depressive symptoms.

In 1988, we reported a few preliminary results of our study of a random sample of 34 families from the general population over a 15-month period to determine their risk for depression (Schwab, Stephenson, & Bell, 1988). We interviewed adults and children in their homes three times and evaluated risk for depression on four instruments, including the Diagnostic Interview Schedule (DIS). At baseline, 40% of the families contained one or more members at risk for depression. During the 15 months, nine families changed from "not at risk" to "at risk"; the 15-month family incidence rate for risk for depression was 26%, and for continued good mental health, 74%. Our finding that the mental health status of 35% of the families changed in some way during the 15-month period suggests that only longitudinal studies can provide a picture of family mental health.

RESEARCH PERSPECTIVES ON DEPRESSION AND THE FAMILY

The possibility that depression is a family illness produced in part by disturbed interpersonal relations or deleterious interactions is based on clinical observations and on Penrose's (1944) finding that spouses (usually wives of mentally ill husbands) were at significantly higher risk for mental illness than those of healthy partners. Kreitman and his colleagues (1962, 1964, 1968) and others have evaluated the following five hypotheses about the development of mental illness in the spouse of a mentally ill person:

1. Both partners are subject to the same stressors that precipitate illness.
2. One spouse's illness is a reaction to the other's breakdown.
3. Treatment for one facilitates the other's obtaining treatment.
4. There is a tendency for persons with similar backgrounds and constitutions to marry (i.e., assortative mating).
5. The spouses exert cumulative, detrimental, interactional effects on each other.

A stressor affecting both spouses has only occasionally been the cause of mental illness in both. Also, there is little evidence to support the reaction hypothesis; however, when one spouse receives psychiatric treatment, it is easier for the other to obtain treatment. The relative importance of the other two hypotheses is disputed.

Assortative Mating

There is persisting controversy about the assortative mating hypothesis. Kreitman, Collins, Nelson, and Troop's (1971) and Hagnell and Kreitman's (1974) studies confirmed the assortative mating hypothesis for psychotically ill affective and schizophrenic patients, but found little assortative mating in patients with neurotic depressions.

Merikangas (1982) concluded from her comprehensive review of studies of morbidity risk for affective disorders in first-degree relatives of couples in which one spouse was affectively ill that there was some evidence for the assortative mating hypothesis. In particular, assortative mating placed wives of affectively ill husbands at increased risk. Recently, Merikangas, Weissman, and Prusoff (1990) reported that in a study of 215 depressed adults, their 165 offspring, and controls, "assortative mating had occurred because increased rates of psychopathology were observed among the relatives of the ill spouses compared with those of the well spouses. . . . It is likely that assortative mating is related both to increased genetic risk and a clustering of environmental risk factors" (p. 97).

The most comprehensive study of assortative mating is Hagnell and Kreitman's (1974) evaluations in Lundby, Sweden, of 269 couples' personality traits and symptoms in 1947 and again in 1957. Evaluations at two points in time enabled the investigators to eliminate the effects of one family member's existing symptomatology on another. Assortative mating was more common in healthy couples than in those in which at least one partner was mentally ill. Thus, the results were in accord with the interactional hypothesis of the etiology of depression and were supported by the finding that wives of sick husbands showed increased morbidity over time that paralleled the duration of the marriage. Remission of upper- and middle-class husbands' illnesses was associated with their wives having short illnesses. Mentally ill wives in the lower social class tended not to improve when their husbands improved, however, probably because they were subjected to many adverse environmental pressures.

Some of the contradictory findings about assortative mating are attributable to investigators failing to specify how they define it. Traditionally, assortative mating has referred to the selective, nonrandom choice of a marital partner whose social, cultural, intellectual, and personality characteristics—other than on Eysenck's (1960) extraversion-introversion scale—matched one's own. Many of the studies of assortative mating in the affectively ill, such as those reported by Merikangas, limit the concept simply to the marriages of two persons who have or have had affective illnesses. According to that narrow definition, there is a tendency for depressives and/or those with depressive relatives to marry (and thus increase the genetic loading and probably cluster environmental risk factors). The restriction of the concept of assortative mating, however, reduces its meaning considerably. Hagnell and Kreitman's study (1974) is especially important, because they had comprehensive evaluations of their subjects' personality characteristics at two points in time and thus could use the broader concept of assortative mating meaningfully.

Marital Interactions and Depression

A number of studies have indicated that deleterious interactions between partners appear to explain, in part, the high risk for depression among spouses of mentally ill persons. These interactions concern mainly communication, the expression of emotions, marital adjustment and satisfaction, role strain, and loss of intimacy.

Communication

Communication between depressed patients and their spouses has been found to be characterized by high levels of tension, negative expressions, self-preoccupation, and diminished nonverbal patterns of support. In *The Melancholy Marriage,* Hinchliffe, Hooper, and Roberts (1978) described the many conflicts in couples where one spouse was depressed, especially when the husband demonstrated an instrumental (i.e., doing, not discussing) communication style and the wife an expressive style (discussing feelings and problems). The strain in the couples' relationships was evidenced by many speech disruptions and pauses, the relative lack of tension releasers and laughter, and their showing less nonverbal responsive "symmetry" than controls. Negative tensions persisted after recovery.

Coyne (1990) reported the effects of depressed persons' interactions on strangers. An interesting finding was that "naive (not depressed) subjects" who spoke for 20 minutes on the telephone with depressed outpatients "showed negative changes in mood and negatively evaluated and rejected the outpatients" (p. 39). The effects of a depressed on a nondepressed person were both subtle and immediate—the negativism picked up in 3 minutes (p. 39).

When a spouse is depressed, disturbances include avoidance of communication as well as tensions and criticism. Weissman, Paykel, and Klerman (1972) found that depressed women were reticent to discuss personal feelings with their husbands. Also MacLean, Ogston, and Grauer (1973) reported avoidance of communication in their study of 20 depressed patients' marriages.

Expressed Emotion (EE). In their studies of EE, Leff and Vaughn (1980, 1987) reported that hostile, negative criticism of depressed patients was correlated with increasing symptom levels and relapse necessitating hospitalization. Also, the combination of independent SLEs (those over which the patient had no control) and high levels of criticism from a person in the home was associated with the onset of a depressive episode.

In her study of 39 depressed patients and their spouses who were followed for 9 months, Hooley (1990) found that high levels of spousal criticism were significantly associated with relapse rates. Wives of depressed husbands made more critical remarks about their spouses than did the husbands of depressed wives. Depressed patients relapsed at lower levels of criticism than were associated with schizophrenic patients' relapse, supporting Hooley's hypothesis that depressives would be more sensitive to high EE than schizophrenics because depressives were self-critical and their cognitive distortions led to exaggerations of the negative aspects of their environments. But depressives usually are criticized by their spouses, whereas schizophrenics are criticized by their parents; spousal criticism may be more threatening than parental criticism.

Inasmuch as EE is a complex construct, Hooley classified the spouses as either high- or low-EE according to the extent to which they made critical, hostile, or emotionally involved remarks about the patient. High-EE couples' marriages were more distressed, especially by spousal criticisms, disagreements, and lack of acceptance of the patients, than low-EE couples' marriages. Hooley (1990) pointed out that the EE interview "may be telling us more about the patient-spouse relationship than about the spouses per se" (p. 75). This view was supported by her finding that the depressed patients' ratings of their spouses' criticisms correlated with the spouses' ratings of level of criticism and with relapse at 0.64, and were not associated with gender or with severity of the depression. Also, the patients' scores remained stable over time.

Hooley (1990) emphasized the predictive value of the EE construct: "Unipolar patients who live with critical or high-EE spouses are significantly more likely to relapse in a nine-month period after hospital discharge than outpatients who live with non-critical or low-EE spouses" (p. 77). The causal link appeared to be from the relative or spouse to the patient, but it is possible that "subtle characteristics of the patient can engender high levels of criticism" (p. 77) from family members or that certain patient characteristics might, in themselves, be associated with relapse. Thus, cause and effect relationships are unclear; however, "EE is a marker of relapse and of poor prognosis inasmuch as EE and marital satisfaction are interchangeable predictors of relapse. . . . [The EE construct] may simply be old wine in new bottles" (pp. 78–79), but it is one of the better predictors of relapse.

Marital Adjustment, Dissatisfaction, and Depression

The possible associations between marital adjustment, dissatisfaction, and depression have been studied repeatedly. The results indicate that tangled, disquieting webs of negative feelings and attitudes were bound up with marital dissatisfactions and depressive symptomatology. Alarcon (1976) reported that two thirds of the depressives who had high negative marriage scores had their first breakdown in the first 19 years of marriage; in contrast, two thirds of those with low negative marriage scores became ill only after 20 or more years of marriage. Neurotic depression was the most common condition associated with poor quality of the marriage; it could lead to marital disharmony, but it is possible that the marital disharmony generated the symptoms. In the Isle of Wight Study, Rutter and Quinton (1977) found that depressed women were five times more likely to have disturbed marriages than controls. G. W. Brown and Harris (1978) reported depression in 38% of women without close marital relationships, in contrast to only 4% of those with close relationships. Depressions were related to emotional deprivation, not just dissatisfaction, inasmuch as both depressed and nondepressed women endorsed similar negative items about their marriages.

Rounsaville, Prusoff, and Weissman's (1980) important longitudinal study of depressed married females during the acute illness and the ensuing 48 months showed that more depressed women than controls were dissatisfied with their marriages over the 48 months. Also, of the depressed women's marriages that improved when the illness remitted, approximately 50% had deteriorated by 48 months. The investigators concluded that basically, marriages tended to be either good or disturbed, and that the quality of the marriage both during depression and at remission was related to its quality before the onset of depression. After argumentative depressed women divorced and remarried, they disputed with their new husbands as much as they had with their previous husbands.

The lack of marital satisfaction and the marital disharmony in families in which a spouse (usually the wife) is depressed has been postulated to be caused in large part by personality factors, especially dependency and excessive demands upon the husband. Bullock, Siegel, Weissman, & Paykel (1972) reported that the wife's "dependency took on a demanding quality which was often a source of irritation and confusion to the husband who fluctuated between being overprotective of her and doubting her need for help" (p. 196). Also, it has been hypothesized that a wife's seemingly helpless dependency may feed her husband's need to be a protector and a rescuer. Feldman (1976) found that husbands were able "to regenerate the cycle of depressive symptomatology" (p. 392) in their wives by undermining their self-worth.

In Ruestow, Dunner, Bleecker, and Fieve's (1978) study of marital adjustment in patients with affective disorders, dependency was related to the affectively ill patient's (not the spouse's) age and sex. The dependency in the affectively ill married persons might have been the result of either recurrent illness episodes or a personality trait that preceded the illness. Ruestow et al. recommended couples therapy directed at dependency, because it was a major area of marital disturbance. Men with bipolar diagnoses often had a good marital adjustment when they were euthymic, but adjustment was strained during mania. Men with unipolar depression had poorer marital adjustment than men with bipolar illness or women with any affective disorder. The spouses' marital adjustment ratings correlated well. Ruestow and his colleagues' (1978) results supported Weissman and Paykel's (1974) findings that recovered depressives reported poor marital adjustment, infrequent intercourse, and disinterest in sex.

Merikangas and her colleagues (1985) reported that marital adjustment was impaired in most areas of functioning in couples in which one spouse had major depression. The similarities between the patients' and spouses' reports supported Ruestow and his colleagues' (1978) findings; marital maladjustment was not simply a result of the patients' symptomatic status but reflected persisting personality characteristics. Distinctive background features in the families of the depressed patients were childhood bereavement, mental illness, and parents' separations or divorces. But, Hirschfeld, Klerman, Clayton, and Keller's (1983) study did not find that personality features were associated with the higher frequency of depression in women than in men.

Many studies have reported that depressed patients' marital relationships were impaired, marital discord was confirmed by their spouses, and that impairments persisted after recovery. Many depressed individuals are highly disillusioned with marriage, but those in Merikangas and her colleagues' (1985) study did not blame their spouses, and few reported that they would marry different persons. It appears that the depressive's negative self-concept influences adjustment to marriage; the marital disharmony may be caused by the depression or by role disputes that seem to lead to depression. Inasmuch as unipolar depressives tend to report serious marital dissatisfaction, both they and their spouses need treatment.

Role Conflicts, Lack of Support, Loss of Intimacy, and Depression

During the past 20 years, many studies (e.g., Radloff, 1975; Weissman & Paykel, 1974) have reported that role strain and role conflicts are at least partly responsible for the high rate of depression in young and early-middle-aged married women, many of whom are in dual-career households. In Krause's (1983) study of a community sample of 273 married women, those with depressive symptoms reported that conflicts in sex-role expectations existed in their marriages. The conflicts stemmed from the spouses' differing attitudes about a woman's role in housework, employment outside the home, extrafamilial activity, financial responsibilities, appearance, and interactions with men. The married women with relatively few symptoms of depression did not report such sex-role conflicts.

The results of Vanfossen's (1981) study of employed husbands, nonemployed wives, and employed wives suggested that everyday social roles that produced low self-evaluation or involved strain were associated with depression, and that non-supportive marital relationships precipitated depression in vulnerable persons. Husbands were likely to be depressed when their spouses were unaffectionate and unaffirming, especially when the husbands' work relationships are unsatisfactory. Unemployed wives were likely to be depressed when their husbands were unaffirming and expressed negative evaluations that increased the wives' dissatisfaction with housekeeping roles. Employed wives were depressed when their husbands were unaffirming, were inequitable, and disagreed about sharing domestic duties.

Reports of role conflicts, lack of support, and negative interactions in marriages in which a spouse is depressed have led to a view of depression as coercive behavior. MacLean et al. (1973) reported coercive communication patterns and an anarchic approach to domestic problem solving in couples in which one spouse was depressed. Studies by Hokanson and his associates (1980) and by Blumberg and Hokanson (1983) showed that depressed persons in high-power roles tended to be exploitative and noncooperative and to communicate self-devaluation and helplessness, whereas the depressed in low-power roles tended to blame their partners. In his study of depressed and schizophrenic patients and their spouses, Hell (1982) found that the spouses (especially husbands) of moderately to seriously ill depressed patients had a tendency to depict themselves as more submissive than did the spouses of schizophrenic patients. Overall, the spouses' well-being correlated with the seriousness of the patients' illnesses and especially the course of either depression or schizophrenia. Hell emphasized that research on family attitudes and environments has greater significance for the rehabilitation of mentally ill persons than for determining the cause of the illness.

The lack of affective involvement in marriage is a loss that may be conducive to depression. Kreitman (1964) found that depressed men spent increased time in face-to-face contact with their wives, but the increased time did not mean greater affective involvement and may simply have reflected a reduction in the time the couple spent away from home. Characteristics of families with a depressed spouse included lack of cooperation, failure to share roles in the marriage, increased husband-wife face-to-face contact, friction about child rearing, restricted social activities, and little positive affection from the mentally ill partner. Kreitman (1962, 1964, 1968, 1971) emphasized that over time, the depressive operates in a progressively shrinking social framework that eventually involves the spouse, who becomes progressively more disturbed.

Other investigators have reported that depressive symptomatology diminishes the expression of affection. Demers and Davis's (1971) study of 14 manic-depressive patients' marriages revealed that spouses expressed less affection when the partner was actively ill than when he or she was in remission. Coleman and Miller (1975) reported that a depressed husband had a more negative impact on marital interaction than a depressed wife. Hinchliffe, Hooper, and Roberts (1978) also found that depressed husbands were more likely than depressed wives to express overt hostile behavior toward the spouse and that, generally, either spouse's being depressed was associated with increased negative affective expression. The association between limited affective involvement in marriage and depression may be related to the quality of the attachment. Henderson's (1981) studies of attachment in adults found that diminished affective involvement was related to increased depression and that there was an inverse relationship between social bonds and neurotic symptoms. Whether and how the problems with attachment stem from difficulties with bonding and attachment early in life deserves study.

Studies of intimacy in the marriages of depressed persons by Waring and Patton (1984) showed that increased severity of depression was associated with a loss of intimacy. Also, the quality of the intimacy appeared to be predictive of the outcome of the depression; those who were depressed at follow-up reported less intimacy than those who had improved. Waring and Patton emphasized that the loss of intimacy is a serious problem for depressed women and can be likened to a grief state.

Many studies have revealed that a lack of emotional support and affection between the spouses, and often throughout the family, is associated with depression. When one spouse was depressed, the marriages were characterized by reduced affective involvement, reduced expression of affection, increased criticism, and struggles for interpersonal control. Also, such marriages tended to be less cooperative and characterized by husband-dominated patterns more often than those of controls.

Stressful Life Events, Social Support, Chronic Depression, and Depression in the Family

For many years, SLEs, especially losses, have been associated with the onset of depression. Paykel and his colleagues (1971) estimated that about 9% to 10% of all exit events are followed by depression and that the relative risk for exit events in depression is 6.5. He and his colleagues (1969) reported that "increase in arguments with spouses" was the event that most significantly differentiated 185 depressive patients from controls.

Research on SLEs and depression is complicated by a number of factors: depressives tend to report more events than controls, and they often have difficulties with recall and the dating of an event. We found that families at risk for depression reported a significantly larger number of total and undesirable SLEs than those not at risk at baseline and both 6 months and 15 months later, but the two groups reported about the same number of desirable-ambiguous events (Stephenson et al., 1990). The most commonly reported SLEs were hospitalization of a family member, death of a close friend, and a minor law violation. We were surprised to find that all of the family members reported only 30% to 35% of the number of SLEs that had occurred. The wife/mother reported an additional 33%, compared to the husband/father's 20% to 24% and the children's 15% to 20%. This lack of agreement about whether major events had occurred within the past 6 months points to a research problem and the importance of W. I. Thomas's (1923) "definition of the situation" (i.e., how a person defines an event and what it means determines whether it and its effects on that person and others will be reported).

In his review of SLEs and depression, Hirschfeld (1981) concluded that SLEs are neither a necessary nor a sufficient cause of depression and that the study of personal resources has been neglected. G. W. Brown and Harris (1978) found that the risk of depression for women in London increased when women had three children under the age of 14 in the home but did not have a confiding, supportive relationship. They and others maintain that marriage can be protective and can moderate the influence of SLEs. Warheit (1979) reported that low socioeconomic status, not being married, and not having friends were better predictors of depression than SLE loss scores. Thus, the deleterious effects of SLEs can be either increased or lessened by marriage and the family.

In African Americans, D. R. Brown and Gary (1987) found that the relationships between social supports, SLEs, and emotional and physical health were not the same for males and females. "Being embedded in a large social support network of nearby relatives" (p. 172) reduced the females' psychological distress and corroborated the importance of the extended family for them. In contrast, the males' depression scores were not related to family or other social support measures investigated. In a later, larger study, however, Gary, Brown, Milburn, Ahmed, and Booth (1989) reported that participation in social organizations was associated with lower depression scores for both black males and females.

The deleterious influence of chronic stressors on individuals and families has been neglected, even though in a study of 2,299 Chicago adults, Ilfeld (1977) reported that the level of depressive symptoms was related less to SLEs than to the number and type of current social stressors. These were defined as the "circumstances of daily social roles that are usually considered problematic or undesirable" and include marital, parenting, occupational, financial, and neighborhood stressors. Marital stressors had the highest correlation with depressive symptoms, followed closely by parental stressors for women and job stressors for men. The stressors accounted for 25% of the variance in the level of depressive symptoms; sociodemographic characteristics accounted for only 8%.

In a random sample of 1,018 African-American adults in Norfolk, Virginia, Gary and his colleagues (1989) found that 34.5% scored high on the Center for Epidemiologic Studies Depression Scale (CES-D). The divorced and separated had much higher scores than the never-married, widowed, or married respondents (pp. 60–65). Both the number of undesirable SLEs in the preceding year and of chronic stressors (related to finances, personal relationships, and alcohol) were significantly associated with high depression scores as well as perceived racial discrimination (p. 72). The investigators emphasized the relationship between daily "hassles" and high depression scores.

Poverty is the most significant stressor. Individuals and families tend to adapt to acute financial losses, whereas chronic poverty is associated with family instability and pathologies. Moreover, the association between low socioeconomic status (SES) and depression has been found consistently in Western society. In the U.S., Holzer and his colleagues (1986) reported that the inverse relationship between socioeconomic status and the frequency of depression was not linear because those in the bottom SES quintile had not just the highest, but an especially high, rate of depression. Also, Warheit, Holzer, and Schwab (1973) found that the very high rates for depressive symptoms in blacks were not significantly higher than those for whites when the two groups were controlled for income, occupational, and educational levels.

Thus, the role of family factors in depression is pervasive. The results of many studies revealed that negative interactions, a loss of intimacy, SLEs and stressors, the lack of a supportive marital relationship, and both separation and divorce have been associated with depression. We and others have reported high rates of depressive symptoms in the divorced, and especially in the separated (Schwab et al., 1979). Tragically, family problems also have recently been associated with adolescents' suicide attempts and deaths (Jennings, 1990).

THE FAMILY LIFE CYCLE

The concept of the life cycle reaches back in history to Ecclesiastes and includes Shakespeare's (1968) immortal "seven ages of man." Studies of the life cycle, however, have flowered mainly in the latter part of this century. Interest in the life cycle stems from the lengthening of the life span and the increasing number of elderly persons and of three- and four-generation families. In his classic study of York, Rowntree (1903) categorized the family life cycle into three stages. The first was that of poverty when a family consisted of the parents and young children. The second, that of prosperity, coincided with the children's reaching the age when they could be gainfully employed and help support the family. The third was that of poverty in old age.

In 1936, Loomis and Hamilton presented "Family Life Cycle Analysis," the first scientific article on the topic. In accord with Sorokin's views, they limited the family to the parents and children and the cycle to four stages, beginning with marriage and ending with the death of one parent if there were no children, or with the death of both parents if there were children. Although historical family life cycle analysis was promising, it was handicapped by the paucity of data about major biological, social, and economic events. Loomis and Hamilton (1936) proposed an alternative cross-sectional approach that entailed interviewing the family to gather information about its size and composition and about the social and economic processes impinging on it. The two approaches yielded different results because the cross-sectional method could not take into account occupational and other shifts and was "non-historical."

For their pioneering Halifax, North Carolina, study, Loomis and Hamilton (1936) found 14 homogeneous "Negro cropper and tenant families," married between 1905 and 1914, that could be studied by the two methods. They concluded that "a relatively accurate picture of the historical [family life cycle]" (p. 231) could be obtained by cross-sectional analysis when there had been few "great changes in social and biological factors affecting the family" (p. 231). But during periods of great or rapid changes in birth and death rates, only historical analysis was sufficient.

Glick (1947) compared 1890 and 1940 census data on three family life cycle topics: The ages at which married couples reach various stages, changes in the composition of the family during the life span, and changes in residence and economic characteristics over the course of the life cycle. The average couple marrying in 1890 was older than the 1940 couple, and marriage in rural areas was later than in urban areas. In 1940, there was a growing trend for more couples to live with a family of origin or other relatives as a result of the hardships of the Great Depression.

Changes in the composition of the family were as follows: In 1890, the average woman bore 5.4 children over a 9-year period of time and gave birth to her last child at age 32; but in 1940, she bore 3.1 children over a 4.5-year period, and her last child was born when she was 27.2. In 1890, the average woman's five children had left home when she was 47 to 55 years old, whereas by 1940 the average woman's three children would have left home when she was 45-50 years old (thus the prominence of the "empty nest" syndrome in the late 1940s and 1950s (Glick, 1947, p. 168).

The mortality data are interesting in view of the shorter length of married life in the 1980s than in the preceding two or three decades. In 1890, a couple had an even chance of surviving together for 31 years, at which time the husband would be 57 years old and the wife 53, and their youngest child would not be expected to marry for 2 more years. In contrast, by 1940, the couple could expect to have 39 years of married life, until the husband was 64 years old and the wife 61, at which time they would have been alone for 11 years. Glick (1947) explained that with smaller family size and longer life expectancy, a couple in 1940 would have "one-fourth of the married life still to come" after the last child left home (p. 168). He emphasized that "this remarkable change since 1890 . . . [is] one of the most significant . . . of all changes in the family cycle in the last 50 years" (p. 168).

Glick's (1947) analyses also revealed the increasing mobility of the American family that Vance Packard would describe in the mid-1950s. In 1940, only 16% of family heads under age 33 were living in the same dwelling in which they had lived 5 years before, but older couples moved less often.

Between 1937 and 1987, the younger age of first marriage, the lower birthrate, the couple's having one fourth of their married life alone, and the lengthening of the life span all have had implications for the instability of marriage and the family since the 1960s. It is possible that the transition "from institution to companionship" (Burgess & Locke, (1945, 1960) had placed an emotional burden on the couple and contributed to the rising rate of family disruption.

Hill's (1970) study of *Family Development in Three Generations* stimulated further interest in the family life cycle. But even earlier, researchers were influenced by Erikson's (1950) classic analysis of the developmental tasks of each stage of the individual's life cycle in *Childhood and Society*. More recently, the individual life cycle has been studied intensively, for example, by Daniel Levinson (1978) in *The Seasons of a Man's Life,* and it has been the main topic of such popular works as Gail Sheehy's (1976) *Passages*.

Glick's (1988) discussion of the family life cycle cited Hill and Rodger's (1964) report that events occurring both inside and outside the family were more important determinants of adults' changing roles than age. Also, the increased marriage-divorce-remarriage cycles were affecting the sequencing of family events and complicating classifications of the life cycle into stages. The term *family life course* has been replacing *family life cycle* inasmuch as the former implies that "family events occur in the context of previous family experiences" (p. 864).

MARITAL AND FAMILY SATISFACTION IN DUAL-CAREER AFRICAN-AMERICAN FAMILIES

The recession that developed in 1990 brought many middle-class families' economic problems into sharp focus and increased the need for them to have two incomes. The number of dual-career middle-class families had grown from 900,000 in 1960 to 3.3 million in 1983, a 267% jump in 23 years (Conference Board, 1985). As was discussed in Chapter 1, common problems in those families stem from the needs for shared child care, housework, and home upkeep, and there is "a sharing gap"; Arlie Hochschild (1989) found that the wives did more work on the "second shift" than the husbands. V. G. Thomas (1990a) reported that in black dual-career couples "the distribution of child care and housework is probably the most critical issue" (p. 58). She notes that most research on dual-career couples had been on white families and raised questions about the possibility that black couples' "problems and concerns" (p. 59) differed.

V. G. Thomas's (1990b) study of 41 dual-career black couples in a metropolitan area revealed that many of their problems sprang from having an "inadequate amount of time to spend with their family" (p. 60), competing work-family demands, and problems finding affordable child care. The issues of equity were as prominent as they were in white families. Black families also had some unique problems: racial discrimination, social isolation, increased competition between spouses, and money management. Thomas recommended that therapists working with dual-career black families use culturally sensitive approaches that have "ethno-therapeutic" relevance. Also, it is necessary to see that black families are not homogeneous and to grasp black men and women's varying "expectations, needs, and experiences" (p. 66).

In the 41 middle-class black couples, on a 5-point ("very unhappy" to "very happy") marital and life happiness scale, 47.6% of husbands and wives reported being "somewhat happy" and 42.7% "very happy." There were no significant differences between the husbands' and wives' ratings (V. G. Thomas, 1990a, p. 175). Percentages reporting being happy with the following aspects of their lives were as follows: marital condition—97.6% of husbands and 85.3% of wives; relationships with children—100% of husbands and 92.7% of wives; and relationships with other family members—92.6% of wives and 78.1% of husbands (a significant difference). About 80% of husbands and wives were happy with their health status and slightly more than 60% were happy with their work and careers, but only 50% were happy about their finances (Thomas, 1990a, p. 175). Multiple regression equations showed that marital happiness was the strongest determinant of global life happiness. On the Moos and Moos (1981) Family Environment Scale, the husbands' cohesion scores correlated most strongly with marital happiness, whereas for the wives cohesion was most strongly correlated with quality of communication.

Thomas (1990a) concluded that, overall, these spouses with multiple roles were relatively happy with their lives. She postulated that the multiple roles provided gratification and security and enhanced self-esteem; both spouses had "a strong sense of purpose." She attributed the greater happiness with relationships than with careers to job stress and the "perception of inequities in the professional work world" (p. 177).

Thomas's research with middle-class African-American couples helps to fill a void in knowledge about the black family in contemporary society. She pointed out poignantly that middle-class blacks "report a great deal of 'cognitive dissonance' because they have a relatively affluent lifestyle and are very much aware of the impoverished state of many other black persons, even close relatives and friends" (p. 177). Her research needs to be extended to black families in the lower socioeconomic status groups.

FAMILY FUNCTIONING

During the past 20 years, family researchers have devoted significant efforts toward developing ways to assess family functioning. One major approach is self-report by the family members to items about decision making, communication, and affectivity on instruments that have been developed to evaluate such aspects of family functioning. The other is observation of videotapes of families performing a specified task and subsequent rating for similar factors indicative of family functioning. The self-report approach is the more parsimonious of the two, but self-reports are variable and subject to many biases. Observer ratings are expensive, time-consuming, and subject to rater bias as well as distortions inherent in the sessions being "experimental" and/or videotaped. Some researchers have used both approaches and obtained fruitful results. In addition to methodological problems, however, the entire topic of family functioning needs to be more precisely defined and conceptualized in view of its complexity and inherent tautologies.

The McMaster Model of Family Functioning

The studies of families that began with Westley and Epstein's pioneering 1969 study *The Silent Majority* led Epstein, Bishop, and Baldwin (1984) to develop the McMaster Model of Family Functioning (MMFF), which is based on a systems approach. According to the model, families have three basic groups of tasks. The first group includes such instrumental tasks as providing food, money, and transportation. The second group consists of the developmental tasks, which concern "crises of infancy, childhood, adolescence, and middle and old age . . . [such as] the beginning of the marriage [and] the first pregnancy" (p. 78). The third area, hazardous tasks, involves managing crises produced by illness, loss of income, and the like. Families that were unable to deal with the three major task areas were those likely to develop clinically significant problems.

The six MMFF dimensions of family functioning are as follows: (a) *problem solving* in terms of both instrumental (e.g., money) and affective (e.g., anger) issues; (b) *communication,* the instrumental and affective "exchange of information"; (c) *family roles,* the "pattern of behavior by which family members fulfill family functions" (e.g., provide resources; p. 84) and role allocation and accountability; (d) *affective responsiveness,* the "ability to respond to a given stimulus with the appropriate quality and quantity of feelings" (p. 86); (e) *affective involvement,* the extent to which members are interested in others' interests and activities; and (f) *behavior control,* a family's way of handling such potentially risky situations as those involved with psychobiological needs and drives and socializing.

The MMFF has been used in a variety of clinical settings, including family practice, psychiatry, rehabilitation medicine, in a family outcome study, and in the selection of "superfunctioning" families for a therapeutic foster placement program. Two assessment instruments developed from the MMFF are (a) the McMaster Clinical Rating Scale (CRS), which is completed by therapists after clinical assessment and consists of seven scales, one for each of the six dimensions of the MMFF and one for overall family functioning; and (b) the McMaster Family Assessment Device (FAD), a 53-item questionnaire completed by family members over the age of 12 years that supplies scores on each of the six dimensions of the MMFF and overall family functioning and thus reflects the family members' perceptions of family functioning. The scores on both instruments discriminate between families with and without psychiatric problems (Miller, Kabacoff, Epstein, Bishop, & Keitner, in press).

Epstein and his colleagues (1984) have used the CRS and the FAD in studies of patients with chronic illness and/or disability and their families. Also, Keitner (1990) has used the FAD to study the effects of depression on family functioning during illness and after remission. The development of the MMFF and its two clinical scales represents a significant forward step in the application of knowledge about family functioning to the real-life problems encountered by persons with chronic physical illnesses, disabilities, and psychiatric illnesses.

The Olson Circumplex Model

In 1979, Olson and his colleagues at the University of Minnesota presented their "Circumplex Model of Marital and Family Systems" that was based on the theoretical foundation developed by Reuben Hill (1949) in his study of *Families Under Stress.* For their major study, "Families: What makes them work," Olson and his colleagues (1983) used that model and conceptualized family functioning on two axial dimensions, cohesion and adaptability. Family adaptability, the "ability of a marital or family system to change its power structure, role relationships, and relationship rules in response to situational and developmental stress," is scored on a four-level continuum ranging from chaotic to rigid (p. 60). Cohesion, the "emotional bonding that family members have toward one another," (Olson, Russell, & Sprenkle, 1983, p. 70) ranges across four levels: disengaged, separated, connected, and enmeshed. On both dimensions, optional functioning was in the central areas ("balanced" families), with either extreme being problematic, if not pathological ("midrange" families were in one central extreme area, and "extreme" families were in the extreme areas on both dimensions). Communication was seen as a facilitating dimension; communication skills were either positive (supportive and sharing) or negative (critical and restrictive).

Scales based on the model include the Family Adaptability and Cohesion Evaluation Scale (FACES II), a 30-item self-report scale that was used in the National Survey of 1,000 families (Olson, Portner, & Bell, 1982). Olson, McCubbin, et al. (1983) reported the results of that highly publicized research on 1,040 couples and 412 adolescents in 31 states. The goal was to study family stresses and coping across seven stages of the family life cycle, ranging from young couples without children to families in retirement. The sample consisted of volunteer families recruited through a fraternal organization with offices in many states. They represented "the middle and upper-middle class of our society. . . . This is a study of intact families, who in conventional terms might be described as 'normal,' 'typical,' 'non-clinical,' or 'ordinary'" (Olson et al., 1983, p. 26). Over 90% were Lutherans and were in their first marriage. The investigators had difficulties with participation even with a selected population; fewer than half of the contacted families agreed to enter the project. Information was gathered from parents and their adolescent children who came to group meetings where a leader explained the research and distributed questionnaires containing 14 scales for the family members (separated from each other in the group room) to complete. There was much less agreement between husbands and wives than is generally assumed, and even less agreement between the adolescents and their parents. Wives saw their families as more cohesive and adaptable than the husbands, and adolescents reported lower levels of family cohesion and adaptability than their parents. About 53% of the couples were balanced family types, 32% were in the midrange, and only 15% were extreme types. Cohesion and adaptability were at low levels during the fourth and fifth (adolescent and "launching") stages of the family life cycle, and at their highest levels at stage one (before the couple had children) and later in life (during the empty-nest and retirement stages).

The chief stressors and strains during the preceding year were intrafamily strains, financial strains, work-family strains, and illnesses.

Marital strains were reported only in the empty-nest stage, and then by only 10% of the respondents (p. 123). Olson and his colleagues (1983) stated that "family stressors and strains associated with financial demands, intrafamily struggles, and work-family difficulties persist across all stages of the family cycle" (pp. 129–130).

Differences in marital and family satisfaction levels across the life cycle, like scores on cohesion and adaptability, were small and followed a shallow U-shaped curve. Satisfaction scores dropped slowly over the first five life cycle stages. The husbands' lowest score was during stage 4 (when adolescents were at home) and for wives it was during stage 5 (the launching stage), but scores increased during the empty-nest and retirement stages. The four satisfaction measures correlated negatively with family stress; couples under stress were dissatisfied with their marriages and family lives (p. 185).

The adolescent years were the most stressful. The adolescents reported difficulties in communicating with their parents, but communication with their mothers was more positive than with their fathers. The mothers reported that communication with their adolescents was more positive than did the fathers. During family life cycle stage 4 (adolescence), 60% of the parents reported stress related to finances; however, only 10% of the adolescents reported stress from finances but 50% reported stress from dealing with the family. Olson, McCubbin, et al. (1983) stated that parents and their adolescent children inhabit different worlds. "From the adolescent's perspective, the major family stressors were the day-to-day 'hassles' with their parents" (p. 228).

The study turned out to have a host of methodological problems, including (a) the homogeneity of the sample of mainly white Lutheran families, which precluded generalizations to most families in America; and (b) the tautologies present in a major cross-sectional study of this sort. Notwithstanding these limitations, the results received wide publicity in popular family magazines in the mid-1980s, and Olson appeared a number of times on the NBC "Today" show. Unfortunately, the methodological problems were compounded by recently revealed conceptual flaws. Beavers and Voeller (1983) reported that Olson's Circumplex Model had logical defects, did not conform to clinical realities, did not integrate systems concepts, and did "not relate family systems to human developmental theory" (p. 46). They maintained that cohesion was confounded and that a linear continuum for cohesion and an infinite one for adaptability fit "clinical realities better than a model integrating two curvilinear dimensions [e.g., the Olson model]" (p. 47).

Green, Harris, Forter, and Robinson's (1991a) recent study of family functioning in 2,440 male National Guard members' families used the

FACES III (Olson, Portner, & Lavee, 1985), a refinement of FACES II that was based on the Circumplex Model. Green and his colleagues (1991a) "failed to confirm the predicted curvilinear relationship" (p. 69).

Cohesion was related in linear—not curvilinear—fashion to such measures of family well-being as scores on the Kansas Marital Satisfaction Scale (KMSS; Grover, Paff-Berger, Russell, & Schumm, 1984) and the Generalized Contentment Scale (GCS; Hudson, 1982), and the adaptability subscale scores were not even related to either the KMSS or the GCS scores (p. 69).

Green, Harris, Forter, and Robinson (1991b) also presented data on 1,780 wives of the men who participated in their previous study (pp. 93–94). Overall, the results were "very similar to those for the men. . . . Clearly, family functioning bore no relationship at all to predictive placement on the Circumplex when respondents' scores from FACES III subscales were calculated in the traditional manner" (p. 80). They noted that Olson had recently revised the scoring procedure so that both cohesion and adaptability subscales would be considered linear measures; higher scores would be indicative of more favorable levels of family functioning than lower scores.

Research by other investigators also indicates the need for the development of the new FACES IV, in which Green and his colleagues will be joining Olson and Thomas. Such collaboration has been needed in family research; the field has been penalized by the failure of investigators to work together.

The Beavers Systems Model

The Beavers Systems Model is a cross-sectional model in which family structure, flexibility (adaptability), and competence are scored on one dimension (the horizontal axis) and the family style of interaction on the other (the vertical axis). Adaptability is on an infinite continuum—the more, the better. Autonomy is a function of the family system's capacity to encourage growth and also is rated on an infinite dimension. But the family's stylistic dimension (i.e., its interactional style) is seen as curvilinear (Beavers & Voeller, 1983, p. 47) and also is centripetal/centrifugal in that satisfactions come either from within the family or from outside the family; both extremes are pathological. Beavers and Voeller (1983) emphasized that the model has a competence continuum that reflects both clinical realities and changes in either health or regression.

Family functioning is on a continuum containing five types of families. At one extreme are the severely disturbed families (those with the lowest level of functioning) who have poor subsystem boundaries, live with confusion, and communicate poorly. Next, the borderline type is characterized by "ineffective efforts to rid the systems of confusion by simplistic and often harsh efforts at control" (p. 50). In the midrange, those families that turn out "sane but limited offspring" have relatively definite boundaries but expect to be controlled. On the healthy side of the continuum, the adequate families have boundaries, but "negotiate with pain, recognize ambivalences reluctantly, and share warmth but struggle for control. At the far end are the optimally healthy that are capable, negotiate, make individual choices, respect ambivalence, and show warmth and humor" (p. 50).

The Beavers Systems Model has demonstrated clinical utility, and the book *Successful Families: Assessment and Intervention* (Beavers & Hampson, 1990) is a major contribution to knowledge about intact, well-functioning families.

Reiss's Problem-Solving Model

Since the early 1970s, David Reiss and his colleagues (1982, 1986) at George Washington University have been developing their problem-solving model of family functioning to provide a classification of families that has clinical utility. Inasmuch as predictors of dropping out of therapy early are general (e.g., low SES, authoritarianism, and therapy being initiated by one spouse rather than by both), there is need for a classification of families that has predictive power.

Reiss, Costell, Jones, and Berkman (1986) reported that families could be classified according to adaptability to new situations in a manner "analogous to a character diagnosis, by measuring family members' behavior in problem-solving situations in the laboratory" (p. 141). The problem-solving situations evaluated two dimensions: configuration, or the extent to which family members use each other's observations and ideas to solve test problems, and coordination, or "the degree to which each family member integrates or dovetails his or her own problem-solving efforts with others" (p. 142). These dimensions provide combinations that place families into four groups. Those high on configuration and coordination are *environment-sensitive,* inasmuch as family members work together to explore and understand the environment and thus are similar to Wertheim's "open-integrated" families. Those high on configuration but low on coordination are *achievement-sensitive* families that explore and master laboratory situations but do so in a competitive rather than a cooperative manner (Wertheim termed such families "externally open-integrated"). Those low in configuration but high in coordination are *consensus-sensitive* families that work closely with each other, but whose high level of cooperation interferes with problem solving because they "thirst for agreement and consensus no matter what the consequences for problem-solving" (p. 142); they are frightened by the outside world and thus become a mutual self-protection group that Wertheim termed "closed-pseudointegrated." Those low on both coordination and configuration are *distance-sensitive* families that work separately and ineffectively, maintain distance from each other, and are pessimistic about obtaining help from others, similar to Wertheim's "closed-disintegrated" families.

Reiss and his colleagues' (1986) controlled 2-year study of 32 families (each with an adolescent on an inpatient unit that had an intensive group-focused treatment program) showed that the family can be considered a unitary entity and classified as such. Their classification system enabled them to make qualitative and quantitative predictions about the risk of treatment failure. Environment-sensitive families turned out to be those with least risk of failure inasmuch as they were conspicuous, had open boundaries, and participated in the therapeutic community. The risks for the achievement-sensitive and the consensus-sensitive families were subtle and qualitative; the members maintained boundaries around themselves and were engaged with each other, but did not enter freely into the therapeutic community. The distance-sensitive families had the greatest risk; they were inconspicuous, felt little cohesion with the group, had poor attendance at group meetings, and were likely to drop out of the research or treatment program (p. 154).

Epstein and his colleagues (1984) compared Reiss's model with the MMFF. They maintained that high configuration reflected empathic involvement and "personal development in 'roles'" and that coordination indicated clear communication and assessed "well-handled systems maintenance, management, and roles" (p. 95). They considered Reiss's four-case family typology to be "premature"; instead of developing a typology, they preferred to identify dimensions of functioning and determine how families are distributed on the dimensions. They concluded that the clinical utility of Reiss's model was "questionable" because it required extensive observations of family behavior and was too time-consuming for clinical work. They also questioned whether the four-family typology had predictive value because it might be "too gross a measure" and left out many aspects of family functioning.

Although their method is complicated, time-consuming, and requires a laboratory, Reiss and his colleagues' (1986) study is important because it is directed toward treatment. Theirs was the first successful use "of a family classification scheme to predict a family's response to a family-oriented treatment program" (p. 141). Their family typology allowed them to make predictions that were not tautological; that is, they could make predictions about a family type according to the way, not just whether, it solved problems. Such predictions are much more scientific than those postulating that various degrees of family function or competence are associated with various outcomes. Also, the model has significant research potential, especially for studying the difficult topic of family interactions. Although it has limitations, the problem-solving model is promising and is a major contribution to the field.

The Moos and Moos Family Environment Scale

The 90-item Family Environment Scale (FES; Moos & Moos, 1981) assesses three dimensions of the family environment—interpersonal, personal growth and development, and systems maintenance—and has 10 subscales that measure cohesion, conflict, independence, moral-religious orientation, control, etc. A family incongruence or discrepancy score can be calculated from the differences in individual family members' scores. The family's scores on the various subscales can be portrayed as a profile, similar to Minnesota Multiphasic Profile Inventory (MMPI) scores. Moos and Moos have reported profiles for their "normal" families, as well as profiles of alcohol problem families, clinic families with various disorders, and so forth. Because we used the FES in our epidemiological study, fairly complete information about it and our results are presented in Chapter 5.

Lewis: Family Competence

In the late 1960s, Jerry Lewis, W. R. Beavers, and their colleagues developed methods to study family functioning primarily in healthy families because "little is known systematically about the processes of healthy family systems" (Lewis, et al. 1976, p. 11). They conducted a pilot study with 11 volunteer white, upper-middle-class families from a local Protestant church, all of which had intact marriages and at least one adolescent child, and families with adolescents at Timberlawn Psychiatric Hospital. The investigators gathered self-report data from scales developed in their clinical work and also observational data by having the families come to the research setting to be videotaped while carrying out family interactional tasks. The pilot study was expanded by adding 33 more middle-class families, some of which were patients' families.

The overall goal was to develop methods to assess family competence on a continuum ranging from the competent to the dysfunctional. Lewis (1989) defined family competence "as the extent to which a family accomplishes two cardinal tasks: producing psychologically healthy children who can function autonomously and enter into enduring relationships outside the family, and stabilizing the parents' personalities while facilitating their continuing development" (pp. 2–3). As the reader has seen, most family scholars have considered those to be the two essential family functions. Family competence in this study had five components: power structure, degree of family individuation, acceptance of separation and loss, perception of reality, and affect. In the 44 volunteer families, there were 10 to 12 healthy families and many more "adequate" families. Lewis and his colleagues (1976) stated that there were no epidemiological data with which to make comparisons: "We simply do not know the relative proportions of optimal, adequate, or various degrees of dysfunctional families in a general population" (p. 205).

Since the early 1970s, Lewis and his colleagues (Lewis et al., 1976; Lewis & Looney, 1983) have reported the results of their ongoing research on the continuum of family competence with patients' as well as volunteers' families. On the continuum that extends from flexible to rigid to chaotic, there are five family types: highly competent, competent but pained, dominant-submissive, conflicted, and severely dysfunctional. The highly competent family is considered ideal. Characteristics of competent but pained families include their "underlying parental conflicts around the issues of closeness and intimacy," but the conflicts do not involve the children, who will probably be psychologically healthy. The dominant-submissive families show high levels of commitment, variable levels of closeness, an absence of intimacy, and skewed power. The rigid family system is controlled by the dominant parent; these families are dysfunctional because of "an increased probability of the development of psychiatric syndromes in either the submissive spouse or the children" (Lewis, 1989, p. 6). Conflicted families are characterized by the spouses' chronically antagonistic relationship; the children often become involved and choose sides, but sometimes manage to distance themselves.

The last type of family, the severely dysfunctional, contains three subtypes. In one, the parents have a symbiotic relationship, with fused identities and often poor levels of individuation. Their children are either incorporated into the symbiotic system or are excluded from it. Another is that in which "one parent dominates the family with his or her psychotic distortions" (Lewis, 1989, p. 7); many of these families have a paranoid outlook on the world. The third is characterized by complete parental alienation and by one of the parents sometimes developing a close relationship with a child.

Much of Lewis and his colleagues' work during the past few decades can be seen as a prelude to the study of how competent family systems develop over time. Lewis (1989) described the background for that research and the theoretical issues, building on Erikson's (1950) theory of the epigenesis of the individual's psychosexual development and response to the specific challenges of each of the eight life cycle stages (from birth to death). An issue that Lewis (1989) regards as fundamental, in accord with concepts of epigenesis and Bowen's theories of individuality and togetherness, is that the psychological health of the parents and the children depends largely on the parental balance between individuality and mutuality. The key processes "in negotiating this relational balance" (p. 25) are commitment, power, closeness, intimacy, and autonomy.

The subjects in the ongoing family development study consist of 40 young volunteer white middle-class married couples in which the wives were in the second trimester of their first pregnancy. After 5 years, 37 of the 40 couples were still participating; data are available from the Time 1 interviews during the second trimester of pregnancy, the Time 2 interviews shortly after the birth of the infant, the Time 3 interviews when the infant was 3 months old, and the Time 4 interviews when the infant was 1 year old. (The seventh interview has been completed as of this writing.) In addition to the self-report data from interviews, observer-based data were obtained from ratings of videotapes of marital interactions in accord with the Beavers-Timberlawn Family Evaluation Scales.

At Time 1, during the second trimester of pregnancy, 8 of the 38 couples were rated as highly competent, 13 as competent but pained, 10 as dominant-submissive, 7 as severely conflicted, and none as severely dysfunctional. According to Lewis (1988), "This type of distribution in which 21 of 38 couples can be understood as either having competent relationships or as manifesting strengths in child-rearing despite marital pain is consistent with our earlier studies of families containing adolescent children" (p. 159). Greater competence was significantly associated with higher socioeconomic status.

Lewis (1988) summarized the results as follows. First, the findings supported the application of the construct of epigenesis to family systems; the resolution of key relationship issues early in the marriage "forms a basic template for the characteristics of the evolving triadic system" (pp. 419–420). Second, the continuum of marital competence demonstrated its utility; the prenatal competence of the parental marriage predicted how well the child would be incorporated into the family at both 3 months and 1 year. Third, the relationship measures were much more important determinants of the incorporation of the infant into the family than individual psychological health measures; "the data support the system construct that the whole is greater than the sum of its parts" (p. 420). Fourth, measures of marital satisfaction had little predictive value. Fifth, there were few associations between changes in the level of marital competence and incorporation of the child into the family. Sixth, there was a "need for more complex models of family development" (p. 420). Seventh, families that function well were underrepresented in "current model building" (p. 420). Eighth, spouses who had not evolved a mutually satisfactory level of closeness were vulnerable to crises. Ninth, couples with traditional, gender-stereotyped marriages may present stable marriages but have difficulty with the transition to parenthood. Tenth, highly conflicted couples were relatively unpredictable. Eleventh and finally, only 2 of the 38 couples had improved relationships 1 year after the birth of the child.

Although Lewis and his colleagues' family research is limited by its being centered mainly on middle- and upper-middle-class white families in Texas and by the tautologies inherent in studies of family competence and mental health, the ongoing *Birth of the Family* (Lewis, 1989) study should be one of the most important family studies of the latter part of this century. As noted in Chapter 2, Lewis and Looney (1983) evaluated the continuum of competence in a small sample of relatively low-income black families. Contrary to their hypotheses, the characteristics of competence in the black families were similar to those previously found in white middle- and upper-middle-class families. Thus, the methodology for the ongoing study had been tested.

Finding that competent families are characterized by a high degree of autonomy and egalitarianism on the part of the parents raises questions about the stability of those marriages over time, inasmuch as there is such a strong trend toward individualism in the United States. That trend, coupled with egalitarianism, could have a destabilizing effect on marriages and families, particularly those without institutional supports. Westley and Epstein (1969) reported that the children from their "father-led" families in Rhode Island had a much greater chance of being psychologically healthy than those from the "equalitarian" families. Thus, longitudinal studies such as that by Lewis (1989) are needed to establish the characteristics of healthful family functioning and of family competence over time, ascertain changes at different times in the family life cycle, and assess the outcomes for the children.

Belsky's Pennsylvania State University Infant and Family Development Project

Belsky, Spanier, and Rovine (1983) reported results of their ambitious, well-focused longitudinal study of 70 volunteer families from last trimester of pregnancy until the infant was 9 months old. Methods included interviews with the couples, questionnaires given to each spouse individually, and observations of the interactions and other behaviors in the home. Spouses and couples that had initially scored high on measures of marital adjustment and functioning tended to do so across the 1-year period of study. The addition of a firstborn or later infant, however, had a negative impact on the marital relationship.

Cohesion scores dropped significantly for women during the postpartum period and declined as well for men, but less so. Romance scores also declined, but not significantly. A "honeymoon period" might extend through the first postpartum month but was no longer apparent by the third month. The addition of the child to the family increased the burden upon the wife, who had to take care of the home as well as the baby. As the marriage became increasingly focused on instrumental functions, there was less emotional expression. The overall quality of the marital interaction was lower for couples having more than one child than for those with only one child.

Belsky and his colleagues concluded that the transition to parenthood, or the addition of another child, affected the marital relationship. The overall level of marital quality declined, but the ranking of individual spouses and couples remained relatively unchanged (i.e., those scoring either high or low in marital functioning in the last trimester of pregnancy had about the same scores both 3 and 9 months postpartum). The investigators hypothesized that the decline in marital quality might be "a function of the increasing instrumental nature of family life associated with child care" (p. 568).

In describing their Pennsylvania State University Infant and Family Development Project, Belsky, Rovine, and Fish (1989) maintained that the family must be viewed as an entity composed of multiple interrelating elements and subsystems, and they emphasized the importance of interdisciplinary studies that look at how children affect marital functioning and how it affects parent-child relationships and child development. The project was a three-cohort longitudinal study of maritally intact, Caucasian working- and middle-class families that were bearing and rearing their first child. Total enrollment consisted of 250 families in the last trimester of pregnancy, of which 173 were in the second and third cohorts. Two thirds of the fathers were college graduates; only

16% had less than a high school education. Average annual income was $24,000. The couples were young—the mean ages were 28.6 for husbands and 26.6 for wives—and the average length of marriage was 3.9 years. The families were studied prenatally and again when the infants were 3 and 9 months of age. Parents in the second cohort responded by mail to questionnaires about personality factors when the infants were 15 months of age.

Belsky and his colleagues (1989) emphasized that the family system is a complex social organization, composed both of developing individuals and of relationships, that cannot be characterized at one point in time. Only limited evidence indicated that adults change in some fundamental way upon becoming parents. Marriages that functioned well prior to the birth of the child continued to function well after the transition to parenthood, although feelings of love for the spouse declined and ambivalence about the marital relationship increased. Joint leisure activity decreased, and the household division of labor became more traditional; conflict increased, while problem-solving communication decreased. The investigators maintained that such changes are reciprocally related and cannot be subjected to linear causal analysis.

Although spousal relationships changed, patterns of parent-infant interaction remained constant. Generally, mothers assumed primary responsibility for the children, and the fathers were secondary parents. The degree of the father's involvement varied with the functioning of the marital relationship; spousal interaction promoted father-infant interaction. The quality of the infant-mother relationship was related specifically to the quality of the marital relationship. Mothers of insecurely attached infants experienced a greater decline in the quality of marital relationships than did mothers of secure infants. Also, the degree of infant–mother attachment security covaried with changes in the mothers' personal opinions of themselves. Overall, the quality of the marriage affected the multiply determined infant-mother attachment bond.

Belsky and his colleagues (1989) maintained that there were two general types of family systems. In *engaged* systems, high levels of interaction took place in all three dyads; in *disengaged* systems, low levels of interaction were observed across all three dyads, or just the mother-infant subsystem was highly interactive. The mother's personality characteristics and the spouses' appraisals of each other distinguished the engaged from the disengaged families prior to the infant's birth.

The investigators stated candidly that they undertook systems research but were doubtful about the extent to which their research was truly systemic in nature. They focused on the family as a system, viewing the family members as the elements of the system and the interacting elements or relationships as the subsystems. They concluded that studying the individuals, the relationships, the interdependence of relationships, and the family triad was only a beginning; it was necessary to find ways to study such characteristics of systems as self-stabilization, self-organization, and hierarchical organization.

Belsky and his colleagues' work has immense promise. Long-term follow-up of their large sample of families from the upper-, lower-, and middle-class strata should show how changes (e.g., accompanying births, divorces, or remarriages) in the composition and structure of families are associated with the adults' as well as the infants' and children's well-being and development. In particular, the families' varied socioeconomic statuses should reveal differential responses to SLEs and to life transitions. Also, the parents' relatively young age will enable the investigators to see how the cohorts are affected by historical and sociocultural events and processes.

CONCLUDING REMARKS

The importance of the family in relationship to mental disorder is being addressed belatedly by the American Psychiatric Association, whose Task Force on Nomenclature and Statistics is preparing a major revision of the current diagnostic and statistical manual (DSM-III-R; American Psychiatric Association, 1987). There is pressure for the new DSM-IV (scheduled for publication in 1994) to contain an added Axis VI for "family and/or relational problems." At present, the International Classification of Disease (ICD-10) contains codes for "relational problems" with major categories for (a) parent-child relational problems (e.g., abuse of child, parental discipline, and high expressed emotion); (b) partner relational problems (e.g., physical and/or sexual abuse); and (c) other relational problems. Also, in 1975 the World Health Organization (WHO) produced a multiaxial classification of child psychiatric disorders that included, for example, abnormal intrafamilial relationships, inadequate or distorted intrafamilial communications, and societal stressors. Both the ICD-10 codes and the WHO classification are being evaluated for the DSM-IV section on relational problems.

During 1990, relational problems began to be assessed in field trials with the Global Assessment of Relational Functioning (GARF) scale. Ratings for both current and past periods consider the affective and instrumental functioning of the relational unit according to problem solving, organization, and emotional climate. The GARF scale is analogous to the DSM-III-R (Axis-V) Global Assessment of Functioning scale and is scored from 0 to 99. Features of ratings in the 81–99 range are that (a) daily routines meet the needs of each family member, (b) there are defined processes for assigning tasks and establishing leadership, (c) there is an optimistic atmosphere, (d) functioning is satisfactory, and (e) there is no need for clinical assistance. In contrast, features of ratings in the 1–20 range are that (a) family routines are negligible, (b) the family is organized in such a way that members may be injured or endangered, (c) despair and cynicism pervade the family, (d) the relational unit is too dysfunctional to retain continuity, and (e) clinical assistance is needed.

In addition to field trials, extensive literature reviews are being carried out to look at the clinical utility and validity of relational (mainly family) problems. It is envisioned that the text for the four relational problems in DSM-IV will include a discussion of essential features of the problem (e.g., criteria for diagnosis), associated features and comorbid disorders, the familial pattern, the course (e.g., onset, persistence, and duration), and the differential diagnosis.

The development of the section on relational problems for DSM-IV is a forward step. The formation of standardized criteria for family and other relational problems will be beneficial to researchers, and the entire process will stimulate study of the family. As the reader has seen, research on the functioning of the family and the well-being of its members began only about 150 years ago and, for many decades, was considered to be "retarded." The inclusion of diagnostic codes for relational disorders in DSM-IV indicates that family research has finally achieved the status needed for proper visibility. Research can build on the foundations established by investigators in the latter part of this century to make significant advances in family theory and therapy, as well as to increase knowledge of the many aspects of the family and the causes, course, treatment, and consequences of the mental disorders.

CHAPTER 5

Our Family Studies

BACKGROUND AND METHODS

Background

In our everyday clinical experiences, many of the concerns about the well-being of the family have appeared in all-too-human form as adults and children in distress. Their problems, the rapidly changing social scene, and our long-standing interest in the epidemiology of the mental disorders combined to stimulate us to undertake a series of family studies. Three other major factors coalesced to increase our interest. One was the influence of James Grier Miller, president of the University of Louisville and a professor in its Department of Psychiatry, and the publication of his definitive *General Living Systems* (1978), which supplied the theory needed for our studies. The second was the development of instruments for community studies of mental disorder, based on the new American Psychiatric Association diagnostic and statistical manual (DSM-III), that were being used effectively in the Epidemiologic Catchment Area (ECA) studies (Freedman, 1984). The third was that after those studies were completed, there would be need for the field of psychiatric epidemiology to make a conceptual and methodological leap forward.

We wanted to develop new approaches to studies of family functioning and mental disorder, as well as to be as comprehensive as possible. Therefore, during the 1980s, we carried out three different types of studies. One was a study of the history of the family in Western society. The second was the major effort, a pilot epidemiological study of a random sample of 43 families in their homes over a period of time. The third, more clinically oriented study was an intensive analysis of samples of the records of child psychiatry clinic patients and their families from 1923 to 1988. We also completed a case-control study of nine child psychiatry patients' families and eight matched same-neighborhood control families. We planned to augment the findings from those complementary historical, community, and clinical studies with our substantial clinical, teaching, and research experiences with families in a variety of office, hospital, and behavioral science settings.

We considered a historical approach necessary because the family is the basic unit of social organization, and its status and well-being in Western society have fluctuated with changes in the social and political currents of history. One of our convictions is that the family is not an isolated social unit but one that influences and is influenced by communities and institutions as well as by sociocultural processes, the events in ordinary persons' everyday lives, and those occurring on the stages where "the captains and the kings" hold forth. Also, historical studies would enable us to place the late twentieth-century concerns about the family in a meaningful perspective and enhance our evaluations and judgments by increasing knowledge and reducing biases.

Our historical research consisted mainly of studies of about 1,000 books, articles from both scientific journals and popular magazines, and newspaper clippings. Also, we carried out an intensive review of studies of the family and of various types of mental disorders. We made a strenuous effort to obtain data from their primary sources. Over a 9- to 10-year period, we compiled abstracts of much of the literature that had been reviewed and collated them into a number of preliminary "rough drafts." Other sources of historical data included those obtained from interviews with authorities on various topics and from television and radio programs.

The epidemiological studies in the families' homes would enable us to look at the family environment, how families functioned in their everyday settings, and how they reacted to stressful events and circumstances. We wanted to have the opportunity to see how families with either adequate or inadequate incomes managed their finances, to assess the quality of their marriages and marital adjustment and satisfaction, and to identify sources of tension and strain, as well as to evaluate possible symptomatology. Miller's (1978) general living systems theory supplied the conceptual basis for our evaluations of families, especially associations between the mental health of individual family members at one level, family well-being at another, and the influences of the community and society at still another level. Therefore, we gathered information about what was happening in the community during the years when we conducted the field studies and collected census tract data to obtain information about the families' neighborhoods and communities. Inasmuch as it appeared that only a few family studies had given attention to historical events and societal influences that impinge on family life, we carried out a retrospective case study of child psychiatry patients and their families from 1923 to 1988. That study was designed to buttress our clinical approach and also to help tie our historical, epidemiological, and clinical efforts together.

Description of Louisville

Louisville is a middle-American city with a traditional city structure (i.e., a center, suburbs, and exurbs). The population in the greater metropolitan area, the setting for our studies, is about 1 million persons. It is an appropriate site for a prospective study of families inasmuch as the community is reasonably stable; there have been no major demographic changes since World War II except for a moderate increase in population. Also, we had reason to believe that the study would be acceptable to the community. For many years, there has been excellent rapport between the university, with its urban mission, and the community. The medical school, the 11th oldest in the United States, is the pride of the city. Also, the increase in adolescent suicides in the late 1970s alarmed the community and its leaders; we felt they would be receptive to a study addressed to what was perceived as a burning social issue. Moreover, previous Louisville studies (Bell & Sundel, 1975; Matheny & Dolan, 1980; Roper, 1950) had good response rates and low attrition.

In 1980, the population of Jefferson County was 685,004; its population was both urban (654,938) and rural (30,066). There were slightly more females (359,392) than males (325,612); the median age was 30.1 years (28.8 years for males and 31.7 years for females). Of the population, 575,304 (about 85%) were white; almost all of the remaining 109,702 were black. The total number of Native Americans, Asian Americans, and Hispanic Americans amounted to only 6,000 persons. The total number of families was 182,954; the mean number of persons per family was 3.22.

During the years (1981 to 1986) when we did our fieldwork, Louisville underwent extensive economic changes. It lost its relatively heavy concentration of industries and 45,000 jobs. The percentage of the labor force in manufacturing dropped from 35% in the early 1970s to 18% in 1985. According to Coomes (personal communication, 1991), "All of the mainstays of economic production that were the fabric of Louisville and which built the city over the decades and created wealth, went down together."

Even though heavy industry moved away, most people did not leave Louisville for jobs elsewhere as they did in many parts of the Midwest. This was probably because, as Coomes (personal communication, 1991) stated, "the population was older and many had job seniority and high wages." Also, many felt "settled" and/or owned homes that had relatively low mortgage payments. Thus, the major economic theme during the years of our study was job loss, which was greater than the national average. Louisville was slow to rebound from 1982–83 "Reagan Rust Belt" recession; we interviewed families at a time when the recession was probably at its worst in this region. The nation began to recover in late 1982, but Louisville did not really begin to do so until 1985.

Methods for the Epidemiological Study

Our major objectives were to develop and test methods for epidemiological studies of families and to evaluate their feasibility by studying a random sample of 50 families over time. The specific aims were to (a) gather, manage, and analyze individual- and family-level data over time; (b) evaluate conceptual, methodological, and analytical issues; (c) assess both ongoing (step-by-step procedural) and overall feasibility; and (d) use the findings to establish a basis for longitudinal family studies.

Developing methods for the epidemiological study of families was an immediate task inasmuch as, to the best of our knowledge, such a study had not been carried out before. We needed to adapt instruments and procedures that we had used in studies of individuals to the study of the family as a unit, not just as a collection of individuals.

We had three major groups of methodological tasks—conceptual, procedural, and analytical. The conceptual tasks included the development of definitions of the family, family functioning, family-level risk factors, and family health and illness. The procedural requirements were the development of sampling procedures and study criteria, the selection of instruments, the construction of the interview schedule, the testing of the field procedures, and the choice of approaches to keep families in the study over time. The analytical tasks involved data management and confidentiality, the methods to be used for the analysis of data over different time periods and for the prediction of risk or symptom status, and the selection of tests for statistical significance.

Conceptual Issues

The foremost conceptual issues were how to define a family for study, how to assess family functioning, and the determination of the major family risk factors for mental disorders. We reviewed conventional definitions of the family but, in accord with the principles of general living systems theory, defined the family system as a set of individuals living in a household who interact and are bound together by common, shared properties (legal, affectional, or other). Thus, we were studying small groups with special ties, not just households.

We developed a model of family functioning that (a) could be measured at the family (not at the individual) level; (b) did not focus just on characteristics or dimensions of the family or on family competence (a value judgment), but on family system processes—namely, performance of the tasks of everyday life; and (c) was not tautological in that family functioning was not equated with health or illness. The description of the family functioning model and the Bell and Schwab Family Systems Assessment Scale, the results of their use, and their associations with symptomatology will be reported in a companion volume.

Family risk factors for mental disorder that we selected were the occurrence and impact of stressful life events (SLEs) and the quality of the family environment. In addition, we looked at the fit between each family's income and characteristics of the census tract in which it lived, particularly illness and crime rates and median family income.

Procedural Issues

We recruited and trained interviewers for the fieldwork. Generally, those who were most able and most acceptable to families were middle-aged women with some college education, experience in the health field, and personality characteristics that enabled them to develop empathic relationships with families.

We sent letters to all eligible families to inform them that they had been chosen from a random sample to participate in a study of health and family life that had been funded by the National Institute of Mental Health (NIMH) and was supported by prominent community and university officials. One week after we mailed the initial letter, two interviewers visited the household to explain the project, obtain written informed consent, and make an appointment for the first interview.

The trained personnel interviewed each child and adult individually in their homes for about 1½ hours. In addition, the families were videotaped in their homes while they completed the "family interview." The videotapes were rated to obtain observer-based as well as self-report data. Families were interviewed in their homes at three times: (a) at baseline with the Time 1 interview, (b) 6 months later with the followup Time 2 interview, and (c) 9 months after that with the Time 3 interview.

The comprehensive interview schedules covered essential personal and family history data, attitudes toward marriage and the family, physical and mental health status, an SLE inventory, and the Moos Family Environment Scale (FES). The adult schedule was modified somewhat for children to include age-appropriate instruments. The various interview schedules contained the following diagnostic and screening instruments:

1. The Diagnostic Interview Schedule (DIS; Robins, Helzer, Croughhan, & Ratcliff, 1979), which assesses symptoms and can yield symptom counts and diagnoses; given to all participants age 16 or older
2. The Center for Epidemiologic Studies Depression Scale (CES-D; Radloff, 1977), a measure of emotional distress during the preceding week
3. The Short Michigan Alcohol Screening Test (SMAST; Selzer, Vinokur, & Van Roijen, 1975)
4. The Diagnostic Interview Schedule for Children (DISC; Costello, Edelbrock, Dulcan, et al., 1984; used for those aged 6 to 15
5. The Child Behavior Checklist (CBCL; Achenbach & Edelbrock, 1983) and the Denver Developmental Screening Test (DDST; Frankenburg, Dodds, Fandal, et al., 1975); used for children under age 6

Videotaping the family interview was technically easier than we had foreseen. Our newly available portable video equipment (with a wide-angle lens and recorder) could be used in the home without special lighting. The family members were asked to arrange themselves comfortably for a family discussion, and the camera was placed in an inconspicuous spot. The interviewers then proceeded with the specific family interview task, which usually took about one hour.

Several types of attrition must be considered in a family study such as ours. One that is inherent in any study over time is the dropout rate. Although 9 (21%) of our 43 families dropped out, only 7 (16%) were true dropouts, most of whom explained after the initial interview that "the study took too much time." The remaining 2 (5%) moved away from the Louisville area. Thus, we did not have a problem with families leaving throughout the study.

Another type of attrition is the addition and/or loss of family members over time. That attrition was more prevalent that we had expected; for example, adult children moved in and out of their parents' homes and sometimes brought their own children with them.

Analytical Issues

The analytical issues consisted, first, of sampling, and second, of finding and using such means as the Scientific Retrieval System (SIR) to manage the immense amounts of data at three levels of complexity—the community, the family, and the individual—at three different time periods.

We used the most recent Louisville and Jefferson County directories as our sampling frame and simple random sampling procedures to identify families that were permanent residents of the Louisville-Jefferson County area. After drawing the sample, we checked telephone listings, postal authorities, neighbors, and so forth to verify that the name listed for a given address was correct before we sent letters to the families. Also, we located the families' residences on a county map to ascertain the representativeness of the sample.

Of the 185 households identified, 82 families (44%) did not meet the study eligibility requirements (i.e., the household must consist of two or more members, and at least two members of the household, including one adult, must agree to participate). Of the remaining 103 eligible families (56% of the sample drawn), 43 (42%) participated and 60 (58%) refused. As the study progressed, the participation rate improved. Examination of the participating and the refusing families' characteristics revealed no major differences except that many more of the refusing than the participating families were couples without children at home.

One of our concerns has been how to develop family-level measures of symptomatology, health, and stress, not just individual members' scores on scales, ratings, and the like. We used such conventional approaches as averaging all family members' scores to arrive at a family mean score but were not satisfied because of the distortions and the loss of information. Consequently, whenever possible, we have used raters' discussions and consensus and found that they supplied a feasible way to move from individual-level to family-level data. Also, we have relied on our clinical experience to evaluate various symptoms and the impact of individual events on the family. Other analytical issues were how to predict risk and mental health status over time and which tests of significance to use for evaluations of risk factors and symptom status.

Fieldwork

To publicize our study, we obtained endorsements from prominent community leaders, and the media gave the project publicity and credibility. Interviewers working with a particular family continued to maintain contact with that family. They made the appointments for the next interview and reviewed the previous interview schedules to make the ensuing interview more personal and to link the interviews. Although participation in a family study involves a substantial time commitment from the family members, many families reported that the interviews were both satisfying and pleasantly thought-provoking. Often, they told us that the previous sessions had stimulated them to think about a variety of issues and how they were dealing with them.

Summary

Our study demonstrated that it is possible to study families over time. But studying a community sample of families is far more complex and requires much more time and effort than studying a community sample of individuals. Prospective studies of families need to take into account changes in the composition and structure of the family as its members, especially adult children, move into and out of the parental home or as persons marry or divorce. Additional methods that probably would be helpful are to request the families to keep a family diary and also to assign a "family friend" to call the families at regular intervals to obtain some basic information about members' physical and mental health and the degree of stress in the home.

SOCIODEMOGRAPHIC CHARACTERISTICS, SYMPTOM STATUS, AND FAMILY RISK FACTORS

In this section, we look at the 43 families' sociodemographic factors and their risk factors for mental illness. We close the section with a short presentation of the findings on life cycle stage and symptomatic status and illustrative family vignettes.

Sociodemographic Characteristics

Family Size and Structure

The 43 families' racial, sexual, educational, and income distributions were closer to the distributions for Jefferson County, Kentucky, than we had anticipated for a small random sample. Their being representative of the county's population is one of the study's major strengths.

Inasmuch as we were studying a sample of families from the general population, the 43 participating families varied considerably. The average family consisted of 3.3 persons ($SD = 1.3$), but there were 15 (35%) with 2 members, 14 (32%) with 3 members, 5 (12%) with 4 members, 5 (12%) with 5 members, and 4 (9%) with 6 members. Of the 43, 34 (79%) were two-parent families, and the remaining 9 (21%) were single-parent families—8 of which (89%) were headed by a female and only 1 (11%) by a male.

Five (12%) of the 43 families were black families, the same racial distribution as in Jefferson County. Of them, 4 (80%) were single-parent families, and 1 (20%) was a two-parent family. In contrast, of the 38 white families, 4 (11%) were single-parent families, and the remaining 34 (89%) were two-parent families.

At Time 1, the families were divided into two groups: the 18 (42%) that were asymptomatic and the 25 (58%) that contained at least one symptomatic member. As a group, the asymptomatic families were smaller, with a mean size of 2.9 ($SD = 1.3$) persons, than the symptomatic families, with a mean size of 3.6 ($SD = 1.3$) persons. Also, the two groups' family structures differed in that only 1 of the 9 (11%) single-parent families was in the asymptomatic group; the remaining 8 (89%) were in the symptomatic group. Of the 5 black families, only 1 (20%) was asymptomatic; the other 4 (80%) were in the symptomatic group.

There were 141 persons in the 43 families, 73 (52%) males and 68 (48%) females; their age-sex pyramid is shown in Figure 5.1. Of the 129 family members who participated, 63 (49%) were males and 66 (51%) were females.

Family Composition and Genograms

Family size and structure were associated with symptomatic status. To learn more about the composition of the family than shown by an enumeration of the persons living in the household and their relationships, we used the *genogram* or graphic representation of the family members and their relationships. It was derived from genealogical studies and has been effectively developed for clinical and research work by Bowen and his colleagues, especially McGoldrick and Gerson (1985). At Time 1, we asked each household head and spouse separately whom he or she considered to be in his or her immediate families. From their responses, we drew genograms of the 43 families, which we then classified into five types.

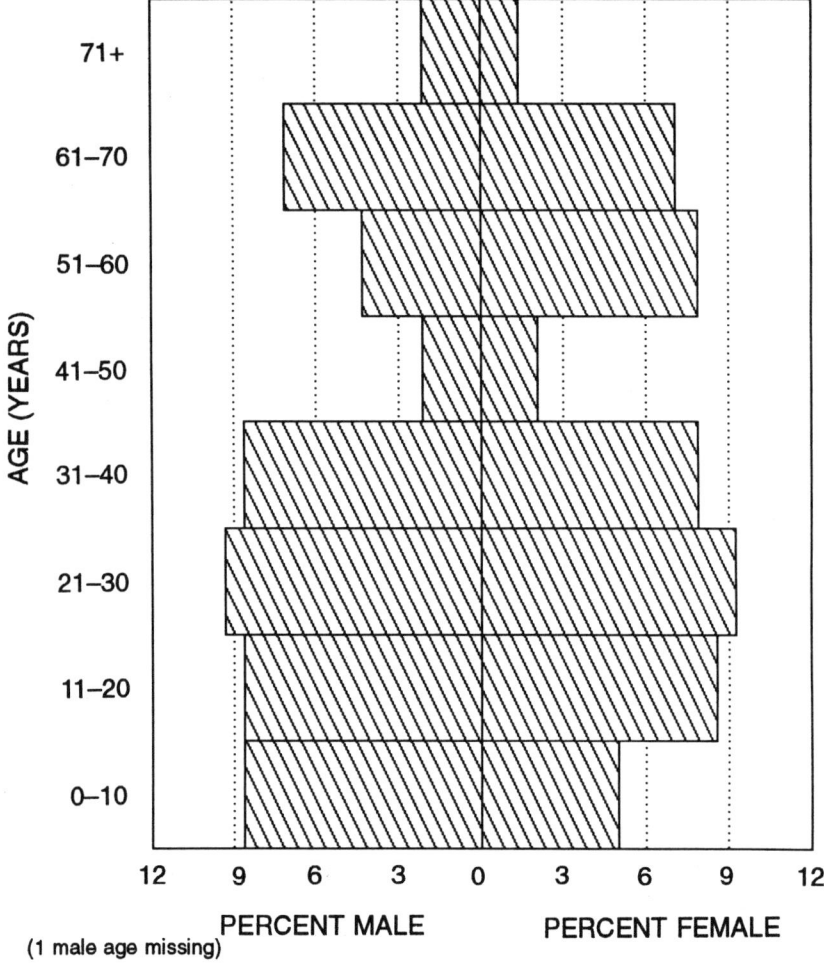

Figure 5.1. Age-sex pyramid for 43 families, 140 persons.

Type I families were the 9 (21%) in which there was consensus as to who was in the immediate family. In 4 (44%), the immediate family consisted only of members of the household; these 4 were "younger" families with children under age 18. In another 4 (44%), the immediate family consisted of older couples, their children, and grandchildren, although only the couple lived in the household. In the 1 (12%) remaining case, the immediate family consisted of a mother and adult daughter, who lived together, and the mother's mother, who lived in a nursing home. Of the 9 Type I families, only 2 (22%) were symptomatic.

An illustrative Type I genogram family was a husband and wife, both age 38, and their 12-year-old son, all of whom lived in a middle-class neighborhood. The husband was a computer programmer who wanted to make a job change. The wife was a substitute teacher who liked to make stained-glass art and had sold some of her work; she was thinking about becoming a professional. Both parents centered a lot of attention on their son. The father referred to several things he and his son had done together. The family seemed to be a close-knit unit and interested in each other. Although there was an underlying feeling that both adults wanted to make some changes in their careers, there was no strong discontent. All three family members were asymptomatic at both Time 1 and Time 3. In response to the question about who was in the immediate family, there was consensus that the immediate family consisted of the father, the mother, and the son.

Type II families were the 20 (47%) that consisted of all members of the household mentioned by everyone, plus various others outside the household who were mentioned by at least one but not all members. Those outside the household were either members of the husband's or wife's family of origin, adult children, and/or spouses and grandchildren. Of the 20 Type II families, 12 (60%) were symptomatic.

One Type II family was headed by a black, 54-year-old woman who had been separated from her husband for several years. Two of her six children—an adult daughter, age 22, and an adult son, age 25—were still at home, but the son did not participate. He managed a 24-hour neighborhood market where his mother was a cashier. The daughter, a university graduate, was unemployed. The family members seemed to interact well and were close to extended family members who were often "in and out of the house." Their home was the center for their active social life. The children were in contact with their father, who had a steady job at a major factory in Louisville. At Time 1, the adult daughter was symptomatic on the CES-D and reported depressive symptomatology. The family broke many appointments and dropped out after Time 1, ostensibly because of the study's time demands.

The mother named all of her children and her 84-year-old mother as the members of her immediate family. The adult daughter named her mother, all of her brothers and sisters, and her father. The genogram illustrated the family situation. As a single-parent family, the mother included her own mother, and the adult daughter appropriately considered her father in her immediate family, even though he and her mother were separated and he did not live at home.

Type III consisted of the 10 (23%) families in which one spouse omitted the other as part of the immediate family while including persons outside the household. The omission of a spouse may reflect the instability of the marital or other relationship, or simply that the other did not consider him or her to be a "blood" relative. Of the 10 Type III families, 7 (70%) were symptomatic.

One Type III genogram family consisted of a 32-year-old husband and his 35-year-old wife who had been married for 3 years and had no children. Both were employed full-time. He was a successful audiologist who also sold life insurance, and she was a junior accountant who liked her job. She had an extensive history of mental illness. She had been hospitalized twice for anxiety and depression, first at age 12 after her grandfather died and then for 16 months when she was a teenager. She was functioning but reported bouts of "depression off and on." Shortly before the Time 1 interview, she had been at the funeral of a close friend (who had been killed in an accident) and was feeling "depressed." The couple was cordial and friendly and were seen as ambitious, orderly, and happy. At Time 1, the wife was symptomatic on the CES-D, and the husband was asymptomatic; at Time 3, however, their statuses were reversed.

The husband included his mother, father, and brother in his immediate family but omitted his wife. She included her husband and also her grandmother, mother and father, aunt and uncle, brothers and sisters, and her husband's parents and siblings. The distinctive features of their genogram were that the husband mentioned his family of origin but omitted his wife; however, she mentioned him and included both families of origin. We speculated that their genogram was unusual because the couple had not yet resolved the developmental task of the first stage of the family life cycle—separating from the families of origin and bonding to form a new family with deep emotional commitments to each other. The "ping-ponging" of symptomatology from Time 1 to Time 3 suggests problems as well.

The 2 (5%) Type IV families were those in which members other than the spouse were omitted even though they lived in the household. Type V families consisted of the 2 (5%) families in which there was only one adult respondent. All of the Type IV and Type V families were symptomatic.

Thus, we can see that the perceived family composition, as well as family size and structure, was associated with symptomatic status. There was a strong tendency for the genogram type to be associated with symptomatology. Only 22% of the families whose genograms depicted consensus about members of the immediate family were symptomatic, in contrast to 70% of the families in which one spouse had omitted the other. It is highly likely that the genogram, as we used it, was an in-depth measure of family cohesion, the extent of which generally is associated with the family's mental health or illness.

Socioeconomic Status

Fewer of the heads of households than their spouses had completed high school, but almost equal numbers had more than a high school education. For the heads, level of education was inversely related to age; mean age of those with less than a high school education was 58.4 years ($SD = 14.9$); those with a high school education, 53.2 years ($SD = 16.5$); and those with more education, 45.9 years ($SD = 15.1$). There has been a trend for persons born after the Great Depression to obtain more years of education than their predecessors.

Almost 70% of the heads and 40% of the spouses were employed either full- or part-time. Although unemployment was not a major problem for them, it was for their adult children, as we discuss in Chapter 6. Throughout the sample, both the heads of households and their spouses were involved in a variety of occupations—a judge, university professors, teachers, nurses, and building contractors, as well as laborers and clerical and service personnel.

Family take-home incomes (reported by 41 of the 43 families) ranged from a low of $310 per month to a high of $7,000 per month; the median monthly income was $1,830 and the mean was $2,074 ($SD = $1,505$). The median annual family income was $20,400 and the mean was $24,571 ($SD = $17,948$); larger families tended to have lower annual incomes than the smaller.

We found significant associations between socioeconomic status (SES) and symptomatic status. Only 2 (11%) of the 18 asymptomatic families were headed by persons who had not had 12 years of education, in contrast to 8 (36%) of the 22 symptomatic families. Also, 13 (72%) of the heads of the 18 asymptomatic families were employed (1 was a full-time student), in contrast to only 12 (48%) of the heads of the 25 symptomatic families. And significantly fewer of the asymptomatic families than the symptomatic families had annual incomes in the lower 2 quartiles under $20,400 (chi-square [3 df] = 10.77, $p = 0.01$). The association between families being of lower SES and having symptomatology was the strongest found in our study.

The median incomes for the census tracts in which the two groups lived was almost the same, $22,417 per year for the asymptomatic group and $21,840 per year for the symptomatic group. Only 45% of the asymptomatic families, however, had annual incomes less than the median annual income for the census tract in which they lived, in contrast to 65% of the families in the symptomatic group.

As discussed in Chapter 4, Le Play's studies of families' budgets revealed that those families that allocated specific amounts for living expenses and also saved money tended to be cohesive and to have a sense of family security and purpose. In contrast, those that spent all available money and/or wasted it (e.g., on alcohol or gambling) were usually families in various types of distress. At Time 1, 40 (93%) of our families completed a monthly family budget that listed monthly family income and 15 categories of expenses; 9 (23%) of them had negative balances—that is, they spent more than they took in. The families symptomatic for mental illness and/or with alcohol-drug problems—which, as a group, had lower incomes than the asymptomatic—tended to spend a greater percentage of their income on food, gasoline, and utilities (utilities chi-square $[40df] = 4.95, p = 0.03$). The asymptomatic families tended to spend a relatively greater percentage than the symptomatic on day care and, as to be expected, had a larger percentage of income allocated to savings. Thus, our results were in accord with LePlay's postulates and data. It is difficult to understand why so many family researchers in this century ignored pioneering research; Zimmerman and his few associates are notable exceptions.

Marital Status

Of the 43 families, 34 (79%) were married couples, with or without children in the home. The remaining 9 (21%) were single-parent families with at least one child; of them, 3 (33%) were separated, 3 (33%) were divorced, and 3 (33%) were widowed. In 1 of the 9, a male partner lived with a divorced mother and her daughters. For the 34 married couples, the number of years married ranged from 2 to 59 years, with a mean of 25.8 years ($SD = 14.9$). In 30 couples (88%), the spouses had been married only once; in 4 couples (12%), one or both spouses had been married more than once. According to Norton and Moorman (1987), in 1980, 23.1% of women 20 to 54 years of age were divorced after their first marriage (p. 4). At a time when there was much concern about the high divorce rate, our sample contained fewer divorced women than expected (6, or 14%).

Family Symptom Status

At Time 1, only 18 (42%) of our 43 families were asymptomatic. Of the 129 participating members in the 43 families, 44 (34%) members in 25 families were symptomatic. In those 25 symptomatic families, 44 of the 81 members, or 1.8 persons per family, were symptomatic.

Although none of the 97 adults given the DIS met full criteria for a definite diagnosis of mental disorder within the past year, several adults

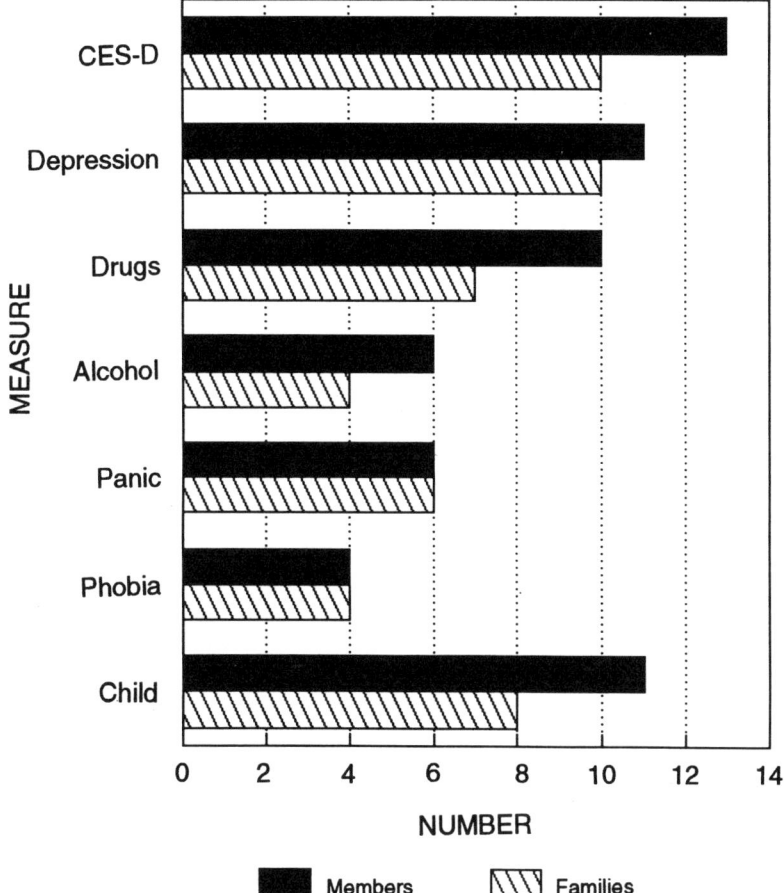

Figure 5.2. Numbers of members symptomatic on the various measures.

and children were suffering from emotional distress and were symptomatic. Figure 5.2 shows the number of members and families that were symptomatic on each symptom measure. There was more than one symptomatic member per symptomatic family for the CES-D, depression, drugs, alcohol, and child measures, but just one symptomatic member per family for the panic and phobia measures. We did not expect that none of the 97 adults would meet criteria for a DSM-III mental disorder, inasmuch as ECA (Wessman et. al, 1984) data indicated that the 6-month prevalence rate for all mental disorders was almost 20%.

An analysis of family symptom status addresses three major areas: (a) who in the family is symptomatic; (b) on what measures; and (c) what the patterns of symptomatology are within families. Family symptom status is a complicated issue, because in some families just a single member was symptomatic on a single measure, whereas in others a single member was symptomatic on more than one measure (multi-measures). In still other families, multiple members were symptomatic on a single measure, and there were also families in which multiple members were symptomatic on multiple measures.

In regard to who in the family was symptomatic, we found that 90% to 100% of the adult sons and daughters in the 25 families were symptomatic. Exactly 50% of the wives/mothers were symptomatic, as were 38% of the husbands/fathers. We were surprised to find that 29% of the young sons/brothers and 60% of the young daughters/sisters were symptomatic. In regard to the family members' types of symptomatology, the husbands tended to report depressive symptomatology or substance abuse/dependency; the wives tended to be symptomatic on the CES-D and/or to report depressive symptomatology, or to report panic symptomatology; the adult sons tended to report substance abuse/dependency problems and/or to be symptomatic on the CES-D; and the adult daughters tended to be symptomatic on the CES-D, to report drug problems, or to have phobic symptomatology.

In regard to patterns of symptomatology within families, we often found husbands and wives to be symptomatic on the CES-D and to have anxiety and depression symptoms, the adult sons to have substance abuse/dependency problems, the adult daughters to be symptomatic on the CES-D, and the young children to be symptomatic on the child measures (the CBCL and/or DISC rating for psychopathology). Symptoms and problems clustered in certain families. Although only 1 (8%) of the 13 families with a single symptomatic member had a member who was symptomatic on two measures, 11 (92%) families of the 12 families with two or more symptomatic members had members who were symptomatic on two or more measures. Wives/mothers and adult sons were more likely than husbands/fathers and adult daughters to be symptomatic on two or more measures. When the wives/mothers were symptomatic on multiple measures, those measures tended to be the CES-D and depression symptoms, and/or panic or phobia. When the adult sons were symptomatic on multiple measures, those measures were alcohol, drugs, CES-D, and depression symptoms. As to be expected, as family size increased, larger percentages of the families were symptomatic; however, there was no relationship between the size of the symptomatic families and the number of symptomatic family members.

Family Risk Factors and Symptom Status

Lifetime Diagnoses of Mental Disorders

At Time 1, 15 (18% of the total sample) members in 12 (28% of total) families had a DSM-III lifetime diagnosis of one or more mental disorders. Of the 9 families (75%) in which one member had a DMS-III lifetime diagnosis, 4 wives had experienced major depression, 2 wives panic disorder, and 3 husbands previous DSM-III diagnoses of alcohol abuse/dependency. Of the 3 families (25%) in which 2 members had previous diagnoses, in one family, a father and adult son had experienced alcohol abuse/dependency; in another, 2 adult sons had done the same; and in the third family, the mother met criteria for major depression, panic, and alcohol abuse/dependency and her adult son the criteria for alcohol abuse/dependency. These diagnoses and their sex distribution are in many ways in accord with the ECA (1984) findings showing that the male-female ratio was about 1:1 when substance abuse problems were counted. As expected, females tended to have depressive and panic disorders, and males to have suffered from alcohol and drug abuse/dependency. Our lifetime prevalence rate of 18%, however, was lower than the ECA 30% lifetime prevalence rate (Robins et al., 1984).

Physical Health Status

Each family was given a general *physical health rating* that took the past histories of hospitalizations, operations, or serious accidents into consideration, as well as *severity of current physical illness* rating. When the raters disagreed, we averaged their ratings. On a scale in which 1 was most healthy and 5 least healthy, the mean physical health rating for the 43 families was 2.3 ($SD = 1.3$). The asymptomatic families were only slightly healthier (mean = 2.3, $SD = 1.4$) than the symptomatic families (mean = 2.4, $SD = 1.2$). But ratings for severity of current physical illness showed a greater difference between the two groups. On a scale in which 1 was least severe and 3 most severe, the mean current severity rating for the 43 families was 1.7 ($SD = 1.0$). The asymptomatic families' mean rating was 1.3 ($SD = 0.9$), much less severe than that of symptomatic families (mean = 2.0, $SD = 1.0$). Thus, the symptomatic group had more current physical health problems than the asymptomatic.

Stressful Life Events and Stress Themes

At Time 1 and Time 3, each adult and child over the age of 11 was given a 28-item SLE inventory. For each event, we asked whether it occurred, who experienced it, when it happened, why it happened, how much difference it made in the family's normal routine, how the family was getting along since the event, and who in the family was most affected by it. We have since presented some findings for the 34 families that completed this study (Stephenson et al., 1990). At Time 3, almost 2 more SLEs per family (5.82 ± 3.70) were reported than at Time 1 (3.97 ± 2.59). We think that methodological factors were responsible for this; over the 15 months of the study, family members began to confide in the interviewers more and to discuss personal events. Also, it appears that some undesirable events were so important that families "forgot" the actual dates of the events and mentioned them on more than one interview.

One such family that was asymptomatic at both Time 1 and Time 3 but reported the same SLE twice consisted of a couple in their late 40s and their 21-year-old son. He was the first person in the family to attend college and his parents had high expectations of his success, but he failed. The parents blamed the university, although the son admitted that he had not done well. He recognized that his parents expected too much of him, but he could not talk to them about it. Apparently, his failure was so traumatic that it stayed with the parents like an open wound, and they referred to it again and again when asked about SLEs during the 15 months of the study.

There was little agreement about the occurrence of SLEs among the family members; in fact, all the family members reported only 35% to 40% of the total SLEs that had occurred. When we examined the couples' reports of SLEs, we found that the wife/mother reported more SLEs (33%) than the husband/father (20% to 24%). In families with children, reports of SLEs by the children added approximately 20% to those reported by the parents. This lack of agreement within the family about SLEs also pertains to the types of events reported by the various family members. The wives/mothers and the children tended to report more undesirable or negative events than the husbands/fathers.

In view of the limitations of individual family members' reports of SLEs, we developed the concept of a stress theme and could present family-level stress scores. We conceptualized a stress theme as a family concern that consisted of a single SLE or of multiple related SLEs. To do so, we examined the family members' reports of SLEs and their impact on the family, ascertained the dominant themes (e.g., work, illness), and then determined whether each theme (composed of one or more SLE and the information about their impact) was positive, negative, or had no impact. We placed the stress themes in three categories: (a) referable only to those within the household (*intrafamilial*), (b) referable to relatives residing outside the household (*other relatives*), or (c) referable to a friend or colleague (*friend*).

We rated the impact of the theme on the family on a scale from -4 (very great negative impact) to $+4$ (very great positive impact). Examples of themes rated negatively were use of drugs, loss of a job and loss of income, school suspension, or academic failures. Examples of themes rated positively were engagement and marriage, a personal achievement, or changing jobs with an increase in income. For each family, we obtained overall intrafamilial, other relatives, and friend stress theme scores by adding the individual stress theme ratings within each of the three categories. We were guided by the DSM-III-R (American Psychiatric Association, 1987) Axis IV Severity of Psychosocial Stressors Scale (p. 11), which ranges from 1 ("no stress") to 6 ("catastrophic stress").

As can be seen in Figure 5.3, work/finances was by far the most common intrafamilial stress theme. This is not surprising inasmuch as the study took place in the early 1980s, when Louisville was hard hit by the recession. Loss of income, being laid off, or being out on strike were common events mentioned by the families. The hospitalization of a family member was another frequent theme, especially hospitalization of other relatives, many of whom were the parents or older relatives of the heads of households and/or their spouses. Generally, more symptomatic families than asymptomatic families mentioned a given theme.

The symptomatic group's mean intrafamilial stress theme rating was negative (-1.8 ± 3.5), in contrast to the asymptomatic group's positive rating (0.6 ± 1.7); these ratings differed significantly, ($t[(34\ df] = 2.29$, $p = .028$). Also, the symptomatic group's mean other-relatives stress theme rating (-0.8 ± 2.2) was more negative than the asymptomatic group's mean rating (-0.1 ± 1.7). The mean friend stress theme ratings for both groups (-1.0 and -1.2) were negative because those themes concerned negative events such as friends dying or moving away.

Inasmuch as the only positive mean stress theme score was the asymptomatic group's intrafamilial score, we wondered whether positive themes protected the family against developing symptoms or whether asymptomatic families had more good things happen to them and remembered them better. We think the stress theme approach has merit and hope that it will be pursued.

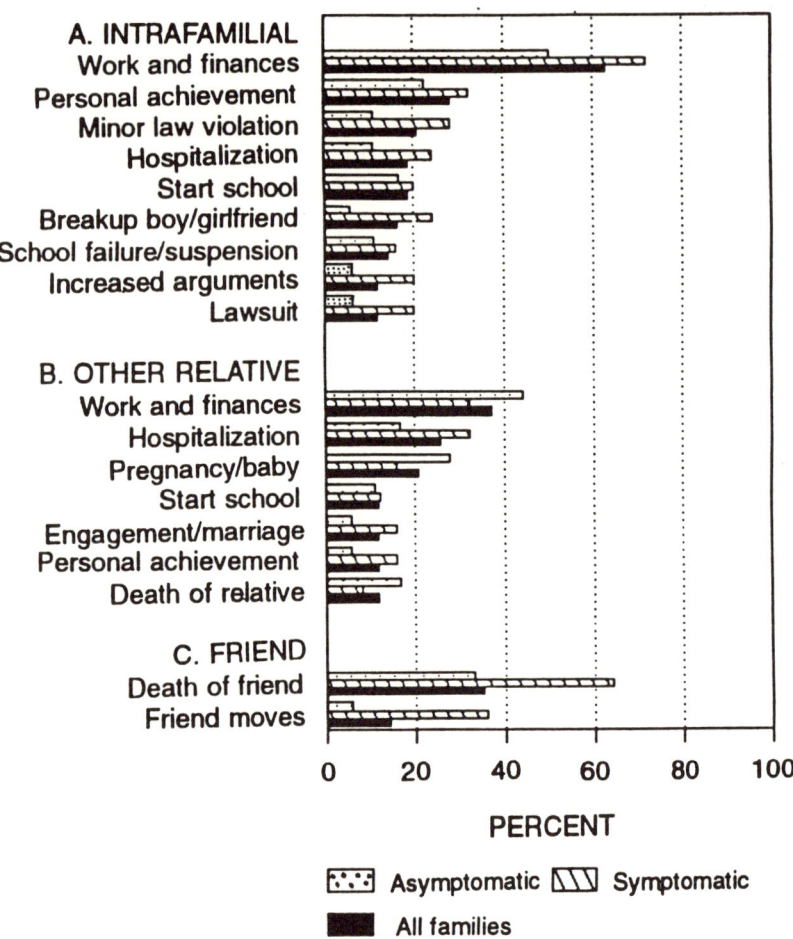

Figure 5.3. Percentages of the most frequently mentioned stress themes by family symptom status.

Social Support

We determined the extent of each family's social support system by rating family members' responses to questions about involvement with relatives, friends, neighbors, churches, and clubs and organizations. As a group we examined, discussed, and rated each member's responses and gave each family a consensus rating on a scale with 0 indicating low and 3 indicating high social support. The asymptomatic families had a higher mean social support rating (mean = 2.1, SD = 0.6), than the symptomatic (mean = 1.8, SD = 0.7). Although the difference between the ratings was not statistically significant, the asymptomatic families reported more involvement and greater satisfaction with their involvement with churches, clubs, and organizations than did the symptomatic group. There were no differences in the two groups' involvement with relatives, friends, or neighbors. As presented in Chapter 4, recent research indicates that active participation in clubs, churches, and other organizations buffers the adversities of SLEs (D. R. Brown & Gary, 1987; Warheit, 1979).

Family Life Cycle Stage, Stress, Symptoms, and Family Vignettes

We developed a family life cycle typology consisting of the following five stages:

1. Beginning families in which there were no children
2. Families in which the oldest child was under age 12
3. Families in which the oldest child was between the ages of 12 and 18
4. Families in which there was an adult child
5. Older families consisting only of married couples

Of our 43 families, only 2 (5%) were beginning or stage 1 families; however, the others were fairly evenly distributed across the other four stages. In the first stage, 1 (50%) of the 2 families was symptomatic; in the second stage, 7 (70%) of the 10 families were symptomatic, as were 7 (70%) of the 10 third-stage families. In the fourth stage, 8 (80%) of the 10 families were symptomatic, but this was true for only 2 (18%) of the 11 families in the fifth stage. The number of symptomatic families in the various life cycle stages differed significantly (chi-square [4 df] = 10.4, p = .03); more families in the earlier stages were symptomatic than in the last stage.

A symptomatic second-stage (children under age 12) family that showed many of the stresses of young families in the United States in the 1980s consisted of a 34-year-old father, a 33-year-old mother, and their 8-year-old daughter. He was a carpenter but had not worked much recently, while the mother had a stand-by job in retailing. Both agreed that their incomes were small and "irregular"; they wanted full-time jobs. Inasmuch as the father had a "tendency to drink," the mother handled all the money. He was a somewhat passive person but had a calming effect on his wife, who was "a worrier." She was expressive, fidgety, and nervous and had many obsessive and phobic symptoms.

Both parents seemed to be close to their young daughter but were concerned about her. On the CBCL, the mother reported that the daughter had many anxieties that were strikingly similar to the mother's fears. We wondered whether the mother had projected her symptoms onto her daughter. At Time 1, the father was positive on alcohol problems, the mother had depression symptomatology, and the daughter had a symptomatic CBCL. At Time 3 the father had stopped "drinking to relieve stress," but the mother was positive on both the CES-D and on depression symptomatology, and the daughter's DISC showed definite evidence of symptomatology. It appeared that the daughter had adopted her mother's symptoms, possibly by contagion (learning) or simply as a constitutionally vulnerable child.

A stage 3 (some children aged 12 to 18) family consisted of a mother and her five children, aged 4 to 16. The father was laid off during the recession and after his unemployment payments ended, the parents separated so that the mother and children would be eligible for Aid for Families with Dependent Children (AFDC). This black family lived in a small rented house that was not as well kept up as others in the poor neighborhood. The furniture consisted only of the bare necessities. Four children slept in one room: the 6-year-old daughter and the 4-year-old son in the bed, the 13-year-old son on the floor, and the 16-year-old son on a couch when he was at home. The 15-year-old daughter slept with the mother in another small room. Soon after our first contact, the 16-year-old son's truancy and continued behavior problems in school resulted in his being placed in an institution for delinquent children. The 15-year-old daughter, who was symptomatic on the CES-D, was mentally handicapped and in special classes in school. The 13-year-old son's DISC was rated as symptomatic. The mother, who was very religious, believed that God would take care of them. All of them were concerned about getting the family back together and about the father's finding employment. When we contacted them for Time 2 reinterviews, the father was living at home. They declined to be interviewed again; we wondered whether they feared that giving us information would jeopardize their receiving AFDC or other benefits for the unemployed.

The transitions encountered by the fourth-stage (at least one adult child at home) families are illustrated by two families that were asymptomatic at both Times 1 and 3. Both had daughters getting married shortly after we interviewed them the first time; however, the families coped with those transitions differently. One family consisted of the 46-year-old father, the 43-year-old mother (who had just started her own business), three children (aged 20, 17, and 16) at home, and an older daughter who was married and living elsewhere. Inasmuch as the children were just about grown, and with the support of her family, the mother started a business that kept her on the road; frequently, she was not home at night. The father adjusted by taking over many of the household tasks, including coping with the two teenage boys. The 20-year-old daughter married after we had first met the family, but her marriage lasted only a few months; she returned home before our study ended.

The other family consisted of the 51-year-old father, the 51-year-old mother, two children (aged 21 and 20) at college, a 15-year-old daughter at home, and a daughter who married after we first interviewed them. The father, who worked two jobs, expressed dissatisfaction with not being very active sexually. The mother, who did not work outside the home, appeared to be living "through her children." The daughter's marriage was intact at the end of the study. Although this second family was asymptomatic and still had children at home, there were some indicators of marital difficulties; we speculated that the husband and wife would have problems in the next few years.

Of the 11 families in the fifth stage (older couples with no children at home), only 2 (18%) were symptomatic. We were surprised that so few were symptomatic, because the twilight years often become a season of loss, and our older families were not free of stress.

The mean intrafamilial stress ratings of the beginning families and those with children under age 12 were positive (1.8 ± 1.8 and 1.1 ± 2.3, respectively). In contrast, the families in the third stage (with children under age 18 at home) had the largest and most negative mean intrafamilial stress rating (-2.3 ± 3.4), followed closely by the fourth-stage (adult children) families (-2.2 ± 2.8) and then the fifth-stage (older couples) families (-1.8 ± 3.7).

The mean other-relatives stress theme ratings for the five groups were all negative and ranged from a low of -0.6 for the fifth-stage families to a high of -1.0 for the first-stage group. The mean friends stress theme ratings for all five groups were also negative; they ranged from a low of -0.9 for the fifth-stage group to a high of -1.4 for the second-stage group.

The associations between the stress theme scores and the various stages of the family life cycle support findings from studies of stress (mainly SLEs) in individuals over the life course. Family members generally report more stress in midlife, especially when there are adolescent or young adult children at home, than either younger or older families. Although "midlife crisis" became a popular topic in the late 1970s, Rashkis (1968) emphasized that parents in their 40s were subjected to stress from above (aging parents and relatives), below (adolescent children), externally (job and financial pressures), and internally (biological and psychological changes).

The greatly increased family stress during the adolescent stage of the life cycle was discussed at length by Olson and his colleagues (1983). Tensions between parents' and their teenagers' differing views of the family were considered to be largely responsible for the high stress in midlife families. Most family studies report that marital satisfaction is at its low point during the adolescent stage of the life cycle.

We were pleased that the results obtained by our stress theme methodology were in accord with those of other studies of stress and satisfaction over the life cycle. Also, the concept of the stress theme and the methods we used have some advantage that others do not. They are comprehensive, take into account the person(s) involved and the impact of SLEs, and yield family-level stress scores.

PERCEPTION OF THE FAMILY ENVIRONMENT

We gave the Family Environment Scale (FES) developed by Rudolph and Bernice Moos (1981) in all three interviews with our families. It consists of 10 subscales that assess families' social environments in three dimensions: (a) the interpersonal relationships among family members; (b) the directions of personal growth emphasized within the family; and (c) the basic organizational structure within the family. A brief description of the dimensions and subscales is presented in Table 5.1.

We averaged the individual family members' subscale scores together to arrive at family subscale scores. Also, we obtained the "family incongruence score," which measures the overall disagreement among family members about their perceptions of the family environment, by summing the absolute difference between each pair of family members' subscale scores on the 10 subscales. We and Boake and Salmon (1983) have found that Louisville families' mean subscale scores differed significantly from the Bay Area norms that had been developed. For example, Louisville scores were higher on cohesion and moral-religious emphasis and lower on conflict and intellectual-cultural orientation than the California scores.

We had three families in the interpersonally effective cluster (Figure 5.4). They had high cohesion and expressiveness subscale scores, the highest mean scores on the intellectual-cultural and the active-recreational subscales, and the lowest mean score on the moral-religious emphasis subscale. They were outgoing and involved in many recreational activities and intellectual-cultural pursuits. Only one of the three

Table 5.1
FES Subscales and Dimension Descriptions

Relationship Dimensions

1. Cohesion — The degree of commitment, help, and support family members provide for one another
2. Expressiveness — The extent to which family members are encouraged to act openly and to express their feelings directly
3. Conflict — The amount of openly expressed anger, aggression, and conflict among family members

Personal Growth Dimensions

4. Independence — The extent to which family members are assertive, are self-sufficient, and make their own decisions
5. Achievement Orientation — The extent to which activities (such as school and work) are cast into an achievement-oriented or competitive framework
6. Intellectual-Cultural Orientation — The degree of interest in political, social, intellectual, and cultural activities
7. Active-Recreational Orientation — The extent of participation in social and recreational activities
8. Moral-Religious Emphasis — The degree of emphasis on ethical and religious issues and values

System Maintenance Dimensions

9. Organization — The degree of importance of clear organization and structure in planning family activities and responsibilities
10. Control — The extent to which set rules and procedures are used to run family life

Source: Reprinted from Rudolf H. Moos and Bernice S. Moos, *Family Environment Scale Manual,* Palo Alto: Consulting Psychologists Press, Inc., 1981, p. 2.

families was symptomatic; in that family, the two children under age 16 had high CBCL scores.

An example of an interpersonally effective family was an upper-middle-class white couple in their early 60s who lived in a spacious, beautifully decorated home. The husband was a professional person who had been financially successful and looked forward to less demanding work in a few years. His parents were uneducated, and he had "pulled himself up by his bootstraps." He and his wife were active in the community and proud to have raised four children who lived in distant states and had their own families and careers. They visited often and planned to do so more often when the husband's work was easier. The wife spent considerable time caring for two elderly relatives. They were engaging, intelligent, busy people who viewed their participation in the research as "our duty." They declined, however, to be videotaped be-

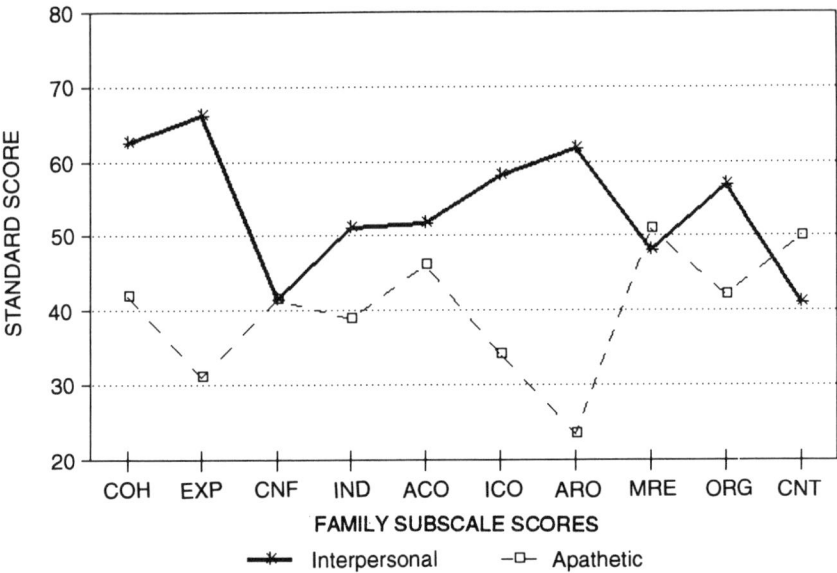

Figure 5.4. Mean FES profiles for interpersonally effective and apathetic clusters. *Key*: COH—cohesion; EXP—expression; MRE—moral-religious; CNF—conflict; ICO—intellectual-cultural; IND—independence; ORG—organization; ARO—active/recreational; ACO—achievement orientation; CNT—control.

cause of his prominent position in the community. They were asymptomatic at both Time 1 and Time 3.

The apathetic cluster (see Figure 5.4) contained the four families with the lowest mean scores on 7 of the 10 subscales —cohesion, expressiveness, independence, achievement orientation, intellectual-cultural orientation, active-recreational, and organization. All four were symptomatic. In one family, consisting of an elderly mother and her adult daughter, the mother was symptomatic on the CES-D and reported depressive symptomatology, and the daughter was symptomatic on the CES-D. In the second, consisting of a mother, her live-in boyfriend, and her two daughters, the mother was symptomatic on the CES-D and reported depressive symptomatology, and both daughters were symptomatic on the child measures; this family was receiving mental health care. In the third, consisting of a single mother and her five children, the mother was symptomatic on the CES-D and reported depressive symptomatology and phobias, her adult son was symptomatic on the CES-D, and the child psychiatrist rated a young son's DISC as showing evidence of psychopathology; the other three children were asymptomatic.

The fourth family is illustrative of the many problems of the elderly who are chronically ill and poor. The husband was 84 years old and the wife was 76. They lived in a rent-subsidized, racially mixed apartment building that was part of a complex composed of two buildings that faced each other across a courtyard. There were no trees in the courtyard and no plantings around the buildings. They had been married many years and had raised seven children, most of whom lived out of town. They especially missed their youngest son, who recently moved to another city; he had been attentive and kind. The wife had diabetes and high blood pressure, and the husband had suffered a stroke and had poor recall and difficulty walking. According to the wife, her husband had a bad temper, had been a "drinker" all his life, and would still drink if he could "get out to buy a bottle." The couple did not get along; she was angry "because his drinking had caused them to lose everything." They had little money, and she felt trapped. She stayed in the back part of the apartment, and he stayed in the front; however, she kept house for them. The wife longed for a porch so that they could sit outside. A visiting nurse came in once a week. At Time 1, the husband scored high on the CES-D and had depressive symptomatology, and the wife was symptomatic on the CES-D. At Time 3, he was still symptomatic on the CES-D, but she was asymptomatic. It appeared as if their lives were winding down and that the outlook for the couple was bleak.

The structure-oriented cluster (Figure 5.5) of 11 families closely resembled Moos and Moos's (1981) "structure-oriented" profile. These families placed their greatest emphasis on organization and also were high on cohesion and moral-religious emphasis. According to Moos and Moos, such "families show a strong emphasis on structuring family activities and on explicitness and clarity with regard to family rules and responsibilities. There is a hierarchical structure of family organization; however, control is not manifested in a rigid, autocratic manner. Family members are strongly committed to the family and feel that they are generally mutually helpful and supportive" (p. 362).

We were surprised to find that 8 (73%) of the 11 structure-oriented families were symptomatic. In four, a single member was symptomatic on a single measure. In one, the wife was symptomatic on the CES-D, and in another, the wife reported panic symptomatology; in the third, an adult son reported drug problems, and in the fourth, a daughter was rated as showing psychopathology on the DISC. In two other families, two members were symptomatic, each on one measure; in one, the father reported depressive symptomatology and the adult son had drug problems, and in the other, the wife reported panic symptomatology and the young son was symptomatic on the child measures.

The two remaining families of the eight were symptomatic on five measures. In one, the mother reported depressive symptomatology, panic symptomatology, and phobias; one adult son was symptomatic on the CES-D, reported depressive symptomatology, and had drug and alcohol problems; and the other adult son had drug and alcohol problems. In the other family, the mother was symptomatic on the CES-D; one adult son reported depressive and panic symptomatology and also had alcohol and drug problems; a second adult son had alcohol problems; and a third son was symptomatic on the child measures.

Our structure-oriented group did not seem to fit Moos and Moos's description of families with that profile. We conjectured that the somewhat low expressiveness and relatively high organization and control subscale scores for these families reflected compensatory efforts to maintain concordance and strengthen boundaries and to lessen conflict, as evidenced by the low conflict score. But it could be that they really did not talk about their problems, that they kept a tight lid on them and through efforts at organization maintained a veneer of respectability that ensured a degree of functioning consistent with their high scores on moral-religious emphasis. Also, it is possible that the structure was so rigid that it contributed to the development of symptomatology.

The fourth cluster, the moral-religious-oriented (Figure 5.5), contained 25 families, more than half of our sample. These families had above average scores on cohesion and expressiveness, but were relatively unstructured. Of the 25 families, 12 (48%) were symptomatic. Only one person was symptomatic in 9 of 12 families: In two families, an adult daughter was symptomatic on the CES-D; in the third, an adult daughter had drug problems; and in the fourth, an adult daughter was symptomatic on the CES-D and reported phobias. In the fifth family, the husband reported phobias; in the sixth, the husband reported depressive symptomatology; in the seventh, the wife reported depressive symptomatology; in the eighth, an adult son had alcohol problems; and in the ninth, a daughter under age 16 was symptomatic. Two or more persons were symptomatic in each of the remaining families: In the tenth, the husband had drug problems and his wife reported panic symptomatology; in the eleventh, the husband had alcohol problems, his wife reported depressive symptomatology, and their young daughter was symptomatic; and in the twelfth family, an adult son and daughter both had drug problems and another adult daughter reported phobias.

In these four clusters, we see some associations between the family environment and symptomatic status. The small interpersonally effective and the large moral-religious clusters contained smaller percentages of symptomatic families than the sample as a whole. In contrast, all four families in the small apathetic cluster were symptomatic. We do not know whether their apathetic (if not demoralized) family environment preceded, accompanied, or followed the onset of their extensive symp-

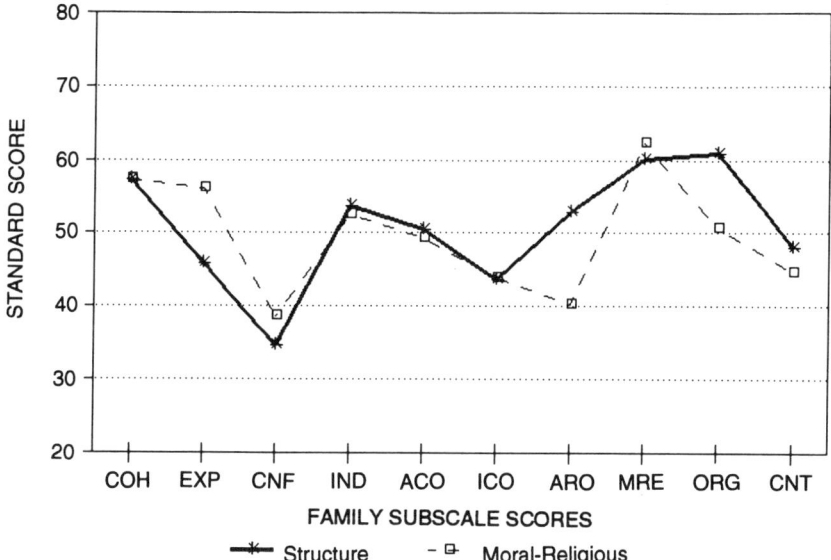

Figure 5.5. Mean FES profiles for structure-oriented and moral-religious-oriented clusters. *Key:* COH—cohesion; EXP—expression; MRE—moral-religious; CNF—conflict; ICO—intellectual-cultural; IND—independence; ORG—organization; ARO—active/recreational; ACO—achievement orientation; CNT—control.

tomatology, but combining a view of their perceptions of their family environments with their many symptoms presents a dreary picture of distress.

FES Profiles of Families with and without Symptomatic Children

The FES profile of the eight families with symptomatic children differed significantly from that of the nine without symptomatic children. Families with symptomatic children had a significantly lower mean independence ($t[41\ df] = 2.1$, $p = .05$) score than those without symptomatic children. Also, families with symptomatic children had a definitely lower mean organization subscale score and higher mean family incongruence score than those whose children were asymptomatic, but the differences were not statistically significant.

FES Profiles of Symptomatic and Asymptomatic Families

As shown in Figure 5.6, as groups, the 25 symptomatic families differed from the 18 asymptomatic families in that they had significantly

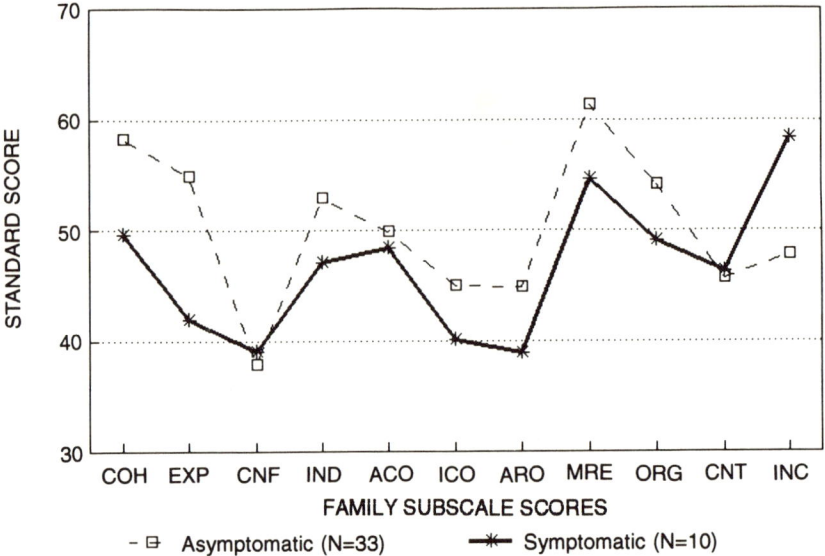

Figure 5.6. Time 1 Family Environment Scale profiles for asymptomatic and symptomatic families (CES-D). *Key*: COH—cohesion; EXP—expression; MRE—moral-religious; CNF—conflict; ICO—intellectual-cultural; IND—independence; ORG—organization; ARO—active/recreational; ACO—achievement orientation; CNT—control.

lower mean scores on the cohesion ($t[41\ df] = 2.8, p = .007$) and expressiveness ($t[41\ df] = 2.2, p = .04$) subscales than the asymptomatic families. The mean incongruence score for the symptomatic group also was higher than that of the asymptomatic group, but the difference was not statistically significant.

In our relatively small sample, there was a remarkable consistency between symptomatology and certain high or low FES subscale scores. Also, the many symptomatic families' high incongruence scores depicted the members' lack of cohesion, discrepant views, and differing attitudes compared to the asymptomatic families. Families with high CES-D scores that indicated current distress also had significantly low mean cohesion ($t[41\ df] = 3.8, p = .001$), expressiveness ($t[41\ df] = 3.2, p = .003$), and moral-religious emphasis ($t[41\ df] = 2.7, p = .009$) scores and a significantly high mean family incongruence ($t[38\ df] = -3.0, p = .004$) score. Those with depression symptoms also had significantly low mean cohesion ($t[41\ df] = 4.9, p < .001$) and expressiveness ($t[41\ df] = 3.0, p = .005$) scores and a significantly higher mean family incongruence ($t[38\ df] = -2.7, p = .010$) score. Thus, the subscale scores in the interpersonal dimension reflected the families' affective distress.

Families with drug problems had significantly lower mean cohesion ($t[41\ df] = 2.2$, $p = .032$) and intellectual-cultural orientation ($t[41\ df] = 2.0$, $p = .047$) scores and a higher mean conflict ($t[41\ df] = 2.2$, $p = .031$) score than those without drug problems. But their incongruence scores were only slightly greater than those of the families without drug problems—indicating, unfortunately, that all the families are perceiving their distress in about the same way, leaving little doubt that the distress is real. The families with panic had lower expressiveness and independence mean subscale scores and somewhat higher mean organization and control subscale scores than families without panic symptomatology. The panic families' relatively low expressiveness and independence and relatively high organization and control subscale scores suggest that the symptomatology is affecting the entire family environment. Panic patients tend to become helpless and to cling to those near them; also, control becomes a vital psychodynamic issue inasmuch as the patients dread and experience the panic attack as loss of control. The panic families' subscale scores probably are indicative of compensatory adjustments in the environment. The families with phobic symptomatology had lower mean cohesion and control scores and higher mean independence and achievement orientation scores than families without phobic symptoms. For both the panic and the phobic families, however, the differences were definite but not statistically significant.

Thus, the FES provided an assessment of family members' attitudes toward each other, a view of their interests and priorities in everyday life (as reflected, for example, by their scores on the active-recreational and moral-religious emphasis subscales), and a glimpse of intrafamily dynamics and differences. As the reader will see later, some information about individualism versus familism could be derived from the subscale scores, and they had surprisingly good predictive values.

Predicting Family Symptomatic Status from the FES Subscale Scores

Even though our sample size was small, we were able to predict family symptom status from the FES subscale and incongruence scores by using discriminant function analyses and also logistical regressions. Both of these multivariate statistical techniques predict group membership (e.g., family status as being either symptomatic or asymptomatic) from a set of independent variables (e.g., the FES scores). Discriminant function analysis, however, requires more assumptions than logistical regression.

Table 5.2
Results of Discriminant Function Analyses Using Time 1 FES Subscale Scores to Predict Family Symptomatic Status

Group Variable	Independent Variables	% Asymp. Classified	% Sympt. Classified	% All Classified
Time 1 symptom status	COH1	83.3	56.0	67.4
Time 1 CES-D status	COH1, EXP1, MRE1	78.9	80.0	79.1
Time 1 depression status	COH1	87.9	80.0	86.1
Time 1 alcohol status	[no scores]	—	—	—
Time 1 drug status	CNF1, ICO1, IND1, ORG1, COH1,	77.8	57.1	74.4
Time 1 panic status	IND1, ORG1, ARO1, EXP1	73.0	66.7	72.1
Time 1 phobic status	ACO1, CNT1, COH1	71.8	75.0	72.1
Time 1 child status	IND1, ARO1, COH1, CNT1, ORG1, ICO1, ACO1, CNF1	100.00	100.00	100.00

Key: COH—cohesion; EXP—expression; MRE—moral-religious; CNF—conflict; ICO—intellectual-cultural; IND—independence; ORG—organization; ARO—active/recreational; ACO—achievement orientation; CNT—control.

Table 5.2 summarizes the results of discriminant function analyses that used the ten Time 1 FES subscale scores to predict family symptom status for all and also for each of the various symptom measures. Except for child psychopathology status, the percentage of all families correctly classified ranged from a low of 67.4% for the Time 1 overall symptom status to a high of 86.1% for the depression status. Generally, the discriminant function analysis classified a greater percentage of the asymptomatic correctly than the symptomatic families, probably because the number of symptomatic families was small and their scores varied more than the asymptomatic families' scores. One exception was the discriminant function analysis that predicted child psychopathology status. It used eight of the ten mean subscale scores to classify correctly all the 17 families with children under the age of 16 into two groups: the 8 whose children showed psychopathology, and the 9 whose children did not.

Low cohesion subscale scores were powerful predictors of overall symptom status, high CES-D scores, and depressive symptomatology. The conflict scores, along with other subscale scores, were predictors of drug problems, and independence subscale scores were the main predictors of panic status and of a child having psychopathology.

Logistical regressions using the ten Time 1 FES subscale and the incongruence scores to predict family symptom status correctly classified from 62.8% to 83.7% of the families on overall symptom status, the CES-D, depressive symtomatology, drug use, and child status. As an independent variable, the mean cohesion score was the most powerful predictor of symptomatic status, high CES-D scores, and depressive symptoms. The conflict score was the main predictor of drug usage, and the independence score of child status. Thus, the same subscale scores were the main predictors in both the discriminant function analyses and the logistical regressions. A comparison of the percentages of families correctly classified by the two methods shows that the results of the discriminant function analysis and the logistical regressions do not differ greatly. The discriminant function analysis correctly classified more symptomatic families than the logistical regression but was less parsimonious in that it used more independent variables (i.e., FES subscale and incongruence scores) to differentiate the groups.

It can be seen that the FES is a powerful multipurpose instrument for evaluating an important aspect of family life—the family environment—and thus assessing families. The scores have both clinical and research implications. Of course, the family environment is complex and defies simple measurement, but the use of the FES is a feasible and effective approach that yields meaningful results.

Areas of Family Responsibility

To gain baseline information about how our families were carrying out the tasks of everyday life and to see if the division of labor was associated with symptomatology, we asked all family members aged 16 and older a series of questions. They were about each person's responsibilities for four family tasks—food and its preparation, cleaning the house, home upkeep, and child care (where applicable)—and whether the interviewee was primarily responsible, shared responsibilities, or was not at all responsible for activities in each of those areas. We obtained information from 96 members: 40 heads of households, 35 spouses, 11 adult male children, and 10 adult female children. In addition, for the 32 married couples, we cross-tabulated the husbands' and wives' responses about responsibility in each area.

The findings indicated that, to a moderate degree, there was a traditional sex-role division of labor in the families. Almost 75% of the females had prime responsibility for food preparation and keeping the house clean, and about 67% of the males had prime responsibility for the upkeep of the house. But, in all four areas, 40% to 60% of the household heads, spouses, or both reported some sharing of the activities. Child care definitely was a shared activity; in 60% of the couples, the husband and the wife reported that they shared the responsibility and that neither had prime responsibility. Of the 21 adult sons and daughters, about 50% to 75% reported sharing some of the household tasks, but from 10% to 20% reported no responsibility for the various tasks.

For each of the four tasks we classified the 32 couples into four groups. Couples were labeled *traditional* if, for food preparation, housecleaning, and child care, the wives had prime responsibility and the husbands had no responsibility and if, for home upkeep, the husbands had prime responsibility and the wives had no responsibility. The *sharing* group consisted of those couples in which both spouses reported sharing the tasks. The *modified/mixed* group consisted of the couples in which there was varying participation in the tasks by the husbands and wives, and the *other* group consisted of the few couples that could not be classified. Some tasks were gender stereotypical; for example, almost 50% of the couples still regarded home upkeep as traditional "man's work." But the spouses shared the tasks of child care (60%) and housecleaning (34%), although there was little sharing of food preparation (19%) and of home upkeep (9%). There was no relationship between sex-role division of labor and family symptom status.

Comment

As discussed in Chapter 3, the companionate family that was seen by family scholars as emerging during the 1920s and becoming a dominant family type in the 1950s was considered to be one in which there was a more equitable division of family labor than in the "outmoded" institution-based family. But the increasing percentage (31% in 1960, 70% in 1990) of married women with children working outside the home (NBC News, 1992), the increasing number of "working poor," and the many dual-career families have smudged the pretty picture of family life that was painted by two or three generations of family sociologists. Our data indicate that families are, probably of necessity, changing by sharing. This sharing is probably an adaptive mechanism for families as they strive to cope with the economic hardships and other adversities accompanying the loss of middle-class status for many and the lower family incomes of 40% of Americans during the Reagan-Bush years, when family income of the top 1% of the population rose 60% (Nasar, 1992, p. A1).

Marital Satisfaction

Of our 43 families, 34 household heads (79%) were married, 3 (7%) were separated, 3 (7%) were divorced, and 3 (7%) were widowed. One divorced head was living with a partner; the couple was considered as married. We obtained information about marital satisfaction from 32 husbands and 34 wives, but only 31 couples, because 3 husbands did not participate and 1 wife did not offer responses.

We began by asking the husbands and wives what they liked and disliked most about their marriages. For both partners, the most frequently reported like was "companionship" or "togetherness." The second was, for husbands, "raising a family," and for wives, "security." The most frequent dislikes for both was "nothing." The husbands' second choice was "responsibilities," and the wives' was "household duties and activities."

Next, we asked each partner to rate his or her degree of marital satisfaction on a scale, ranging from excellent to bad. Almost all of the 32 men and 34 women rated their relationships as either excellent (41% of the men and 50% of the women) or good (53% of the men and 44% of the women); only 2 (6%) men and 2 (6%) women rated their relationships as fair, and none rated a relationship as either poor or bad. Slightly more women (17, or 50%) rated their relationships as excellent than did the men (13, or 41%).

There were no significant associations between symptomatic status and reports of marital satisfaction. Of the 32 men, 5 (16%) were symptomatic; 1 rated his marital relationship as excellent and 4 as good. Of the 34 women, 10 (29%) were symptomatic; 4 rated their relationships as excellent, 4 as good, and 2 as fair. Marital satisfaction is a relatively vague outcome measure that reflects each spouse's feelings about the relationship. It is largely an indicator of content or discontent, but persisting discontent and dissatisfaction can lead often to symptomatic distress, and thus in many ways affect the stability of the marriage and personal or even spousal well-being.

Agreement About Marital Satisfaction

We then looked at the level of agreement about marital satisfaction. In 20 of the 31 couples, both partners agreed: Each partner in 10 couples (32%) had rated the relationship excellent, and in another 10 couples (32%) each had rated it good. There was a one-level difference in the partners' ratings in 9 of the other 11 (36%) couples, and two levels of difference in only 2 couples.

There were no statistical associations between symptomatic status and the level of husband-wife agreement about satisfaction. Of the 20 couples in which both agreed, there was symptomatology in 6 (30%); in 2 couples, only the husbands were symptomatic, in another 2, only the wives were symptomatic, and in the remaining 2, both partners were symptomatic. Of the 11 couples in which the husbands and wives disagreed, there was symptomatology in 4 (36%); in 3, the wives were symptomatic, and in the fourth, both the husband and wife were symptomatic.

Changes in Marital Satisfaction

We next assessed possible changes in marital satisfaction over time. Each partner was asked, "Do you get along better, the same, or worse now than 1 year ago?" In 20 of the 31 couples (65%), the partners had similar perceptions of their marital relationship in that 6 couples (30%) viewed their relationships as better and 14 (70%) as being the same as a year earlier. Of the 11 couples (35%) in which there were differences, in 5 (45%) the husbands saw the relationship as better and the wives saw it as about the same; in another 5 (45%) the wives saw the relationship as better than it had been and the husbands saw it as about the same. In one couple (3%), the husband viewed the relationship as worse than a year before, while the wife saw it as about the same.

We found less symptomatology among the couples who had similar perceptions of changes in their marital relationship during the past year than among those whose perceptions differed. Of the 20 couples with similar perceptions, only 5 (25%) of the families were symptomatic—the husband only in 1 case, the wife only in 3 others, and both the husband and wife in the fifth. In contrast, of the 11 couples whose perceptions differed, 5 (46%) of the families were symptomatic—the husband only in 1 case, the wife only in 2 others, and both husbands and their wives in the fourth and fifth. Overall, the couples reported that their marital relationships were good, and in many instances better than a year previously. The responses were skewed toward a degree of satisfaction that is not consistent with the many reports of relationship problems we hear and read about daily.

Effect of Relationship on Physical Mental Health

Each partner was asked about the effect of the relationship on his or her physical and mental health. We found only a few weak associations between reports of the effects of the 31 couples' relationships on their physical health and symptomatic status. Of the 22 couples in which both partners reported that the relationship was either beneficial to or had no effect on their physical health, there was symptomatology in only 6 (27%) families—2 husbands only, 2 wives only, and 2 couples. Of the 9 in which the husbands reported that the relationship was "beneficial" but the wives reported no effect, however, 4 (44%) families were symptomatic—the wife only in 3 couples, and both the husband and wife in the fourth. No one reported that the relationship had a deleterious effect on his or her physical health.

We found greater husband-wife differences about the effect of the relationship on the mental health of the 31 couples. Of the 18 in which both partners reported either that being married was beneficial or that it had no effect on their mental health, only 3 families (17%) were symptomatic—1 husband only, 1 wife only, and 1 couple. But of the 7 couples in which the husbands reported that being married was beneficial to their mental health while their wives reported no effect, 3 families (43%) were symptomatic—the wives only in 2 couples, and both the husband and wife in the third. Of the 3 other couples in which the husbands reported that being married had no effect on their mental health and the wives reported that it had a beneficial effect, in 1 family (33%) the wife was symptomatic. Of the couples in which the husbands reported that the relationship had either a beneficial or no effect on their mental health but the wives reported it was deleterious, all 3 families (100%) were symptomatic—1 husband only, 1 wife only, and 1 couple.

Thus, reports of the effects of the relationship on mental health were definitely associated with symptom status. Such findings are in accord with the results of many epidemiological studies of marriage and physical and mental health. Generally, men report that marriage has a beneficial effect on both their physical and their mental health; in contrast, women often report that marriage has a deleterious effect on their mental health (Radloff, 1975). Results of other studies support some of the reports of the beneficial (or at least protective) effects of marriage on men's physical health. For example, Parkes (1972) found significantly higher morbidity and mortality rates in widowers 1 year after bereavement compared to controls; although the widows' morbidity rates were higher than the controls, their mortality rates were not higher.

In our sample, 10% of the wives reported that their marriages had an adverse effect on their mental health. Generally, women have been more likely than men to express satisfaction with their relationships and also more likely to report that their relationships had an adverse effect on their mental health. We have no ready explanation for such an apparent paradox. In practice, however, we repeatedly see separated or divorced wives who tell that they were satisfied with their marriages and thought that their husbands were also satisfied, but were surprised when the husbands suddenly announced that they wanted divorces. Some fundamental considerations may be applicable; men are notoriously less sexually and maritally stable than women, who in contrast emphasize the need for a stable relationship and, until recent years, have often endured hardships, sufferings, and even abuse to maintain their marriages and families.

Sexual Satisfaction

To evaluate sexual satisfaction, we first asked each partner whether his or her sexual relationship was "somewhat important" or whether he or she "could have gotten along without it." Of the 29 couples in which both husbands and wives reported, 21 (72%) agreed that it was "somewhat important." Overall, about equal percentages, 25 husbands (83%) and 34 wives (76%), reported that it was "somewhat important."

Agreement about the importance of sexuality was associated with symptom status. Of the 21 couples who agreed that sex was "somewhat important," 6 families (29%) were symptomatic—1 husband, 2 wives, and 3 husbands and wives. None of the husbands or wives in the 2 couples in which the partners agreed that they could do without the sexual relationship were symptomatic. But of the 6 couples (29%) that gave mixed reports about the importance of sex in their relationships, 4 families were symptomatic—1 husband and 3 wives. The respondents' ages were not related to their reports about their sexual relationships.

Each partner rated sexual satisfaction on a 5-point scale ranging from "very satisfied" to "very unsatisfied" and rated his or her opinions of the spouse's level of satisfaction. The vast majority of husbands (92%) and wives (86%) reported that they were satisfied or very satisfied; only 2 husbands and 3 wives were "uncertain," and only 1 wife was sexually dissatisfied.

The wives more often than the husbands perceived their spouses' level of sexual satisfaction accurately; the husbands tended to perceive their wives as having a lesser degree of sexual satisfaction than the wives reported. There were no associations between these perceptions and symptom status. In the 25 couples in which both spouses reported, 6 (24%) were symptomatic—1 husband, 4 wives, and 1 husband and wife. In 3 of those 6 symptomatic couples, both partners correctly perceived the other's sexual satisfaction; in 2 couples, however, only one partner correctly perceived the other's sexual satisfaction, and in another neither partner correctly perceived the other's satisfaction. We were surprised by the extent of agreement about sexual satisfaction and wondered whether it was attributable to the greater openness about sexuality since the 1960s or whether the sexually dissatisfied were among the 6 couples on whom we did not have complete reports.

Twenty-four husbands and 27 wives reported how often they had intercourse. Of the 24 husbands, 3 (13%) reported that they had intercourse more than one time per week; 7 (29%) one time per week; 8 (33%) one or two times per month; and 6 (25%) less than once per month. Of the 27 wives, 7 (26%) reported that they had intercourse more than 1 time per week; 8 (30%) one time per week; 4 (15%) one or two times per month; 4 (15%) less than once per month; and still another 4 (15%) that they did not have intercourse at all.

There was agreement about the frequency of intercourse in 7 of the 23 couples on whom we have complete reports. In another 9, the husbands reported a greater frequency than the wives, and in the remaining 7, the wives reported a greater frequency than the husbands. Of the 25 husbands, 15 reported that they were satisfied with the frequency, 9 wanted more frequent intercourse, and 1 wanted less. Of the 29 wives, 26 reported they were satisfied with the frequency of intercourse, and 3 reported that they wanted intercourse more often.

Thus, there were no major differences in the husbands' and wives' reports about their sexual relationships. Also, there were no significant associations between the perceived importance of sex, sexual satisfaction, frequency of intercourse, and symptom status. Generally, however, symptomatology was found more often in couples not in agreement, especially about the importance of sex in the relationship, than in those that agreed.

CHANGES IN SYMPTOMATOLOGY OVER TIME

Introduction

We interviewed the families three times: at the beginning of the study (Time 1), 6 months later (Time 2), and 9 months after Time 2 (Time 3). At the end of the 15 months, 9 (21%) of the 43 families that participated at Time 1 had withdrawn, and 34 (79%) continued. Of the 9 families, 2 (22%) had moved away, and 7 (78%) had dropped out after the Time 1 interview. Those that moved told us that they would have liked to continue in the study; the 7 dropouts stated that the study took too much time.

We are not reporting Time 2 data, because they are not comparable to Time 1 and Time 3 data. We modified some procedures at Time 2 inasmuch as the research was a pilot study designed to develop methods and test feasibility. At Time 2 we tested procedures that the Time 1 experiences led us to think should be evaluated, and we experimented to refine others. The Time 2 interview, therefore, was devoted to testing innovative approaches and was shortened to reduce the amount of time required of family members. We abbreviated the Diagnostic Interview Schedule (DIS) so that we would be looking mainly for gross changes in symptomatology since Time 1, and we gave the stressful life event (SLE) inventory to the family as a group while they were being videotaped, instead of to each member individually as at Time 1.

The yield from the changes made at Time 2 was minimal, and 6 months turned out to be too short a period to see much change in the families. Consequently, although the Time 3 interviews incorporated some modifications indicated by the Time 2 testing, in most ways they were similar to the Time 1 baseline interviews, and we used them with confidence gained from the Time 2 experiences. Thus, we are reporting only the Time 1 and the Time 3 data and the changes that occurred during the 15 months between them.

Sociodemographic Characteristics of the Dropout and Completing Families

As shown in Table 5.3, the 9 families that withdrew differed significantly on some sociodemographic characteristics from those that completed the study. The dropout group contained 6 of the 9 single-parent families and 4 of the 5 black families. Only 3 (33%) dropout families were married; 6 (67%) were separated, widowed, or divorced. In contrast, 31 (91%) families that completed were married, and only 3 (9%) divorced or widowed. Also, the dropout families were larger and had older parents with lower educational levels than those that continued. The dropout group had about a 20% lower median monthly family income, 40% lower median monthly expenses, and 80% higher median monthly disposable income than the completers, but these figures are somewhat misleading because 2 dropout families' monthly incomes were much higher than those of the other 7.

One dropout black family that was having financial problems and intergenerational difficulties consisted of a 57-year-old father and 27-year-old son. The father was a manual laborer who was carrying the burden of the household expenses and worrying about money. He spoke about his son as if he were lecturing, admonishing him to find work,

Table 5.3
Marital Status, Race, and Education of Families That Withdrew From and That Completed the Study

Characteristic	Withdrew From Study		Completed Study		Total	
	N	%	N	%	N	%
Marital status[a]						
Married	3	33	31	91	34	79
Separated	3	33	0	0	3	7
Divorced	2	22	1	3	3	7
Widowed	1	11	2	6	3	7
Race[a]						
White	5	56	33	97	38	88
Black	4	44	1	3	5	12
Education[b]						
Less than high school	5	63	5	16	10	25
High school	2	25	11	34	13	32
More than high school	1	13	16	50	17	42

[a]Percentages are based on the 9 families that withdrew from the study and 34 families that completed the study.
[b]Percentages are based on the 8 families that withdrew from the study (1 of the 9 did not report educational level) and 32 families who completed the study.

share responsibility for the home, and help the family get "closer to God." The son, who was obese and had long hair and possibly gynecomastia, seemed bored and tired. It appeared that conflict and chaos pervaded the home. At Time 1, the father reported depression symptoms, and the son had drug problems. When we contacted them for the Time 2 interview, the father was seriously ill with prostate cancer and declined to participate; also, he reported that his son had moved away and that he was alone.

A different kind of dropout family was one that lived in a large, expensively furnished house in an upper-middle-class suburb. The family consisted of the 50-year-old father (who did not participate but did not object to the others doing so), the 46-year-old mother, and their four sons (ages 24, 22, 19, and 13), only three of whom participated. The father was a successful businessman, but he worried about money and hoped that the economy would soon improve. At Time 1, the mother was symptomatic on the CES-D, and all three participating sons were symptomatic: The 22-year-old had alcohol problems; the 19-year-old reported depression and panic symptomatology and had drug and alcohol problems; and the 13-year-old's Diagnostic Interview Schedule for Children (DISC) showed psychopathology. Family members vigorously denied that anything was wrong. We think that the family dropped out to avoid having to admit that they had problems.

Dropout Families' Time 1 Symptom Status

Of the 9 dropout families, 8 (89%) were symptomatic; 2 (25%) had one symptomatic member (an adult child in both cases), whereas in the other 6 (75%), two or more members were symptomatic. The other 6 families had extensive symptoms and problems. In 3 of them, all of the participating members were symptomatic; in 2 of the remaining 3 families, only the mothers were asymptomatic, and in the third only the young children were asymptomatic. Two families consisted of a single parent and an adult child; in each case, both of them were symptomatic.

Of the 21 participating members in those 6 families, 16 (76%) were symptomatic. They were the one participating husband/father, all five adult sons, all three adult daughters, three of the four young sons, three of the five wives/mothers, and one of the three young daughters. The husband/father reported depression symptoms, the adult sons problems with alcohol and drugs, and the daughters current distress (CES-D) and phobias. The three mothers were symptomatic on the CES-D, and two of them reported depressive symptomatology and one panic symptoms as well. Of the seven children under age 16, four (57%) were symptomatic on the CBCL and/or DISC rating.

All of the symptomatic dropout families contained at least one young and/or adult child who was symptomatic. They are discussed in detail in Chapter 6.

Some Comparisons of the Symptomatic Dropout and Completing Families

A significantly larger proportion (8, or 89%), of the 9 dropout families were symptomatic than the 17 (50%) of the 34 families that completed the study. Also, a smaller percentage (25%) of the symptomatic dropout families contained only one symptomatic member, and a larger percentage (75%) contained two or more symptomatic members than the completing families, in which 65% had only one symptomatic member and 35% had two or more. Additionally, more members in the symptomatic dropout families were symptomatic on multiple measures than in the symptomatic completing families.

Overall, disproportionately more members of the dropout families (18, or 64%) were symptomatic than the members of the completing families (26, or 26%). The high percentage of symptomatic adult children and young children in the dropout families (82%) compared to the percentage in the completing families (32%) is a poignant finding that may well be an indicator of multigenerational distress and of high mental illness rates in the next generation. The dropout families were under considerable stress in many areas; the time, the necessity to be together, the surfacing of problems, and the introspection required by the study probably added even more stress, causing them to withdraw.

The dropout families' mean intrafamilial stress theme rating (-3.2) was significantly more negative than the completing families' rating (-0.3; $t[34\ df] = -2.6, p = 0.015$). There were no significant differences in the two groups' mean other-relatives stress theme or mean friends stress theme ratings. Although there were no statistically significant differences between the dropout and the completing families' mean FES subscale scores, the dropout families tended to have lower mean cohesion, expressiveness, intellectual-cultural orientation, and moral-religious emphasis subscale scores and higher conflict, control, and family incongruence scores than the completing families' mean scores.

We and others have found that lower scores on the cohesion and expressiveness subscales and higher scores on the conflict subscales tend to be associated with symptomatology. The dropout families' lower intellectual-cultural orientation subscale scores reflect their lower socioeconomic status and thus also are associated with symptomatology. The higher control scores often are indicative of compensatory efforts to maintain a family system that is low in cohesion and lacks the communication needed to work out the differences among family members (as revealed by the relatively higher family incongruence scores).

Completing Families at Time 1

Sociodemographic Characteristics and Symptom Status

The 34 families that completed the study tended to be slightly smaller families with younger (mean age 50.7 years) and better-educated heads than those that withdrew. Almost all, 31 (91%) of the 34, were married; only 3 (9%) had been divorced or widowed, and only 1 (3%) was black. The completing families' median annual income was $20,400, slightly lower than the median ($21,926) in the county. They had a 1983 median monthly disposable family income of $240. Their sociodemographic characteristics are shown in Table 5.4.

Table 5.4
Sociodemographic Characteristics of Families That Withdrew from and That Completed the Study

Characteristic	Withdrew (N=9)			Completed (N=34)			Total		
	Median	Mean	SD	Median	Mean	SD	Median	Mean	SD
Family size (number of persons)	3.0	3.7	1.7	3.0	3.2	1.1	3.0	3.3	1.3
Age of head (years)	54.0	53.8	13.1	52.0	50.7	16.3	52.0	51.4	15.6
Monthly family income	$ 1,500	$ 2,416	$ 2,455	$ 1,830	$ 1,988	$ 1,205	$ 1,830	$ 2,074	$ 1,505
Monthly family expenses	$ 791	$ 1,037	$ 801	$ 1,335	$ 1,332	$ 487	$ 1,302	$ 1,269	$ 570
Monthly disposable income	$ 430	$ 1,277	$ 1,815	$ 240	$ 655	$ 1,095	$ 240	$ 780	$ 1,268
Annual family income	$18,000	$28,995	$29,465	$20,400	$23,498	$14,376	$20,400	$24,570	$17,948
Median 1980 census tract family income	$18,174	$22,801	$11,460	$21,968	$21,926	$ 3,498	$21,271	$22,109	$ 5,896

At Time 1, 17 (50%) of the 34 families were asymptomatic, and 17 (50% were symptomatic. In 11 (65%) of the symptomatic families one member was symptomatic, and in the other 6 (35%) two or more members were symptomatic. In the 17 symptomatic families, of the 14 fathers who participated, 5 (36%) were symptomatic; of the 17 mothers, 9 (53%) were symptomatic. Of the 4 adult sons, 3 (75%) were symptomatic, as were all 3 (100%) of the adult daughters and 6 (35%) of the 17 young children.

In the 11 families with one symptomatic member, 31% of the 35 participating members were symptomatic. In 6 of them, the symptomatic member was a child (an adult child in 4 families and a young child in 2); in the other 5 families, the symptomatic member was a parent. All 3 of the adult daughters, 1 of the 2 adult sons, 1 of the 4 fathers, and 3 of the 11 mothers were symptomatic. Of the 4 young daughters, 2 were symptomatic, but none of the 7 young sons was symptomatic.

In the 6 families with two or more symptomatic members, 15 (75%) of the 20 participating individuals were symptomatic. All of the mothers, adult sons, and young daughters, 50% of the fathers, and 33% of the young sons were symptomatic. In 2 of the 3 families in which the husband/father was symptomatic, all of the other family members were also symptomatic (the wife in one family, and the mother and the young daughter in the other). In the third family, the mother was symptomatic in addition to the father, but their two young sons were not. In the 3 remaining families, the mother and children were symptomatic. All of the asymptomatic members of those 6 families were males (a father, a live-in boyfriend, and two young sons).

In the 17 symptomatic families, 3 (75%) of the 4 adult sons were symptomatic on more than one measure, usually alcohol, drugs, and/or depressive symptomatology. None of the 3 adult daughters was symptomatic on more than one measure, but 2 (67%) were symptomatic for current distress (CES-D), and 1 (33%) had drug problems. Of the 17 wives/mothers, 9 (55%) were symptomatic on more than one measure, usually panic symptomatology and/or depression symptoms. Of the 14 husbands/fathers, 5 (36%) were symptomatic on more than one measure, but no syndrome predominated. There were 7 young daughters under age 16 in the group; 5 (71%) were symptomatic on the child measures. In contrast, only 1 (10%) of the 10 young sons was symptomatic. The disproportionately large percentage of symptomatic girls under age 16 reflects the tendency for girls to become affectively symptomatic after puberty; there has been a trend in recent years for increasing numbers of girls in their preteen and early teen years to need mental health care. Traditionally, more boys than girls are in treatment in child psychiatry clinics and practices, but that male-female ratio has been changing during the past decade.

One family with three members symptomatic on six different measures illustrates, in extreme form, the combinations of symptoms and problems we often saw. The family consisted of an elderly couple and two adult sons. The mother reported depressive, panic, and phobic symptomatology; the 29-year-old son was symptomatic on the CES-D, reported depressive symptomatology, and had alcohol and drug problems; and the 28-year-old son had alcohol and drug problems. The mother had been treated for severe alcohol and drug problems in the past.

Asymptomatic and Symptomatic Completing Families' Sociodemographic Characteristics

At Time 1, the 17 (50%) completing families that were asymptomatic tended to be smaller and had older (median age 58 versus 43 years) and better-educated heads, much larger annual incomes (median $24,000 versus $15,450), greater expenses, and more disposable income than the 17 (50%) symptomatic families. Although the 17 symptomatic families had a large, negative mean intrafamilial stress theme rating (−1.0) compared to the 17 in the asymptomatic group, who had a positive rating (0.8), that difference did not quite reach statistical significance. The families symptomatic only on depression, however, had a significantly more negative mean intrafamilial stress theme rating than the families without depressive symptomatology (−3.5 versus 0.5, $t[25\ df] = 3.1$, $p = 0.005$). Also, families with members symptomatic for alcohol had a significantly more negative intrafamilial mean stress theme rating than families with no alcohol problems (−5.0 versus 0.1, $t[25\ df] = 2.6$, $p = 0.016$), and families with symptomatic children had a significant negative intrafamilial mean stress theme rating compared to the asymptomatic families with children (−1.3 versus 1.7, $t[12\ df] = 3.1$, $p = 0.010$). The most common stress themes were work issues and financial problems.

Both the asymptomatic and symptomatic groups' other-relatives mean stress ratings were negative (−0.2 and 1.3, respectively), but the difference was not statistically significant, probably because of the small number of symptomatic families and the large standard deviations. The families symptomatic for depression, however, had significantly greater and more negative mean other-relatives stress ratings than the families without depressive symptomatology (−2.8 versus −0.3, $t[21\ df] = 3.0$, $p = 0.008$). Also, those symptomatic on the CES-D had significantly greater and more negative mean other-relatives stress ratings than the asymptomatic families (−3.2 versus −0.5, $t[21\ df] = 2.5$, $p = 0.023$).

Thus, the stress theme ratings revealed that our symptomatic families had been under much greater stress, as they perceived it, than the asymptomatic families. Although the important and troubling stress themes were intrafamilial, the overall degree of stress in the families symptomatic for depression merits attention. Families with depressive symptoms had high negative stress scores on the other-relative stress themes, as well as on the intrafamilial scores. Only a few SLEs referable to friends were reported; we had too few friends stress theme ratings on which to present data.

FES Profiles of Asymptomatic and Symptomatic Completing Families

As shown in Figure 5.7, at Time 1, the mean FES profile of the symptomatic completing families was statistically different than that of the asymptomatic families. The symptomatic had significantly lower

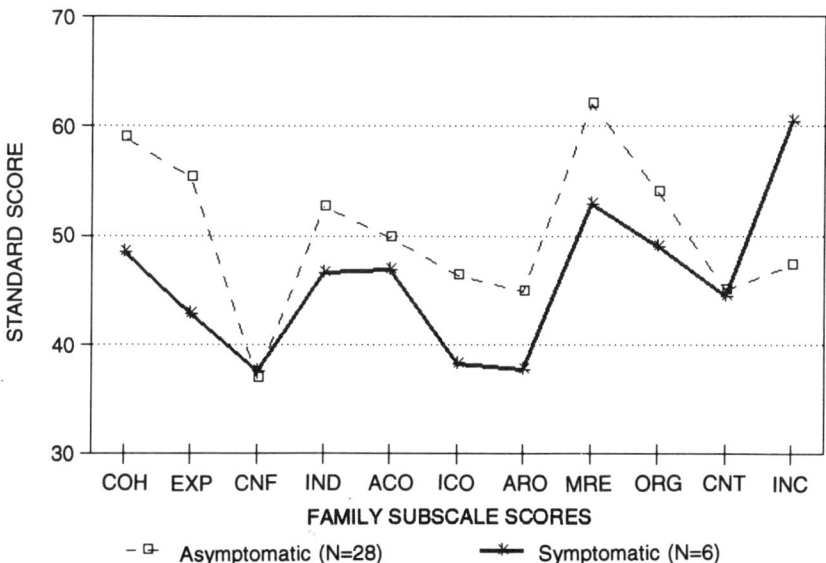

Figure 5.7. Time 1 Family Environment Scale profiles for asymptomatic and symptomatic completing Families (CES-D; $N = 34$). *Key*: COH—cohesion; EXP—expression; MRE—moral-religious; CNF—conflict; ICO—intellectual-cultural; IND—independence; ORG—organization; ARO—active/recreational; ACO—achievement orientation; CNT—control.

mean cohesion ($t[32\ df] = 2.2$, $p = 0.034$) and independence ($t[32\ df] = 2.4$, $p = 0.021$) scores than those that were asymptomatic.

The mean FES profiles of the completing families with members symptomatic on the CES-D were significantly different in five respects from those of the completing families with no members symptomatic on the CES-D. The symptomatic had significantly lower mean cohesion ($t[32\ df] = 4.2$, $p < 0.001$), expressiveness ($t[32\ df] = 2.6$, $p = 0.014$), intellectual-cultural orientation ($t[32\ df]\ 2.5$, $p = 0.019$), and moral-religious emphasis ($t[32\ df] = 3.1$, $p = 0.004$) subscale scores and a higher mean incongruence ($t[32\ df] = -3.4$, $p = 0.002$) score than the families with no members symptomatic on the CES-D. Also, the completing families whose members reported depressive symptomatology had a significantly lower mean cohesion score ($t[32\ df] = 3.9$, $p < 0.001$) and a significantly higher conflict ($t[32\ df] = -2.2$, $p = 0.036$) score than the asymptomatic families.

Even though the numbers of families in the various specific syndrome groups were small, the symptomatic families generally tended to have lower cohesion and expressiveness and higher family incongruence scores than the asymptomatic. Finding that the families with one or more members reporting depressive symptomatology problems had high conflict scores is in accord with results of other investigations and clinical experience. The often divisive effects of a symptomatic person on the family are shown by the high family incongruence scores in instances of depressive symptoms and/or alcohol-related problems. Such findings indicate that differences between symptomatic and asymptomatic families and even between those with various syndromes are associated with the family environment. But data from a larger study are needed to ascertain the sequences involved (i.e., whether problems in the family environment precede, accompany, or are effects of the symptomatology).

Completing Families at Time 3

Symptom Status

There were some changes during the 15 months from Time 1 to Time 3 in the symptom status of the 34 families that completed the study. At Time 3, more of the families (19, or 56%) were asymptomatic and fewer (15, or 44%) were symptomatic than at Time 1, when there were 17 (50%) asymptomatic and 17 (50%) symptomatic families. At Time 3, in the 15 symptomatic families, 4 (33%) of the 12 participating husbands/fathers were symptomatic, as were 6 (40%) of the 15 wives/mothers, 2 (50%) of the 4 adult sons, both (100%) of the 2 adult daughters and 6 (50%) of the 12 young children (twice as many girls as boys).

In 10 of the 15 symptomatic families, one member was symptomatic; in the others, two or more members were symptomatic. In the 10 with one symptomatic member, there were 26 participating members, of whom 10 (39%) were symptomatic. In 7 (70%) families, the symptomatic member was a parent (4 fathers and 3 mothers), and in the remaining 3 (30%) families, the symptomatic member was a child (1 adult son and 2 young daughters). Thus, the 10 symptomatic members were 4 (57%) of the 7 participating husbands/fathers, 3 (30%) of the 10 wives/mothers, none of the adult sons but 1 (25%) of the 4 young sons, and both (100%) of the 2 adult daughters but none of the younger daughters.

In the 5 families with two or more symptomatic members, there were 19 participating members, of whom 10 (53%) were symptomatic. They were 3 (60%) of the 5 mothers, 2 (67%) of the 3 adult sons, 1 (50%) of the 4 young sons, and all 4 (100%) of the young daughters; none of the fathers was symptomatic, and there were no adult daughters. In 3 (60%) of those 5 families, the symptomatic members were the mothers and children (2 adult sons and 1 young child). In the other 2 (40%) families, only the young children were symptomatic. All 5 of the families with two or more symptomatic members also had asymptomatic members—all 5 of the fathers, 2 of the 5 mothers, 1 of the 3 adult sons, and 1 of the 2 young sons.

At Time 3, the adult and young daughters were the family members most often symptomatic, the adult daughters for current distress (CES-D and depression) and the young daughters for the child symptom assessments. Parents were most often symptomatic on the CES-D and/or reported depressive symptomatology. In accord with concepts of females tending to internalize distress, both the wives and daughters tended to be symptomatic on measures of current distress, especially dysphoria and depression.

Overall, the change toward reports of fewer symptoms at follow-up than at Time 1 has been found repeatedly in epidemiological studies. This regression toward the mean was reported even for the 1-year ECA follow-up interviews (Eaton et al., 1989).

Asymptomatic Versus Symptomatic Families

Although there were no statistically significant differences between the asymptomatic and symptomatic families' sociodemographic characteristics at Time 3, the symptomatic families tended to have heads who were somewhat less well educated and had smaller annual incomes (median $15,600 versus $24,000) than those of the asymptomatic families.

Also, the symptomatic families had less monthly disposable income (mean $145 versus $425) than the asymptomatic families.

The Time 3 symptomatic families' mean intrafamilial stress theme rating (−0.8), was more negative than the asymptomatic group's rating (−0.2), but the difference was not statistically significant. The symptomatic families' mean other-relatives stress theme rating (−1.3) was significantly larger and more negative, however, than the asymptomatic families' positive comparable rating (0.3, $t[23\ df] = 3.0$, $p = 0.006$). There were no significant differences in the two groups' mean friends stress theme ratings.

The stress found often in symptomatic families, especially those with low incomes, thus was both intrafamilial and the result of other relatives' illnesses and interpersonal and financial problems. Those external stressors often compounded the family's problems and also indicated that the social support that members outside the immediate family might supply can be burdensome rather than salutary.

Figure 5.8 presents the Time 3 asymptomatic and symptomatic families' FES profiles. The symptomatic families had significantly lower mean cohesion scores ($t[19\ df] = 2.6$, $p = 0.019$) and also lower mean expressiveness and higher mean incongruence scores than those that were asymptomatic.

Changes in Symptom Status Over Time

We divided the 34 completing families at both Time 1 and Time 3 into asymptomatic and symptomatic groups and are presenting the changes from Time 1 to Time 3 in the number of symptomatic families, the specific family members who were symptomatic, the measures on which they were symptomatic, and the combinations of symptomatic members and patterns of symptomatology we found.

At Time 1, 17 (50%) of the 34 families were asymptomatic, and 17 (50%) were symptomatic. At Time 3, 15 months later, a larger number (19, or 56%) were asymptomatic, and fewer (15, or 44%) were symptomatic. Also, at Time 1, there were 11 (62%) families in which one member was symptomatic and 6 (38%) in which two or more members were symptomatic, but at Time 3, 12 (80%) families had one symptomatic member and only 3 (20%) had two or more. There was little difference from Time 1 to Time 3, however, in the number of families with members symptomatic on more than one measure. At Time 1, of the 17 symptomatic families, 11 (65%) had members symptomatic on only one measure, and 6 (35%) had members symptomatic on two or more measures; at Time 3, of the 15 symptomatic families, 10 (67%) had members

OUR FAMILY STUDIES

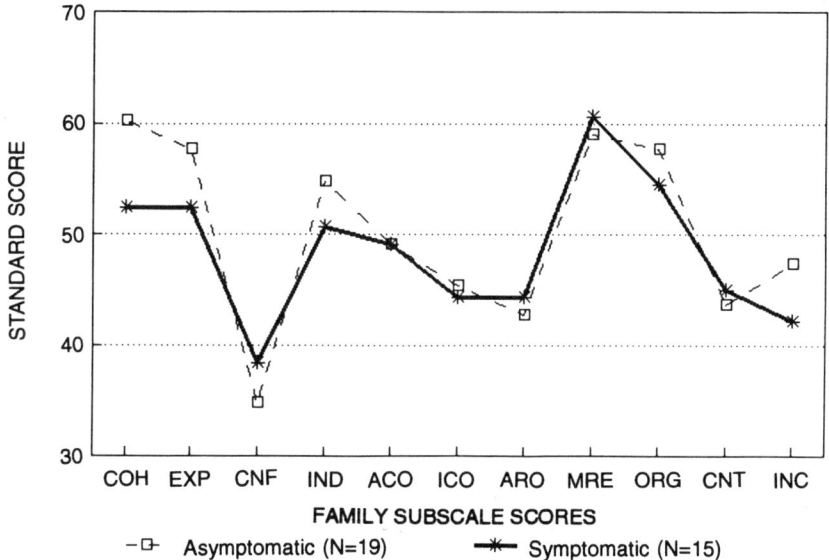

Figure 5.8. Time 3 Family Environment Scale profiles for asymptomatic and symptomatic families. *Key:* COH—cohesion; EXP—expression; MRE—moral-religious; CNF—conflict; ICO—intellectual-cultural; IND—independence; ORG—organization; ARO—active/recreational; ACO—achievement orientation; CNT—control.

symptomatic on one measure, and 5 (33%) had members who were symptomatic on two or more measures.

We classified the 34 completing families into four groups according to symptom status at Time 1 and at Time 3. There were 14 (41%) that were asymptomatic at both times (*healthy* or *asymptomatic* families), 12 (35%) that were symptomatic at both times (*chronic* families), 5 (15%) that were symptomatic at Time 1 but not at Time 3 (*remission* families), and 3 (9%) that were asymptomatic at Time 1 but symptomatic at Time 3 (*incidence* families). Thus, for the 15 months, the good health rate was 41%, the chronicity rate was 35%, the remission rate 15%, and the incidence rate 9%.

Asymptomatic Families

Of the 14 families that were asymptomatic at both times, 4 (29%) had children under age 16 at home; 1 (12%) was a couple in their 40s with an adult child at home; and 9 (64%) were "older" families (i.e., the couples were in their mid-50s or older), of whom 2 had adult children at home.

A typical asymptomatic family group consisted of a 58-year-old mother who was a nurse and her two adult daughters (ages 28 and 24), of whom one also was a nurse and the other a government clerk. They lived in the family home in an older middle-class neighborhood. The house was well kept, and the yard was immaculate. Although the three worked different shifts and were not together much, they cared for each other. Their independent functioning but emotional closeness were prominent features of their lives. The mother was proud of her daughters and of her two married sons, who lived in nearby cities.

Chronic Families

Of the 12 families that were symptomatic at both times, 5 (42%) had children under age 16 at home; 1 (8%) was a couple in their 30s without children; and 6 (50%) were older families, 4 of whom had adult children at home. In those 12 families, of the 24 symptomatic members, 7 (29%) were symptomatic only at Time 1, 5 (21%) were symptomatic only at Time 3, and 12 (50%) were symptomatic both times. The family members most likely to be symptomatic were the daughters; all of the adult and 80% of the younger daughters were symptomatic at both Time 1 and Time 3. Adult sons (67%) were the next largest group symptomatic at both times, followed by the fathers (50%), mothers (25%), and younger sons (0%).

Among the 12 families, there were 3 (25%) in which the same member was symptomatic at both times (one husband and two adult daughters). In 3 (25%) other families, the symptomatic member changed from Time 1 to Time 3. In one family, at Time 1 the wife was symptomatic, but at Time 3 she was asymptomatic and the husband was symptomatic. In the second, the wife was symptomatic at Time 1, but at Time 3 she was asymptomatic and the adult son was symptomatic. In the third, at Time 1 the adult daughter was symptomatic, but at Time 3 she was asymptomatic and her mother was symptomatic.

In 4 (33%) families, there were members who were symptomatic at both times and also members who were symptomatic at Time 1 only. In one family, the husband was symptomatic at both times and the wife at Time 1 only. In the second, the wife and young daughter were symptomatic at both times and the husband at Time 1 only. In the third, two young daughters were symptomatic at both times and the mother at Time 1 only. In the fourth, the mother and one adult son were symptomatic at both times and a second adult son at Time 1 only.

In the last 2 (17%) families, some members were symptomatic at both times and others symptomatic at Time 3 only. In one, a young daughter was symptomatic at both times and a young son at Time 3 only. In the other, an adult son was symptomatic at both times and his mother

OUR FAMILY STUDIES 279

One chronically symptomatic family consisted of a 73-year-old husband, his 63-year-old wife, and their two adult sons (ages 29 and 28). They lived in a single-family house in a lower-middle-class urban setting. The family had the home paid off; their income was from social security and retirement benefits. The husband had a nice-sized vegetable garden and a one-hole "golf course" with a flag in a can. He was hard of hearing and bothered by arthritis, but although he was retired, he stated that he would like to work if there was a job he could do. He had little education and tried to answer the questions "right"; he did not seem to mind that it took 3 hours to complete the interview. His wife was an English war bride who had raised seven children in the United States. She was overweight and had a history of alcohol and drug problems. The family stayed in touch with one another; on Sundays, all of the children were invited to the family dinner, which was served at noon. One son, who was homosexual, expressed concern about sexually transmitted diseases; the younger son, who was not married, talked a great deal about his girlfriends.

At Time 1, the wife was symptomatic for depression, panic, and phobia; the homosexual son for CES-D, depression, drugs, and alcohol; and the younger son for drugs and alcohol. At Time 3, the wife reported depressive symptomatology, and the younger son was symptomatic on the CES-D (but not for drugs and alcohol). When the family was asked why they participated, the wife said, "100 families picked out of the entire Louisville area—[we] thought it was important." Being chosen was meaningful to her, and she made her family participate.

At Time 3, the family was concerned about the 28-year-old, who had mangled his hands in an accident at work. He had not been able to return to work and was suing for compensation. The 29-year-old homosexual son had changed his sexual behavior because of worry about AIDS; he did not engage in sex as often as before and masturbated more often. The husband continued to be troubled by arthritis and hearing difficulties. The wife had completed therapy at a mental health clinic and had an improved outlook on the future.

Remission Families

All 5 of the families that were symptomatic at Time 1 but not at Time 3 had children under age 16 at home. One such family consisted of a 47-year-old husband, his 44-year-old wife, a 16-year-old daughter, a 14-year-old son, and an 11-year-old son. The husband, whose parents were immigrants, was authoritarian and definitely in charge of the family; he owned a small business and was concerned about getting enough work. The daughter, who would soon be leaving home to go to college, was the focus of family interest. The family was upwardly mobile and in transition. The members showed many of the stresses and strains between the father and the children typical of first-generation Americans. The mother, who was obese, seemed to be the mediator between the father and the children. At Time 3, the daughter was away at college, but the family had taken in a niece from France and thus "replaced" her. Although this family exhibited tensions often seen in immigrant families, symptomatology was minimal. At Time 1, the daughter was symptomatic on the CES-D, but no one was symptomatic at Time 3.

Incidence Families

Three families were asymptomatic at Time 1 but symptomatic at Time 3. One was a retired couple in their mid-60s with grown children with whom the parents stayed in close touch. The family had weathered many stressors: Between Time 1 and Time 3, the husband had become ill with back, stomach, and nervous problems, and at Time 3 he reported depressive symptomatology. The couple had an unusual genogram that included their deceased daughter's husband who had remarried, their grandchild by that union, and also the child of the former son-in-law and his new wife. They were concerned about the possibility that the former son-in-law and his wife would divorce and that the children, including the one who was not a relative by birth, would be adversely affected. Also, they worried about another son's grown unmarried daughter, who had lived with various men, and about their daughter, who had experienced a postpartum depression. We postulated that the close emotional involvement with their children enabled this couple to remain healthy, cheerful, and active, or that they had a plenitude of inner resources that sustained them. The husband volunteered that his wife had been kind when he had "felt so bad"; the interviewers saw the relationship between the husband and wife as becoming warmer.

The second family consisted of a father and mother, both age 34, an 11-year-old daughter, and a 3-year-old son. They were a well-functioning middle-class family. When we first met them, both parents were working, and the father was going to night school. The daughter, however, had been making poor grades, and as a consequence the mother had stopped working. The daughter's grades soon improved, and the whole family seemed to be happier and functioning better than when the mother was working. The maternal grandfather died shortly before our Time 3 interview, however, and both the mother and daughter had symptoms of unresolved grief. The mother was symptomatic on the CES-D.

The third family that was asymptomatic at Time 1 but symptomatic at Time 3 was a couple in their late 20s who had a comfortable, middle-class life-style. The husband was a seminary student, and the wife a teacher; both were ambitious, hardworking, and optimistic about the future but in conflict about when to have children. In the interval between Time 1 and Time 3, they sustained considerable stress: The husband's father died of cancer; the couple was apart for 6 months while he studied abroad; and the wife became pregnant. Also, the wife and her sister confronted their mother about their anger and unhappiness about how they had been raised. As a result, the wife's mother and father entered therapy in which the couple themselves occasionally participated, even though they had to travel to a distant state to do so. The wife saw herself as "healing."

At Time 3, they were delighted with their 4-month-old baby, although they were much less well off financially because the wife had taken unpaid maternity leave. She and her husband were in the throes of learning to parent and to share parenting. At Time 3, she was symptomatic on the CES-D. Although the couple had seemed to be functioning well and was asymptomatic at Time 1, each partner had unresolved childhood conflicts that, compounded by current stressors, produced the wife's depressive symptomatology; she did not have just the "baby blues." Even though she was markedly symptomatic, her prognosis was good. Both partners had definite personality strengths, and there was a solid bond between them.

Changes in Symptomatology and Symptom Patterns

In 3 (25%) of the families that were symptomatic at both times, when one family member became asymptomatic, another developed symptoms. This "ping-ponging," which is also seen in practice, was described by Jackson (1957); we thought it interesting to see it emerge in a community sample. Also, the distribution of symptoms among family members was in accord with the results of many epidemiological studies in that the wives tended more often than the husbands to be the symptomatic family members. Our consistent finding that many of the adult children in the families were symptomatic, however, has a new emphasis. Although epidemiological studies since our initial report (Schwab, Warheit, & Holzer, 1973) have reported that surprisingly large percentages of the young adult respondents were symptomatic compared to those in other age groups, our current finding that so many adult children in the parents' homes were symptomatic has, to the best of our knowledge, not yet been reported.

Analysis of the number of families symptomatic on the various measures at Time 1, at Time 3, and at both times showed that certain symptom patterns remained, developed, or cleared up. CES-D and depression were the symptom patterns that remained and/or developed over the 15-month period, whereas panic, phobia, and drug and alcohol problems tended to clear up.

Analyses of Symptoms and Stress Theme Ratings Over Time

We carried out an analysis of covariance (ANCOVA) to determine the effect of the families' Time 1 and Time 3 symptom status on their Time 3 mean intrafamilial stress theme rating; the Time 1 mean intrafamilial stress theme rating was the covariate. After allowing for the effects of the Time 1 rating, the main effects of the Time 1 and the Time 3 symptom statuses were not significant. Thus, the Time 1 intrafamilial stress theme rating was a more important predictor of the Time 3 rating than the families' symptom status at Time 1 or Time 3. There were too few cases to examine the change over time of the other-relatives and friends stress theme ratings.

To the best of our knowledge, the unfortunate consistency of the *intrafamilial* stress theme ratings from one time to another has not previously been reported in a study of family stress. Finding that the Time 1 stress theme ratings predicted the Time 3 ratings points to the continuing stress, usually complicated by symptoms, that affects some families.

Analyses of Symptoms and FES Subscale Scores

Although we found few changes in the families' FES profiles from Time 1 to Time 3, we carried out separate ANCOVAs to determine the effect of Time 1 and Time 3 symptom status on each of the Time 3 FES subscale scores and on the family incongruence score. The respective Time 1 FES subscale scores and family incongruence score were the covariates. After controlling for the Time 1 FES subscale scores, the main effects of Time 1 and Time 3 symptom status were not significant. Thus, the most powerful predictors of the families' Time 3 FES subscale scores were the Time 1 FES subscale scores, indicating that the family environment (healthful or deleterious) tends to be remarkably stable even as family members' symptoms of mental disorder continue, develop, or resolve over time.

Predicting Time 3 Symptom Status From Time 1 FES Subscale Scores

We used the Time 1 completing families' FES subscale scores in a stepwise discriminant function analysis to predict their Time 3 symptom status. A linear combination of the Time 1 cohesion, expressiveness, independence, moral-religious emphasis, organization, and control subscale scores correctly identified 79% of the Time 3 asymptomatic families and 87% of the Time 3 symptomatic families. At Time 3, 82% of all the families were correctly classified as either asymptomatic or symptomatic just by their Time 1 FES subscale scores.

The completing families' Time 1 FES subscale scores also were used in a stepwise logistical regression to predict Time 3 symptom status. The only variable to meet the stepwise criteria was the Time 1 cohesion subscale scores which correctly predicted 61.8% of the completing families' symptom status, but a larger percentage for the asymptomatic (73.7%) than the symptomatic (46.7%) families.

Such analyses indicate that the quality of the family environment is associated with symptomatology and can be predictive of symptom status over a 15-month period of time at a reasonable level of accuracy (i.e., more than 80% of the time). This finding from the discriminant analysis suggests that a healthful (normal) family environment is associated with a family's not being symptomatic and, conversely, that a family environment characterized by relatively low cohesion, expression, independence, and moral-religious emphasis is conducive to the onset of symptomatology. The effects of stressors and the combination of SLEs revealed by our stress themes need to be factored into such findings.

In the next chapter, we examine in detail the findings with regard to the children in the study; in later chapters, we discuss the meaning and implications of our results.

CHAPTER 6

The Younger and Adult Children

The plight of millions of children in the United States in the 1980s finally began to be acknowledged by government officials and politicians in the early 1990s as political candidates struggled with issues that could be used for political gain. Children have no voting power, and those that are in grievous distress too often are living with a disturbed, disadvantaged, or demoralized parent(s) who is/are so alienated that he/she/they do not vote. Consequently, the status and well-being of the children in our society have depended on shifting humanitarian sentiments and our national leaders' often fragile social consciences. The tragedy of children who are hungry, homeless, and/or ill-cared for (if not harmed) has stirred some advocates, who point to the sad statistics about the lack of well-being of children in America and hope that the 1990s will be the decade of our children.

In this chapter, we discuss the results of our study that apply to the families with children. We have divided the chapter into two parts because the interview schedule given to children under age 16 was different from that given to those age 16 and older. Thus, the first part deals with the younger children, and the second with the late adolescents and young adults.

YOUNGER CHILDREN

Sociodemographic Characteristics

At Time 1, there were 20 families with a total of 34 children under age 16, but inasmuch as 2 families with 2 (6%) children did not participate, we excluded them from these analyses. Thus, the sample analyzed 32 children under age 16 in 18 families. The mean number of children per family was 1.68; there were 13 girls (mean age 10 years) and 19 boys (mean age 7.9 years). Of the 32 children, 8 (25%) were less than 6 years old and not in school; 13 (41%) were in the first five grades; 5 (16%) were in the sixth through eighth grades, and 6 (19%) were in the ninth or tenth grades. The families ranged in size from 3 to 6 persons, with a mean size of 4.2 ($SD = 1.2$). There were two parents in 16 (89%) of the 18 families; the other 2 (11%) were single-parent families headed by the mothers. In many ways, the parents fit the general expectations of the norm (inasmuch as none of them was a teenager and we did not have elderly parents with young children), but there was a smaller proportion of single-parent families than the 19.7% in the United States in 1980 (World Almanac, 1990, p. 842).

Developmental Histories

To obtain the children's developmental histories, we asked the mothers about (a) any unusual problems encountered between ages 2 and 5; (b) concerns about the possibility of the child's being "slow" and/or consulting a physician about the child's development; and (c) holding the child back in school (e.g., to repeat kindergarten). At Time 1, the mothers in 7 different families reported that 7 (23%) of the 30 children (5 boys and 2 girls) between the ages of 2 and 15 had experienced unusual problems in their preschool years. But none of the parents consulted a doctor because of concern about the child's development possibly being somewhat slow, and only 1 child (a boy) had repeated kindergarten.

Thus, there were some concerns about the early development of about 25% of the children. This percentage is about the same as that for children seen clinically. Also, finding that only 1 child repeated kindergarten fits in with expectations for the population as a whole. We considered these children's developmental histories to be consistent with those in the general population.

Social Histories

For the 29 children over the age of 3, we obtained information about their social histories from the mothers' responses to four questions comparing their children to others of the same age: (a) how well the children got along with their brothers and sisters, (b) how well they behaved with their parents, (c) how well they were able to play and work by themselves, and (d) how well they were doing in school. Responses for the first three questions were "better," "about the same," or "worse," and for school performance, "above average," "average," or "below average."

The mothers reported that 6 (27%) of the 22 children with siblings were getting along better with their siblings than others their age, 14 (64%) were getting along about the same, and only 2 (9%) were getting along worse. Those in the last category were sisters, ages 7 and 14, who were living with their mother and her boyfriend; both of the girls were in treatment for various emotional and behavioral problems. Almost all of the children were having normal sibling relationships.

Only 2 (7%) children, in 2 different families, were reported as behaving worse with their parents than other same-age children. One was a 14-year-old boy who, along with his older sister, lived in a single-parent family. The mother, who was planning to remarry and move away from Louisville, expressed some ambivalence about the marriage and the move. Although we perceived that the boy's older sister was more reluctant than he to move away from her Louisville relatives and friends, the mother reported that the boy was behaving worse with her than other boys his age. The other child reported as behaving worse was a 14-year-old girl mentioned above who was not getting along well with her 7-year-old sister.

The question about how well a child plays or works by himself or herself is an age-related question; therefore, we asked the mothers to take the child's age and perceived maturity into account. All 18 mothers reported that their children played and worked by themselves as well as other children the same age.

In regard to how well the children were doing academically, of the 26 children who were attending school or preschool, 9 (35%) were reported by their mothers to be doing above-average work; 16 (62%) were doing average work; and only 1 (4%) was below average (the 14-year-old girl who was also having problems with her parents and younger sister and was in therapy).

We concluded from the limited data on the children's social histories that they were doing well; also, there were only slight gender differences. There were no relationships between the children's developmental and social histories and their families' symptomatic status.

Parents' Expectations and Values

We asked the parents in the 16 two-parent families about their expectations, values, and discipline of the children; 14 couples responded, as did 2 mothers whose husbands did not participate. Of the 14 couples, the parents agreed about expectations 71% of the time. This percentage of agreement is much higher than that usually seen in clinical populations of disturbed children and their families. In the few instances when the parents were not in agreement, the fathers had greater expectations of the children than the mothers.

Of the 16 mothers, 14 (88%) reported that they and their spouses shared the same values, and 2 (12%) reported that the values were somewhat shared. No mother reported that she and her husband did not share any values pertaining to their children. Of the 14 fathers, 12 (86%) agreed that they and their wives shared values; 1 (7%) reported that they agreed somewhat, and 1 (7%) reported no parental agreement. Thus, there was remarkable agreement on values between the parents.

We regard shared parental values, like expectations, to be important determinants of healthy child development. When there is parental conflict about values, children tend not to do well because of the resulting inconsistencies in child rearing. We found no relationship between parental and/or child symptom status and the parents' sharing or not sharing of expectations and values.

Parental Discipline

We asked each parent about differences between them regarding discipline of the children. Of the 16 mothers, 13 (81%) reported that they agreed with their spouses on discipline, 2 (13%) that they were stricter, and another 1 (6%) that the husband was stricter. But of the 14 fathers only 8 (57%) reported agreement with their spouses; 3 (21%) reported that they were stricter, and another 3 (21%) that the spouse was stricter. Of the 14 couples, 8 (57%) agreed on discipline; in 3 (21%) couples both spouses reported that the husband was stricter, and 3 (21%) other couples disagreed about who was stricter. Thus, about 40% of the couples disagreed on disciplining the children. Although we commonly see differences in clinical populations between parents about disciplining the children, we were surprised to find this much disagreement in a nonclinical population.

In regard to punishment, 13 (72%) of the 18 mothers reported that they had punished their children during the past week, and 5 (28%) that they had not. Of the 14 fathers, 5 (36%) had disciplined their children during the past week, and 9 (64%) had not. The mothers tended to be the disciplinarians much more often than fathers, but the parents agreed that the fathers were stricter than the mothers.

Reasons for Punishment

Each parent was asked independently to name three things for which the children were punished; mothers reported five times as many reasons for punishing the children than fathers. The reasons mentioned most often by the mothers were not following rules, not doing what was expected, talking back, not doing homework, and destructive behavior. The fathers reported the same reasons for punishment; thus, there was a healthy consistency between the parents about the reasons for punishing their children. We found no relationships between the discipline and punishment of the children and parental and/or child symptom status.

The age-old child rearing axioms seemed to apply: Obey the rules; do what your mother and father say; work; and get your destructive impulses toward people and property under control. But it appears that the burdens of child rearing were being borne mainly by the mothers, who generally spend much more time with the children than do the fathers and thus observe the children's infractions of rules and regulations.

Types of Punishment

The mothers reported that the four most common punishments meted out to their children were sending them to their rooms, verbal reprimands, paddling or spanking, and restriction of privileges. Fathers named the same punishments, but did not mention spanking. It appears that the recommendations of modern child development specialists have been followed in that physical punishment was not first on the list.

Time Spent With Children

In response to questions about the amount of time they spent with their children and how satisfied they were with that amount, of the 18 mothers, 6 (33%) reporting spending "quite a lot" of time, 9 (50%) a moderate amount, and 3 (17%) spent relatively little. Of the 14 fathers, 2 (14.2%) spent quite a lot of time with their children, 8 (57%) spent a moderate amount, and 4 (29%) relatively little. Of the 18 mothers, 11 (61%) were satisfied or very satisfied with the amount of time they spent with their children, 5 (28%) were somewhat satisfied, and 2 (11%) were very unsatisfied. Of the 14 fathers, however, only 3 (21%) were satisfied or very satisfied, 3 (21%) were somewhat satisfied, and 8 (57%) were dissatisfied.

The fathers' reports of not spending enough time with their children are not surprising in light of the emphasis in recent years on the importance of fathers devoting time and care to their children. But we did not anticipate that so many of the mothers would report being satisfied with the amount of time spent with their children in view of the widespread publicity about increasing numbers of latch-key children and also concern about child abuse in day care centers.

Parental concern about the mother's working outside the home is illustrated by the following vignette. When we interviewed her family at Time 1, the mother of an 11-year-old daughter and 2-year-old son had taken a job outside the home to increase the family income. We found evidence of emotional distress, and the daughter's grades were dropping. A few months later, the parents agreed that the mother should give up her job and that they should adjust to a smaller family income, because too much responsibility for the care of the 2-year-old was being placed on the daughter. At Time 3, the family showed no evidence of emotional distress.

What Parents Did With Children

In response to questions about the three things they did most often with their children during the week prior to the interview, the mothers reported many more items than the fathers. Both the mothers and fathers, however, reported the same broad categories of activities: eating together, playing and working together, helping with homework, chauffeuring, sharing interests and leisure pursuits, shopping, and spiritual activities. The mothers' and fathers' specific activities varied somewhat in accord with traditional male-female parental roles. Also, the mothers tended to take part in more shared activities with the children (e.g., helping with school projects or piano practice) than the fathers, who often were only spectators at the children's school functions, sports events, and recitals. Thus, the families reported that they did what ordinary middle-class families usually do, namely, eat together, spend both working and leisure time together, share interests, shop, and go to church together.

Symptomatic Status

Child Behavior Check List

At Time 1, 18 mothers completed the Child Behavior Check List (CBCL, Achenbach & Edelbrock, 1983) for each of their 29 children between the ages of 4 and 15 (3 children were below the minimum age). The CBCL is a list of children's and adolescents' common symptoms that have been divided into "internalizing" and "externalizing" groups. These symptom groups are subdivided into eight symptom clusters: The internalizing clusters are anxious/obsessive, somatic, schizoid, and depressed/withdrawal symptoms, and the externalizing clusters are immature/hyperactivity, delinquency, aggression, and cruelty.

Inasmuch as the number of children was small and none had sufficient symptoms to be identified according to the eight symptom clusters, we did a simple symptom count for each child. Of the 29 children, the 5 (17%) that had 30 or more symptoms were considered to be symptomatic. These children were members of three families; in two families, 2 children in the same family were symptomatic, and in the third family, the only child was symptomatic. Four (80%) of the 5 were girls, 2 of whom were school-age and 2 teenage; the 1 (20%) boy was a teenager.

Our finding two families in which more than one child was symptomatic, unfortunately, is not unusual. Having two or more children symptomatic in a family suggests serious parental problems and that the family is dysfunctional. Such families often have multiple problems, and a parent(s) as well as the children may be symptomatic. In the families in which the two children were symptomatic on the CBCL, one mother was symptomatic for depression and panic, and the other mother was asymptomatic; both fathers were asymptomatic. In the family in which the only child was symptomatic on the CBCL, both parents were symptomatic—the mother on the CES-D and for panic, and the father for alcohol problems. Thus, in two of the three families with symptomatic children, a parent(s) also was symptomatic.

DISC Ratings

To supplement the information gathered from the parents about their children with data from another source, a senior child and adolescent psychiatrist (who was blinded to other family data) evaluated all of the Diagnostic Interview Schedules for Children (DISC, Costello et al., 1984) that had been administered to the children aged 6 to 15 at both Time 1 and Time 3. The version of the DISC that we used was lengthy and covered a wide range of emotional and behavioral problems; cutting scores had not been established. The evaluations fell into four categories: positive mental health (e.g., a child who was mature emotionally and socially, intelligent and accomplished, had excellent interpersonal skills, possessed better than average coping and problem-solving skills, had a reasonably stable value system, and had good impulse control), normal (e.g., a child with no problems but who was not outstanding, endorsed age-appropriate concerns about school and friends, had mood swings and some performance anxiety, and had mild but no significant problems with authority), at risk (e.g., a child who did not have enough symptoms to warrant being given a diagnosis, but who would bear watching), and definite psychopathology (e.g., a child who endorsed sufficiently severe symptoms to be in need of therapy).

At Time 1, 24 of the 32 children in 17 of 18 families met the age criteria (6 to 15 years) to be given the DISC. Of those 24, 1 (4%) was rated as having positive mental health, 13 (54%) as normal, 3 (12%) as at risk, and 7 (29%) as being in need of treatment. The one with positive mental health was a 14-year-old boy; the three other groups did not differ much by age or gender. The 29% rated as having definite psychopathology is a higher percentage than that in the Institute of Medicine (1990) report, in which 12% of all children and 20% of those in poverty and in urban settings had diagnosable mental disorders. Rater bias is a possible explanation for the finding that 29% of the young persons showed definite psychopathology, but it is unlikely inasmuch as the rater had worked for more than 30 years with children and adolescents who had definite and often extremely serious psychopathology. Bias thus would be expected to be in the opposite direction (i.e., toward regarding the community sample children's complaints as minor).

Of the 24 children for whom we had both the CBCL scores and the psychiatrist's DISC ratings, in 16 (67%) cases there was agreement, and in 8 (33%) there was disagreement. In those 8, the mothers of 3 (38%) children reported them to be symptomatic on the CBCL, but the psychiatrist rated their DISCs as showing no psychopathology. In the other 5 (63%), the mothers placed their children in the normal range on the CBCL, whereas the psychiatrist saw evidence of psychopathology on the DISC. Such disagreement between the results of the mothers' reports on the CBCL and the DISC ratings is consistent with clinical and research experiences. Many parents tend not to see their children's distress, or the children may tend to conceal emotional distress from their parents unless asked specifically about problems and feelings. Of course, sometimes parents tend to do just the opposite, seeing their children as more disturbed than they really are (probably because they project some of their own distress onto them). Other common reasons for large discrepancies between parents' and children's symptom reports are a child's denial of distress or his or her difficulty understanding the questions on semistructured instruments. Child psychiatrist researchers emphasize the importance of obtaining information about children from the child and either a parent or a teacher, and preferably from all three sources.

Thus, at Time 1, of the 30 participating children (2 children were below the minimum age), 20 (67%) were asymptomatic and 10 (33%) were symptomatic. Of those 10, 3 (30%) were symptomatic on the CBCL only, 5 (50%) had DISC ratings of psychopathology, and 2 (20%) were symptomatic on both the CBCL and DISC ratings. The symptom pictures varied, but most of the children had anxiety, phobic, and/or depressive symptoms and presented the "mixed neurotic" picture that is not unusual in childhood. One child had a definite learning problem, and another was oppositional and also had attention-deficit disorder.

Dropout Families

After Time 1, 3 of the 18 families—with 7 of the 32 young children—dropped out of the study. Of those 7 children, 4 (57%) were symptomatic; 2 children in one family reached symptomatic status on the CBCL, and 1 child in each of the two other families had DISC ratings of psychopathology. One of the three dropout families illustrates the discrepancy between a mother's report of symptomatology on the CBCL and a DISC rating of no psychopathology. The family consisted of a 36-year-old single mother and her two children, a 15-year-old daughter and a 14-year-old son. The family dropped out after Time 1 because the mother remarried and they moved from the area, but they stated that they had wanted to continue in the study. The mother reported over 30 symptoms for both of the children; however, the child psychiatrist's reviews of the children's responses to the DISC items led to his rating them as normal; in fact, he viewed the 14-year-old boy as "super normal." It appeared that the mother, who was asymptomatic, had responded positively to the CBCL items about the children's symptoms because she was admittedly ambivalent about the upcoming marriage and move away from Louisville, where they had a large extended family and friends. We conjectured that she projected her ambivalence and anxieties onto the children, who also were reluctant to move.

The second dropout family consisted of a couple and their four sons (the father and one son did not participate). In addition to the young son being symptomatic, the mother was symptomatic on the CES-D, an adult son reported depressive and panic symptomatology and also had drug and alcohol problems, and the other adult son had alcohol problems. Thus, all three of the participating children—two adult children and one young child—were symptomatic.

The third family was a symptomatic family consisting of a black 34-year-old mother and her five children (ages 16, 15, 13, 6, and 4). The parents had separated so that the family would be eligible for welfare benefits. The mother was symptomatic on the CES-D and also had depressive and panic symptomatology. The 16-year-old son was symptomatic on the CES-D; soon after our Time 1 interviews, he was taken from the home by the courts because of truancy and behavior problems in school and placed in a children's home. The 15-year-old daughter, who was "slow," was in special classes, and the 13-year-old son's DISC showed psychopathology. (This family was described in greater detail in Chapter 5.) The poignancy of such family situations is heightened by our realizing that in the 1980s, we were living in a society that demanded so much of its poor and disadvantaged that parents had to separate in order to obtain welfare benefits for their children. The antifamilism of the 1980s exacted a terrible toll on the poor and the politically weak.

Completing Families

Time 1 Status. Fifteen families with 25 children under age 16 completed the study. At Time 1, 6 (24%) children in 5 (33%) of the families that completed the study were symptomatic. Of the 6, 1 was symptomatic on the CBCL only, 3 had DISC ratings of psychopathology, and 2 were symptomatic on the CBCL and also had DISCs rated as showing psychopathology. There were no age and gender differences in the symptomatic children.

In 2 (40%) of the 5 families, the child was the only symptomatic person. One of those families consisted of a couple and their 15-year-old symptomatic daughter, who was the youngest of six children and the only one at home. The other family consisted of a couple and their three children (aged 10, 8, and 5). The father of this family was deeply religious and described himself as a Christian who practiced daily family devotions at home and believed that all activity was directed by God. The 10-year-old symptomatic daughter had a learning disability, anxiety symptoms, some fears and worries, and showed obsessive traits; it is possible that she had an attention-deficit disorder as well. The two younger children were asymptomatic.

In the remaining 3 (60%) families with a symptomatic child or children, other family members also were symptomatic. One family consisted of a couple and their 9-year-old son. The mother, who had been having anxiety attacks since her teens, reported panic symptomatology, and the son was rated as having anxiety and phobic symptoms. The second family consisted of a 32-year-old mother, her 33-year-old live-in partner, and her two daughters, aged 14 and 7. The daughters had such acting-out problems as not getting along with one another and school problems; also, the 14-year-old ran away twice in a 6-month period. The mother reported that she felt trapped and wanted to get out of the relationship with her live-in partner, but could not afford to do so because she was going to school in the evenings and working at a low-paying job during the day. The live-in partner, who was more committed to the relationship, had a fairly well-paying job and contributed significantly to the household expenses. At Time 1, the mother was symptomatic on the CES-D and reported depressive symptoms; both daughters were symptomatic on the CBCL, and the younger child's DISC was rated as showing psychopathology. At Time 3, both daughters were symptomatic on both the CBCL and their DISC ratings. The third family consisted of a couple and their 8-year-old daughter. The mother had depressive symptoms and also numerous fears and worries about the child's safety; the daughter expressed many of the same anxieties and fears. In addition, the father had alcohol problems. Thus, all three of the family members were symptomatic—the mother with depressive symptomatology, the daughter with many symptoms on the CBCL and a DISC rating of psychopathology, and the father with alcohol problems.

Time 3 Status. At Time 3, there were 6 (24%) symptomatic children in 4 (27%) of the 15 completing families with children under age 16. Of the 6 children, 1 (17%) was symptomatic only on the CBCL, 3 (50%) had DISC ratings of psychopathology, and the other 2 (33%) were symptomatic both on the CBCL and the DISC rating. These percentages are just about the same as those at Time 1, and as at that time, there were no gender or age differences in the children with symptomatology.

In 3 of the 4 families, the only symptomatic members were the child or children. In the fourth family, both the mother and her young daughter were symptomatic. At Time 1, all 4 families had been symptomatic, but the members who were symptomatic changed from Time 1 to Time 3.

Time 1 and Time 3 Comparisons. We divided the 15 families with young children into four groups: the 4 (27%) families that were asymptomatic at both Time 1 and Time 3, the 5 (33%) that were symptomatic at both times, the 5 (33%) that changed from being symptomatic at Time 1 to being asymptomatic at Time 3; and the 1 (7%) that was asymptomatic at Time 1 but symptomatic at Time 3. The first group—families that were asymptomatic at both times—contained 6 children. These were child-oriented families, and the members were strongly familistic. The parents had struggled and sacrificed to provide a meaningful family life and future for the children.

One such family consisted of a couple and their 8-year-old son. The father had been laid off from work and had taken a lower-paying job. He worked during the day and was home in the evening, whereas the mother, who was a nurse, worked the evening shift. The parents had arranged their schedules so that one of them was always with the son. A second family consisted of a couple and their 12-year-old son. The father was a computer programmer, and the mother a homemaker who made stained-glass art. Both parents centered a great deal of attention on their son. The third family consisted of an upwardly mobile black couple, their two children, and the wife's son by an earlier marriage. The father was unemployed at the time of the first interview, but subsequently found a job; the mother worked two jobs. The parents cared deeply for the children; they agreed to participate in the study because the mother was "curious." It was the only black family to complete the study. The fourth family consisted of a couple and their four children (ages 22 to 15); only two of the children participated, because the other two were away at college. The big event for this family was the 22-year-old daughter's marriage, which took place shortly after we interviewed them the first time. After she married, the 15-year-old daughter was the only child at home. Family life revolved around the children, who were intelligent, motivated, and independent. The parents sacrificed to send them to college; the father worked two jobs, and the mother was the homemaker.

In the second group, the 5 families symptomatic at both Time 1 and Time 3, there were 10 children. In one of those families, the parents and 1 of the 3 children were asymptomatic at both times, but the second child was symptomatic at both Time 1 and Time 3, and the third was symptomatic at Time 3 only. In another family, the mother and the only child were symptomatic both times, but the father was symptomatic only at Time 1. In another two families, the mothers were symptomatic at Time 1 but not at Time 3. In one of them, 1 of the 3 children was asymptomatic at Time 1 but symptomatic at Time 3, and the other children were asymptomatic both times; in the other family, the 2 children were symptomatic at both times, and the mother's boyfriend was asymptomatic. In the fifth family, the father was asymptomatic at both times, and the mother was asymptomatic at Time 1 but symptomatic at Time 3; their child was symptomatic at Time 1 but not at Time 3. In these families, the predominant parental pathology was maternal depression; the children had mainly anxiety, fears, and depressive symptoms.

The following vignette illustrates some of a typical symptomatic family's problems. The family consisted of a couple (both age 26) and their three sons (ages 6, 4, and 1). The husband did not participate in the study because his job required him to travel 4 days per week. In view of her husband's work schedule, the wife had practically all of the responsibility for the household and the children; at Time 1, she reported depressive symptomatology. The oldest child had school problems between Time 1 and Time 3; the teacher reported that he was hyperactive and causing trouble in class and that she did not know what to do with him. The mother was upset, but she discovered by talking to other parents that their own children were receiving the same reports. Apparently the teacher was pregnant, not feeling well, and not in control of the class. After the teacher took maternity leave, the child was happier in school, although he still had many worries and anxieties. The two younger children were asymptomatic at Time 1 and Time 3. At Time 3, the 6-year-old son's DISC showed evidence of psychopathology; the mother was asymptomatic.

In the third group, which consisted of the 5 (33%) families that changed from symptomatic status at Time 1 to asymptomatic status at Time 3, there were 7 children. In three of these families, only the parent(s) had been symptomatic at Time 1. In the fourth family, the symptomatic member had been an adult daughter, age 16; her two younger siblings were asymptomatic. In the fifth family, both the mother and the child had been symptomatic. This family, consisting of a couple in their 30s and their 9-year-old son, was typical in many ways of the families in the group. The parents were mainly the family members with symptomatology, but no single symptom pattern predominated. The father was a schoolteacher who was suffering from burnout but was not severely symptomatic. The mother had a history of chronic physical symptoms and had suffered anxiety attacks since her teens. At Time 1, she reported panic symptomatology, and the son was rated as having anxiety and phobic anxiety. At Time 1, the mother had just been laid off from her job; however, this did not seem to be upsetting to her because it allowed her to spend more time with her hobby, which was ceramics. The son, an only child, was a high achiever in school. The family began spending more time together and sharing household duties, and at Time 3, all 3 members were asymptomatic.

The fourth group, which was asymptomatic at Time 1 but symptomatic at Time 3, consisted of only 1 family with 2 children. The maternal grandfather had died about a month before the Time 3 interview, and both the mother and one of the two children were having grief reactions. The mother's symptoms were severe.

At both Time 1 and Time 3, in 5 families, we had CBCL reports and DISC psychopathology ratings for 2 siblings. One family was asymptomatic at both times. In the second, the 16-year-old daughter reported symptomatology at Time 1 but not at Time 3; the parents and two younger siblings were asymptomatic at both times. In the third family, the symptomatology shifted from one sibling at Time 1 to the other at Time 3; the parents were asymptomatic at both times. In the fourth family, both siblings were symptomatic at both times, whereas the mother was symptomatic only at Time 1. In the fifth family, the mother was symptomatic at Time 1 but both children were asymptomatic; however, at Time 3, one child was symptomatic, and the mother and other child were asymptomatic.

Among such families as these five, it is not unusual to see one family member get better with or without treatment only to see that another develops symptoms, or that when the child's symptoms clear up, long-suppressed marital problems surface. Some of these families appear to need to maintain a pathological equilibrium. How to resolve such complex problems is a challenge to child and family psychiatrists, as well as other mental health workers.

Summary

We think that the findings about parental expectations, values, and discipline, coupled with the reports of what the parents did with their children, suggest a generally favorable but somewhat guarded outlook for the future of the children in this study. Although the parents' agreeing on expectations and values for their children is conducive to healthy growth and development, finding that only about 60% of the parental pairs agreed on discipline suggests some potential difficulties. In clinical populations, parental disagreements about discipline are associated with childhood psychopathology. But our finding that the mothers and fathers reported agreement on reasons for punishment, even though about 40% disagreed on other points about discipline, is a favorable indicator.

Although the fathers were stricter than the mothers, they disciplined less. Perhaps the fathers' spending less time with the children than the mothers explains this seeming contradiction; at least, it is an explanation frequently heard clinically. This finding is in accord with the advice given to parents in recent years to deal with the child's problem on the spot, rather than waiting until "Dad comes home." An equally valid alternative hypothesis is that it has been the mother's job to raise the children, including setting limits and disciplining them.

The fathers expressed dissatisfaction more often than the mothers about the amount of time they spent with their children. Although such reports run counter to the tradition that the mother raises the children and takes care of the home and the father "brings home the bacon," the data reflected the redefinition and sharing of parental roles that is being given so much attention. These redefinitions became prominent with the baby-boom generation and are consistent with the rapid social change following the historical events of this century (e.g., the world wars and the women's movement), as well as with the economic difficulties that have made it necessary for both parents to work outside the home to maintain a family.

The fathers and mothers reported that they were doing the things with their children that have always been done and we hope will continue. Sharing activities and the parents' serving as role models perpetuate the family as the most viable social unit yet developed for carrying on the necessary functions that preserve human life on this planet.

We do not know why we did not find associations between family/child symptomatic status and parental values, expectations, discipline, modes of punishment, or time spent with the children. It may be that our sample size was too small or, perhaps, our methods for studying these issues may have been too general to detect the more subtle points and associations. Those issues are important aspects of child rearing and in clinical situations are often seen as sources of intrafamilial conflict.

Our results support others' reports of considerable psychopathology in parents and their children that often is unrecognized and untreated. In fact, we found that 29% of the children and young adolescents had symptoms of emotional distress, usually the mixed "neurotic" anxiety and depressive syndromes often seen in children receiving mental health care. Also, symptomatology was more common in the children in the poorer and the single-parent families than in those living in middle-class circumstances and in the traditional husband/wife households. Also, living in a family in which there is mental illness either in a parent or a child is a mental health risk. Yet, parental psychopathology does not necessarily lead to psychopathology in the children.

OLDER ADOLESCENTS AND ADULT CHILDREN

In the early 1980s our interviewers were surprised to find so many "adults" living at home with their parents. Since then, the trend for adult children to remain or return home to live with their parents has become one of the phenomena of the 1980s. According to Glick (1988), as a result of the Great Depression, in 1940 the percentage of adult children living with their parents was high, but it dropped steadily to a low in 1960. Although it has not yet reached the 1940 level, there were more young adults living with their parents in the second half of the 1980s than in the 1960s. Some factors responsible for the increase in the 1980s were high unemployment rates, the later age of marriage, more frequent divorces (with difficulties in adjustment after divorce), and unwed parenthood. Concurrently, there has been a decline in the "proportion of young adults, especially males, who maintain their own homes as householders or as spouses of householders" (p. 869).

Economic, educational, and marital considerations seem to be the primary determinants of this kind of family structure. Yvonne Eaton (1991) noted that "young single men are living with their parents in record numbers according to a recently released 1990 Census Bureau study" (p. H1). Of young adults aged 25 to 34 years, 32% of single men were living with their parents, in contrast to only 20% of single women. Many young persons had returned home because of difficult economic times, later marriages, and their need to obtain more education. Living with their parents provided financial advantages and comforts that they could not afford on their own. After interviewing more than a dozen such families, Eaton (1991) reported that the sons who had returned home generally retained some degree of independence. Financial arrangements varied widely; some adult children paid no room and board, while others contributed $150 or more per month toward the household expenses. Many of the young adults described the advantages "of having Mom do their laundry, keep the house clean, and cook their meals" (p. H1).

According to social scientists at the University of Louisville, in the past, young persons often lived at home until they married, but with the increased prosperity after World War II, they began to leave home soon after finishing high school or college. "The issue is, you don't have the high paying jobs for those under 24 you once had" (Eaton, 1991, p. H6). Eaton cited authorities who reported that many young men also were living at home because men in our society are socialized to think that they need a woman or a mother and are insecure about making a home for themselves. In contrast, women seem to be able to form social support systems and make connections more easily than young men; also, young women today appear to be more open and to be much more willing to share living quarters with roommates than young men. Young women tend to feel "confined at home. . . . Mothers and fathers are much more overprotective of daughters than of sons" (p. H6).

Some parents reported that having their sons at home gave them a sense of security and enabled them to develop peer relationships with them. On the negative side, having adult sons at home interrupted the parents' privacy and their schedules, and everyone lost some autonomy. Many of the young adults reported that they would move out of the parental home after they had become better established financially. One 25-year-old son stated: "I'd like to move out, but I don't have enough stuff. . . . I'd rather buy the things I want than spend it on an apartment. I have a TV. I am still working on my compact disc collection" (Eaton, 1991, p. H6). Some of those who returned home were newly divorced and had lost a significant amount of their property in divorce settlements. Sometimes, adult children return home with their own small children; one mother stated that her returning son and his children, added to her children still at home, now made at total of seven. They were having many quarrels and hard feelings, and "we apologize a lot, but it's not bad" (p. H6).

Sociodemographic Characteristics

There were 29 adolescents and young adults age 16 or older (17 males and 12 females) living at home in 16 of our 43 families; finding more male than female adult children at home is in accord with Eaton's (1991) report. Of the 29 adolescents and young adults, 22 (76%) in 16 families participated in the study, but 7 (24%; 6 males and 1 female) did not—3 were at college, 1 lived on a farm some distance from Louisville, and 3 had schedule conflicts. Of the 22 participants, 19 (86%) were single, and 3 (14%) were divorced. One of the divorced individuals was a 38-year-old female; the others were both 32-year-old males whose children did not live with them.

There were two parents in only 9 (60%) of the 16 families with one or more adult children and/or teenagers living at home. Of those 9 families, 3 consisted of a couple and an adult child, 1 had two adult male children at home, and 1 had one parent and one adult child in two locations—the mother and daughter in the small family home in Louisville, and the father and son on a farm about 50 miles away. The remaining 4 families were couples with younger as well as adult children at home. The younger children ranged in age from 13 years to their early 20s; the older ones were still finishing school.

The family that lived apart consisted of a 52-year-old father, 52-year-old mother, 22-year-old son, and 23-year-old daughter. The family was symptomatic at both Time 1 and Time 3. At Time 1, the father and son lived on a farm about 50 miles from Louisville, and the mother and daughter lived in the city. The family had recently sold a small store in which all of them had worked; financially, however, they seemed to be having problems. At Time 1, the mother stated that she did not know what their income was and that no one was gainfully employed, but that they had some income from dividends, farming, and unemployment compensation. Her husband was an alcoholic and she attended Al-Anon, but her daughter did not say whether she herself attended any meetings. The mother liked the security of being married; her parents had separated when she was 11, and her father had been murdered. Perhaps for this reason, although she did not like the farm, at Time 3 she was living there; however, she returned to Louisville every month or so for a few days. The daughter, who was obese and had a slight speech defect, was the only symptomatic family member; she was symptomatic on the CES-D at both Time 1 and Time 3. She refused to move to the farm and maintained that the Louisville home would not be sold because she was living there. Also, she maintained that their family life was satisfying because they "stuck together."

The other 7 (44%) of the 16 families with adult children at home were single-parent families; 6 were headed by mothers, and 1 by a father. In 2 of them a single parent and the adult child lived together (a mother and daughter, and a father and son). In 3 others, a single-parent mother was living with two adult children. In the sixth, the single-parent mother was living with three adult children and two teenagers, and, in the seventh, the single-parent mother was living with her 16-year-old child and four younger children. Thus, the adult children and older adolescents lived in a variety of family types.

It appears that the parents' health or marital status was not a determinant of an adult child's staying or returning home. The adult children in our study were not at home to take care of their parents; the opposite was the case. They were home because of their own financial and/or marital problems, and they seemed to be wanting and getting care from their parents.

We grouped the 22 young adults into three categories. The first contained the 7 adolescents and young adults who were still in school or otherwise preparing for the future; 2 were daughters who were planning to be married in the next 6 months. The second group consisted of the 6 that we designated as experiencing "extended youth." They were somewhat older than the first group, and in the 1960s, would have already been living away from home, but during the 1980s they had stayed with their families. The third group contained 9 "returnees" who had left home at least once to be out in the world, but for a variety of reasons had returned to live with their parents.

Education

There were no gender differences in the adolescents and young adult children's educational attainments. Although the adult children generally tended to be better educated than their parents, it was disturbing to find that 2 of the females in the "preparing" group and 2 of the male returnees had not completed high school. Thus, 4 (18%) of the young people were, by any standards, poorly educated and were not in school. All 4 of them were symptomatic; 3 used drugs and 1 had phobic symptomatology. Generally, adults who have not completed defined educational stages tend more often to have symptoms of mental disorder than others.

Employment Status and Occupation

The current employment status of the older adolescents and young adult children in the three groups generally was not good. Of the 7 in the preparing group, 1 was unemployed, 1 was employed part-time, and 5 were students. Of the 6 in the extended-youth group, 1 was unemployed, 3 were employed part-time, 1 was employed full-time, and 1 was a student. Of the 9 returnees, 4 were unemployed, 1 was employed part-time, and 4 were employed full-time. Thus, of the 22 persons overall, 6 (27%) were students, another 6 (27%) were unemployed, 5 (23%) were employed part-time, and only 5 (23%) were employed full-time.

The occupational categories of the employed were as follows: professional or technical fields—3 persons, 1 of whom was a craftsperson; clerical work—4 persons; and laborers or housecleaners—3 persons. Of the 5 males with only a high school education or less, 2 were unemployed, 2 were employed, and 1 was still in school; of the 6 females, 2 were unemployed, 3 were employed, and 1 was still a student. Neither educational level nor employment status was related to age or gender.

Our interviewing was done at a time when Louisville was in the throes of the serious 1981-1984 recession. Many young people, particularly those who were not well-educated and were without skills, experienced economic difficulties, and many families could not afford to help their children meet educational expenses. Difficulty obtaining full-time employment and lack of funds for continuing their educations were major reasons why most of these adult children remained at home or returned to their parental homes.

Physical Health Status

As expected, these adult children were a physically healthy group of young adults. The exceptions were two sons in the returnee group who had been seriously hurt in accidents.

Feelings About Current Marital Status

Of the 22 adolescent and adult children, 19 (86%) were single and 3 (14%) divorced; 4 (18%) had lived with someone in the past as married, and 18 (82%) had not. Thus, most had never been married nor lived "as if married." The 18% who had lived as married is a larger percentage than those that had cohabited in their parents' generation. All the divorced and those who had lived in the past as married were in the returnee group.

We asked the adult children to list the three most important likes and dislikes of their current marital status. The single adults in all three groups (preparing for the future, extended youth, and returnees) listed personal freedom as the feature of their current marital state that they liked the most, followed by the ability to spend on themselves and the freedom to date. The singles in the preparing and extended-youth groups liked not having children and liked home life with their parents, while those in the returnee group reported liking the "freedom to be themselves." The divorced adult children also emphasized that they liked this freedom; we wondered whether they found marriage (with its commitments, sharing, and responsibilities) to be too difficult.

In response to the question about what they disliked about their current marital status, most of the adolescents and young adult children in all three groups reported nothing; they reiterated that they liked their current marital status and did not want to change it. A few in all three groups, however, reported a sense of loneliness and a desire for a secure relationship. The divorced adult children disliked most their inability to see their children. But there were no reports of unfulfilled sex, too much or too little responsibility, difficulty coping with children, or lack of help with the chores of living by those in any group.

It appears that individualism, not familism, is the order of the day for these single or divorced young adults who had never left home or had returned there. Freedom, being themselves, the ability to spend money on themselves, no responsibility for children, and dating were what the returnees liked. Thus, these young adults, both those who had stayed and those who had returned, appeared still to be in the process of "finding themselves" and remaining uncommitted while they explored the world of sexuality. In psychiatric jargon, they were still seeking narcissistic gratification and were continuing to be preoccupied with the normal developmental issues of adolescence, even though most of them were adults.

Time 1 Symptomatic Status

At Time 1, of the 22 adolescent and young adult children in the 16 families, 16 (73%) were symptomatic—9 (60%) males and 7 (40%) females. In the preparing-for-the-future group, there were 7 adolescents and young adults in 6 families; of them, 2 (28%) in 2 families were asymptomatic, but 5 (72%) in 4 families were symptomatic on one or more measures. Of the 5 who were symptomatic, 4 (80%, 3 females and 1 male) were symptomatic on one measure: 2 scored high on the CES-D, 1 had drug problems, and 1 had phobic symptomatology; 2 of the 3 females were sisters, and their brother in the returnee group also was symptomatic. The fifth person was a young male who was symptomatic on four measures (depressive and panic symptomatology and alcohol and drug problems); his younger brother in the extended-youth group also was symptomatic.

In the extended-youth group, there were 6 young adults in 5 families; 2 (33%) in 2 families were asymptomatic, but 4 (67%) in 4 families were symptomatic. (One family with two adult children is mentioned twice, because one adult child was symptomatic and the other was not.) Of the 4 individuals (3 daughters and 1 son) who were symptomatic, 3 (75%) were symptomatic on one measure: 1 on the CES-D, 1 with drug problems, and 1 with alcohol problems. The fourth person (25%) was symptomatic on two measures, the CES-D and phobic symptomatology.

In the returnee group, there were 9 adult children in 7 families; 2 (22%) in 1 family were asymptomatic, but 7 (78%) in 6 families were symptomatic. Of the 7 (6 sons and 1 daughter) who were symptomatic, 5 (72%) were symptomatic on one measure (1 on the CES-D, 1 had alcohol problems, and 3 had drug problems); 1 (14%) was symptomatic on two measures (alcohol and drugs); and another 1 (14%) on four measures (CES-D, depression, alcohol, and drugs).

We were surprised to find that such large percentages of these adolescents and adult children in all three groups were symptomatic—72% in the preparing group, 67% in the extended-youth group, and 78% in the returnee group. Inasmuch as those in the three groups were in different life stages, we anticipated that they would have different symptomatic rates. The similarity of these rates indicates, as reported by many epidemiological studies, that just being a young person in the United States at this time in history is associated with high risk for mental illness.

Of the 11 participating males, 9 (82%) were symptomatic, and of the 11 participating females, 7 (64%) were symptomatic. This 20% gender difference is similar to that found in child psychiatric populations and is strikingly different from that found in adult psychiatric populations (in which females outnumber males by a large margin, often at an almost 2:1 ratio). Depression symptoms were reported often by the young adults in the preparing and extended-youth groups, whereas significant drug and alcohol usage was reported often by those in the returnee group. The only report of panic was by a male who was in the preparing group; phobias were reported by two females (one in the preparing and one in the extended-youth group).

Of the 19 young persons who were single, 13 (68%) were symptomatic; all 3 of the divorced adult children were symptomatic. Almost all of the symptomatic adult children were either unemployed or working in a job that would be considered below their educational level; in contrast, those in the asymptomatic group did not show as great a discrepancy between educational level and employment status.

Downward social mobility—"drift" down the social scale following chronic and/or serious mental illness—has been documented in numerous epidemiological studies (Goldberg & Morrison, 1963; Myerson, 1940). But in the current sociocultural climate, in which so many young persons appear to be anomic, apathetic, and/or emotionally distressed, it is difficult to see this group as one that has already experienced such drift. They are not crippled by recurrent or progressive illness. It is possible that some of them are vulnerable persons who have been battered by the harshness of everyday life for those who are not advantaged; also, some may have been "damaged" by alcohol or drugs. Perhaps symptoms were a stress reaction to unemployment or to low-status jobs. Coupland (1991) described underachieving as being a feature of the young in the United States in 1990, especially the "Twentysomethings." Also, distinctive periodic and cohort effects are likely to be responsible in part for the high frequency of symptomatology in these young Americans.

Dropout Families

After Time 1, 7 of the 16 families, representing 10 of the 22 adolescent and young adult children, dropped out of the study. All 7 of the dropout families and all 10 of their adolescents and young adults were symptomatic. Table 6.1 shows the distribution of adolescent and young adult children in the dropout and completing families by group and symptomatic status.

In 3 (43%) of the 7 families, an adult child/children was the only symptomatic member. In one of these, the 32-year-old returnee son had alcohol problems. The family consisted of an elderly couple; the son had

Table 6.1
The Distribution of Adolescents and Young Adults in the Dropout and Completing Families by Group and Symptomatic Status at Time 1

	Dropout				Completers				Total			
	Asx		Sx		Asx		Sx		Asx		Sx	
	N	%	N	%	N	%	N	%	N	%	N	%
Preparing for the future	0	0	4	40	2	33	1	17	2	33	5	31
Extended youth	0	0	2	20	2	33	2	33	2	33	4	25
Returnee	0	0	4	40	2	33	3	50	2	33	7	44
Total		0		10		6		6		6		16

just been divorced and was living with his parents "temporarily." The father had become a nondrinking alcoholic after he had developed diabetes a few years earlier. This family dropped out of the study ostensibly because of the time involved and because it interfered with their work schedules. In another family, the daughter was symptomatic on the CES-D and also phobic. This black family consisted of a divorced mother and two of her six children who still lived at home; one of the two, an adult son, did not participate. The family broke appointments and then dropped out of the study because of work and schedule conflicts. In the third family, the returnee son and the two preparing-for-the-future daughters were symptomatic. The family consisted of a 51-year-old mother and her five children (ages 32, 19, 18, 16, and 15 years). The 32-year-old son had returned home after sustaining severe burns on his hands in an explosion. One of the younger daughters, age 19, was pregnant and unmarried. The family lived in poverty in a dark, roach-infested apartment. The mother was divorced and received Aid for Families with Dependent Children (AFDC) payments and food stamps. She was symptomatic. The three participating adult children also were symptomatic—the 32-year-old son and the 19-year-old daughter had drug problems, and the 18-year-old daughter had phobic symptomatology. The 15- and the 16-year-old children did not participate. The family seemed to be "plugged" into the welfare system; they knew how and when to apply for various benefits.

In the remaining 4 (57%) dropout families, both the adult children and other family members were symptomatic. In one family consisting of an elderly mother and her 38-year-old daughter, the mother was symptomatic on the CES-D and also reported depressive symptomatology, and the adult daughter was symptomatic on the CES-D. The daughter had been divorced about 1 year previously, had quit her job in the East, and had moved home to live with her mother. She wanted her mother to sell the home so that they could move to Florida; however, the mother did not want to move because her own mother, age 91, was still alive in a nursing home in Louisville. Their reasons for dropping out were that the study took too much time and that they might move; however, it seemed that they wanted to deny symptoms and avoid problems that probably would have been opened up for discussion.

The second symptomatic dropout family was an unusual black family consisting of a 57-year-old retired father and his 26-year-old returnee son. The father had raised all of his seven children alone after his wife had left when the children were small. He told how his wife drank excessively and sometimes was violent. He was an active Seventh-Day Adventist who was disappointed that his children did not go to church. A daughter, who was in the army, contributed to the family income; a son was in prison for possession and dealing in drugs. The son who was living at home was unemployed and had a police record for drugs. The father had depressive symptomatology, and the son had drug problems. When we contacted them for the Time 2 interview, the father was seriously ill with prostate cancer and declined to participate. Also, he said that his son had moved away and that he was alone.

The third family consisted of a mother and her five children (aged 16 to 4). She was symptomatic on the CES-D and also reported depressive and panic symptomatology. The 16-year-old son was symptomatic on the CES-D, and the 13-year-old son's DISC showed psychopathology. The mother and father had separated so that the family could receive AFDC help. The fourth family consisted of a couple and their four sons; the father and one of the sons did not participate. The mother was symptomatic on the CES-D; one adult son reported depression and panic symptomatology and had drug and alcohol problems, the other adult son had alcohol problems, and the 13-year-old son's DISC showed psychopathology.

As can be seen, the plight of these dropout families was distressing. They appeared to be overwhelmed by a mass of social pathologies and symptoms of mental disorder, as well as financial and other problems common among the disadvantaged. In such families, often their deprived (if not traumatic) childhoods and the relative absence of adolescence as a meaningful developmental stage lead to personality and other disturbances in early adult life and, too often, to poverty, alcohol, drugs, and the "cycles of disadvantage" described by Rutter and Madge (1976).

Completing Families

Nine families with 10 adolescents and young adults completed the study. Of the 10, there was 1 in the preparing group, 4 in the extended-youth group, and 5 in the returnee group. At Time 1, there had been two asymptomatic daughters in the preparing group who were married between Time 1 and Time 3 and moved from their parents' homes. At Time 1, of the 12 adolescents and young adults then in the study, 6 (50%) were symptomatic—1 (33%) in the preparing group, 2 (50%) in the extended-youth group, and 3 (60%) of the returnees. At Time 3, of the 10 adolescents and young adults remaining, 4 (40%) were symptomatic. The only adolescent daughter remaining in the preparing group was asymptomatic. The extended-youth group contained 4 young adults—2 (50%) asymptomatic sons and 2 (50%) symptomatic daughters, one on the CES-D and the other for depression). There were 5 young adults in the "returnee" group, of whom 3 (60%) were asymptomatic and 2 (40%) were symptomatic, one for drugs and the other on the CES-D.

Of the 10 adult children in the 7 families that completed the study, only 4 (40%) of the adult children in 2 families were asymptomatic at both Time 1 and Time 3. Four (40%) children in 4 families were symptomatic at both Time 1 and Time 3, and 2 (20%) children in 2 families were symptomatic at Time 1 but not at Time 3. (Our numbers show one extra family because in that family, one child was symptomatic only at Time 1, and the other was symptomatic at both times.) Thus, 6 (60%) of the 10 adult children who completed the study were symptomatic at Time 1, and 4 (40%) were symptomatic at Time 3.

In summary, the data on the symptomatic status of the adult children indicate that 73% of them (both dropouts and completers) were symptomatic at Time 1. Males outnumbered the females 9 to 7, and as expected, more of them had problems with drugs and alcohol than the females, who were more likely to be depressed. The symptomatic females tended more often than the males to be in the preparing group, and the symptomatic males were more often in the returnee group. The drug and alcohol usage was confined almost entirely to the adult children in the returnee group. These young adults' problems with drugs and alcohol are a troubling finding that portends ill for the future. Was substance abuse a major reason for their returning to their parental homes, or did their disturbed development make them vulnerable to drug and alcohol abuse? Of course, economic and other sociocultural factors, the antifamilism expressed by the political and other leaders in the 1980s, and the disregard for children's well-being all were contributory to their employment problems, emotional distress, drug use, and consequent return home.

Most of the adult children who were symptomatic at Time 1 were either unemployed or worked in jobs below their educational level. Finding that all 10 adult children in the 7 families that dropped out of the study after Time 1 were symptomatic suggests that those families were burdened by more problems and stressors than most families. Their adult children at home seem to have been an added stressor to an already badly strained family system.

Overall, the extent of symptomatology and alcohol/drug problems in adult children matches or exceeds the frighteningly high mental illness and substance abuse rates currently being reported for young persons in the United States. The high rate of symptomatology that we found showed that these young people were at least subclinical cases at high risk for definite mental illness. Some probably needed some degree of parental care.

Adult Children in the Home and the Family Environment Scale

To learn about possible differences in the perception of the family environment in families with adult children in the home, we first compared the FES profiles of the 16 families with adult children with those of the 27 families without adult children (Figure 6.1). The families with adult children had lower mean cohesion ($t[41\ df] = 2.0, p = 0.06$), expressiveness ($t[41\ df] = 2.0, p = 0.05$), and intellectual-cultural orientation ($t[41\ df] = 2.1, p = 0.04$) scores and also a higher mean incongruence ($t[38\ df] = -2.6, p = 0.01$) score than the families without adult children.

For each family with adult children, we calculated the mean dyadic differences within the family on each of the ten FES subscales and ranked them from the least (a rank of 1) to the greatest (a rank of 5) difference. The dyads were husband-wife, father-son, father-daughter, mother-son, mother-daughter, and adult child–adult child. The mother-daughter dyads had the lowest sum of ranks indicating that, overall, those dyads had the least disagreement across the 10 FES subscales. The dyads with increasingly larger levels of disagreement were the father-son, mother-son, husband-wife, and adult child–adult child dyads. Although we had only two father-daughter dyads, we included them for the sake of completeness; obviously, however, they are too few to be meaningful.

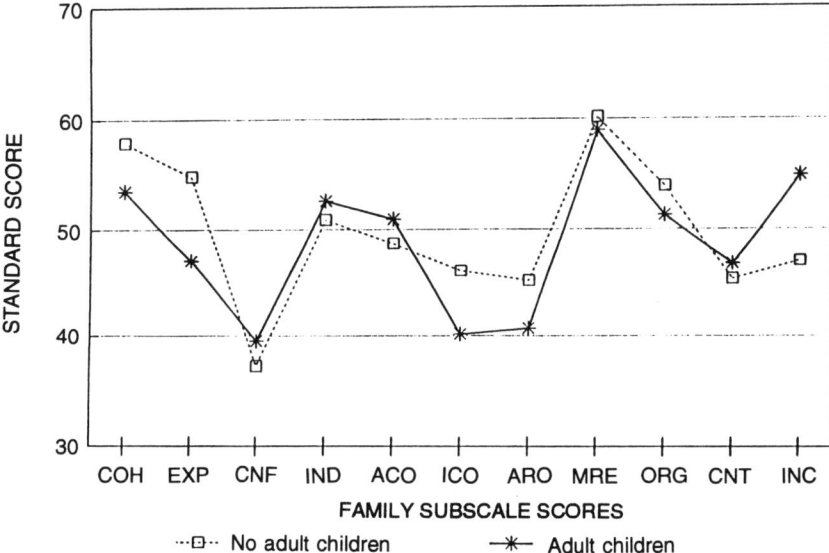

Figure 6.1. FES profiles of families with and without adult children. *Key:* COH—cohesion; EXP—expression; MRE—moral-religious; CNF—confict; ICO—intellectual-cultural; IND—independence; ORG—organization; ARO—active/recreational; ACO—achievement orientation; CNT—control.

The magnitude of the differences in the sum of ranks was greater than we anticipated, ranging from the least difference (mean 21.5) for the mother-daughter dyads to the most difference (34.5) for adult siblings. The husband-wife difference of 33.5, close to the greatest difference and near that of the adult child–adult child dyads, suggests parental disagreement that borders on "sibling rivalry" and has ominous implications. We were concerned about the possibility that the parents were being "split" by the adult child or children in the home and/or that the parents had grown apart; generally, older parents whose children have left home tend to report increasing satisfaction with their marriages and to prize their togetherness. Our husband-wife dyads had only slight differences on the conflict, independence, and especially cohesion subscale scores, indicating that some of their attachments were still firm; but their differences on the expressiveness, control, and achievement subscale scores may have reflected divided opinions about the adult children and, sadly, the likelihood that they could not talk to each other as meaningfully as they wished.

The low mother-daughter differences are in accord with many reports of closeness between mothers and their adult daughters that is conducive to the continuity of family traditions and values. That closeness can be a source of needed social stability in a society that is changing as rapidly as ours. We were surprised, however, to find smaller father-son than mother-son dyad differences. The father-son dyads' large differences on the conflict subscale scores smacked of Oedipal rivalry, but their differences on the organization, control, and expressiveness subscales were small. It is possible that those fathers and sons were developing meaningful adult, peerlike relationships.

In many ways, the mother-son dyads' relatively large differences may be good for all concerned in the long run. It appears that these adult sons were just not being "mama's boys"; thus, the seeming greater closeness to their fathers, despite conflict, may indicate continuing identification that is important for healthy development. We found it interesting that both the father-son and mother-son dyadic differences on independence had a midrange sum rank of 2.5, indicating less difference than the relatively high mother-daughter sum rank of 4.0 and the large but anticipated sibling-sibling sum rank differences of 5.0. The females having more discrepant independence scores than the males probably reflected women obtaining greater equality and independence than they had in the past. The extent of the differences between the adult sibling pairs was to be expected and probably was less deleterious than highly discrepant attitudes and perceptions of the home environment between the adults and the adult children would have been.

We think that these dyadic analyses are important. They have a potential for increasing researchers' and clinicians' understanding of families, and we urge others to use them.

Some Possible Individual and Family Reactions to Adult Children

We can only speculate about the young adult children's reactions to once more living in their parental homes. Such situations can be difficult for all concerned. Nevertheless, regression to a state of being cared for gives the returnee time to heal from the wounds suffered in the wider world. It can be a type of regression in the service of the ego described by Ernst Kris (1952), but such regression becomes pathological when the individual remains in a protected situation and does not make mature commitments to love and work. A person may like a narcissistically gratifying and dependent life without many responsibilities; however, in the long run its cost may be the forfeiture of a meaningful adulthood.

When adult children have stayed at home or are returnees, the parents are called upon to carry out tasks and take on responsibilities they thought had belonged to the past. Also, they are compelled once again to share resources, space, and time with the child, only now it is a grown child (by age at least) who should be able to fend for himself or herself. The changes in the home increase the parents' worries about the children and have an immense potential to produce resentments and to stress the family system as it attempts to adjust.

One possible attempt at adaptation is the returnee's trying to preempt the role of the same-sex parent. Although doing so can maintain the adult child's self-esteem temporarily, the parent could not help but be resentful and protest this recurrence of the Oedipal situation that had been played out twice before during the child's growth and development. Another troublesome problem is the returnee's defiance of the rules, values, habits, and standards of conduct expected in the parental home. A healthy adjustment would be for the returnee to assume an adult role in the family, sharing responsibility for family functioning and thus relieving his or her aging parents of some degree of care. That adjustment is the norm in societies in which extended family systems are functional.

The adult children had a great deal of symptomatology; whether this was responsible in part for their either not leaving or returning home is not known. Also, we do not know whether and how staying at or returning to the parental home is related to the development of psychopathology. In the dominant society, the nuclear family is expected to rear the children, who will then leave home and begin their own nuclear families. We are individualists, not familists. But if the current trend continues, we may need to develop a new kind of extended family, perhaps one based not on blood relationships but on shared goals, values, and interests as well as economic factors. Some experiments in the past with differing family structures have been reasonably successful, at least for short periods of time. In addition to the extended three- and four-generational families seen in such semi-isolated groups as some Eskimo communities, others have been short-lived experiences with communal living (e.g., the Oneida community) and still others have been tragic (e.g., Jonestown).

In the 1990s, the numbers of adult children staying or returning home are likely to increase greatly. In view of the extensive symptomatology we found, they and their families will need the attention of mental health professionals. It will be necessary to help them with their continuing personality development and to treat their emotional distress. Also, it will be necessary to help their parents maintain their own well-being while supporting the growth and development of their adult children.

CHAPTER 7

The Historical-Clinic Chart Study

BACKGROUND AND HISTORY OF THE CLINIC

Concern about the family throughout the century, culminating in the crisis in the family in the 1980s, prompted us to conduct a review of records of children seen at our Bingham Child Guidance Clinic since the early 1920s. We thought that information about the children's sociodemographic characteristics and presenting problems and about their families' (and especially their parents') problems over most of this century would enlarge our historical perspective and add a clinical component to our extensive literature reviews and epidemiological study. We were particularly interested in change in the family over time. Therefore, we reviewed a random sample of records of children seen at the clinic from 1923 to 1988 to determine possible changes in children's and families' presenting problems and in family factors that influenced the children over the greater part of this century.

The Bingham Child Guidance Clinic began in 1913 as a school for "atypical" children. A few years later, a psychological laboratory was added to diagnose and classify unusual children, whether gifted or retarded. In 1921 the school was incorporated as the Psychological Clinic of the Louisville Society of Mental Hygiene, and in 1931 it affiliated with the University of Louisville School of Medicine Department of Psychiatry. A child fellowship program and other educational programs were started, and in 1949 it became the Louisville Child Guidance Clinic. In

This chapter written with the assistance of Bingham Child Psychiatry Fellows Kris D. Houser, Lisa B. Graziano, and Katherine A. Raymer.

1958, the first family treatment program in the South was initiated in the clinic, which later was named in honor of a prominent citizen of Louisville who had generously funded research programs. At present, it is the child outpatient facility for the University of Louisville School of Medicine Child and Adolescent Psychiatry program.

STUDY SAMPLE

Inasmuch as it is the fourth oldest child guidance clinic in the United States, the Bingham clinic is a rich source of data. Reasonably complete records date back to 1922. We sampled the records at 5-year intervals that covered most of the significant historical periods from 1923 to the present, including the Roaring Twenties, the Great Depression, World War II, and the Vietnam era. For each of the 14 years (1923, 1928, . . . 1983, 1988) we tabulated the total number of cases seen in the clinic. We then used systematic sampling methods with a random start to identify 24 to 36 cases from each of the 5 years, for a total of 455 cases.

Although such records are an excellent data source and provide information that is not otherwise available, we are aware that they are secondary source data and that research with such data has limitations. The investigator has no control over the data collection and is limited by definitions and criteria that were used by others and may have changed over time. Also, often the records are incomplete because they were compiled by a number of persons who may at times have omitted such vital points as the subject's age, and the data usually lack uniformity. Despite these limitations, information from secondary source data has added significantly to knowledge about mental illness and, historically, supplies continuity with the past that can enlarge and deepen perspectives on various aspects of the human condition (in this instance, the family and mental illness).

STUDY PROTOCOL

Three child psychiatry residents were trained to review the charts that had been selected and to complete the data-gathering instrument that we had developed. It covered five major areas: (a) the child's sociodemographic characteristics (age, gender, race, and grade in school); (b) referral sources; (c) the child's family (with whom he or she lived, size of family, parents' marital status, age, education, occupation, employment status, number of siblings, family income, and religion); (d) the child's presenting problems; and (e) the family's problems.

RESULTS

The results of the historical-clinic study fall into three main areas—changes over time in the children's and their families' sociodemographic characteristics, the children's presenting problems, and their families' problems.

Sociodemographic Characteristics

There was a fairly stable 2:1 male-female ratio in the number of children coming to the clinic from 1923 until recently, when there has been a slight upward trend in female patients, especially those in early adolescence. This gender difference in the child psychiatry clinic patients is vastly different from that seen in most adult clinic populations, where females usually outnumber males by a 2:1 ratio.

Since the 1960s, a larger number of blacks have sought treatment at the clinic than in earlier years. That change probably is a result of such factors as busing, as well as the clinic's emphasis on serving the entire community. In the earlier decades, especially before 1950, more children were school dropouts than in recent decades. That change may reflect the clinic's special work with "atypical" children and its providing psychological testing services to schools, especially between 1920 and 1950. In addition, there have been changes in the number of years of schooling that are compulsory, and more rigorous enforcement of school attendance.

Since 1923, the average age of the children brought to the clinic for psychiatric care has changed from a high of 10 to 12 years in the 1920s and 1930s to a low of 6 to 8 years in the 1940s and 1950s. It rose again to 9 to 10 years of age in the 1960s and has climbed to 10 to 11 years in the 1980s. The relatively late age in the 1920s and 1930s probably reflects delayed recognition of children's problems, and the younger mean age in the familistic post–World War II era very likely was indicative of the greatly increased attention given to children and to principles of child rearing throughout our society. The later age during the 1960s and especially in the 1980s, unfortunately, can be attributed to the increased turmoil and family disruption that has been pervading our society. The instability and distress of recent decades have been accompanied by the disappearance of adolescence and the precocious maturity of latency-age children that Friedenberg (1964) wrote about in the 1950s. The increased number of older children being brought to the clinic in recent years thus appears to be a result of the family and societal confusion of the Vietnam and the antifamilistic Reagan-Bush eras.

Overall, mean family size declined from about 5.2 in 1923 to 4.1 in 1988. Although it dropped sharply (about 33.3%) in the depression years, it rose slowly during the late 1940s and 1950s to a peak of about 5.8 in 1968 and then declined quickly during the next two decades to a low of about 4.0 in the 1980s. Those changes reflect the brief familistic trend in the 1950s and early 1960s, followed by the sharply rising divorce rate in the late 1960s that persisted well into the 1980s.

Drastic changes over time have occurred in the children's biological parents' marital status. Since 1963, the percentage of children whose parents were married has shrunk from 74% in that year to 19% in 1988, and the percentage of never-married parents increased steadily from 3% in 1968 to 23% in 1988. As would be expected, the percentage of divorced parents rose from 12% in 1963 to 28% in 1988.

As shown in Figure 7.1, the changes in the parents' marital status were accompanied by changes in the percentage of children living with two parents; it dropped from 53% in 1963 to 17% in 1988, while the percentage living with one parent increased from about 16% in 1963 to about 27% in 1988. Other trends were an increase in the number of children living with relatives since 1973, and the marked rise since 1978 in the number of children living in institutions. From 1923 until 1948, 15% to 28% of the children lived in institutions (orphanages), but during the 1960s and early 1970s, only a small percentage did so. Since 1978, however, that percentage has again been in the 15% to 20% range although the type of institution has changed from the orphanage to the foster or group home.

We were surprised to find that the three major referral sources—self-referral (family, relatives, and friends), physicians/hospitals, and schools—have been reasonably constant. The number of children referred by agencies was high in the 1923–1948 years, relatively low from 1953 to 1968, then rose to about 30% in 1988. The large percentage, about 20%, referred from the courts in 1923 reflects the clinic's association in its early years with the judicial system.

Children's Presenting Problems

Table 7.1 presents the children's top ten presenting problems. Inasmuch as school and home are the arenas for most of the child's activities, it is not surprising to find that academic and other school difficulties

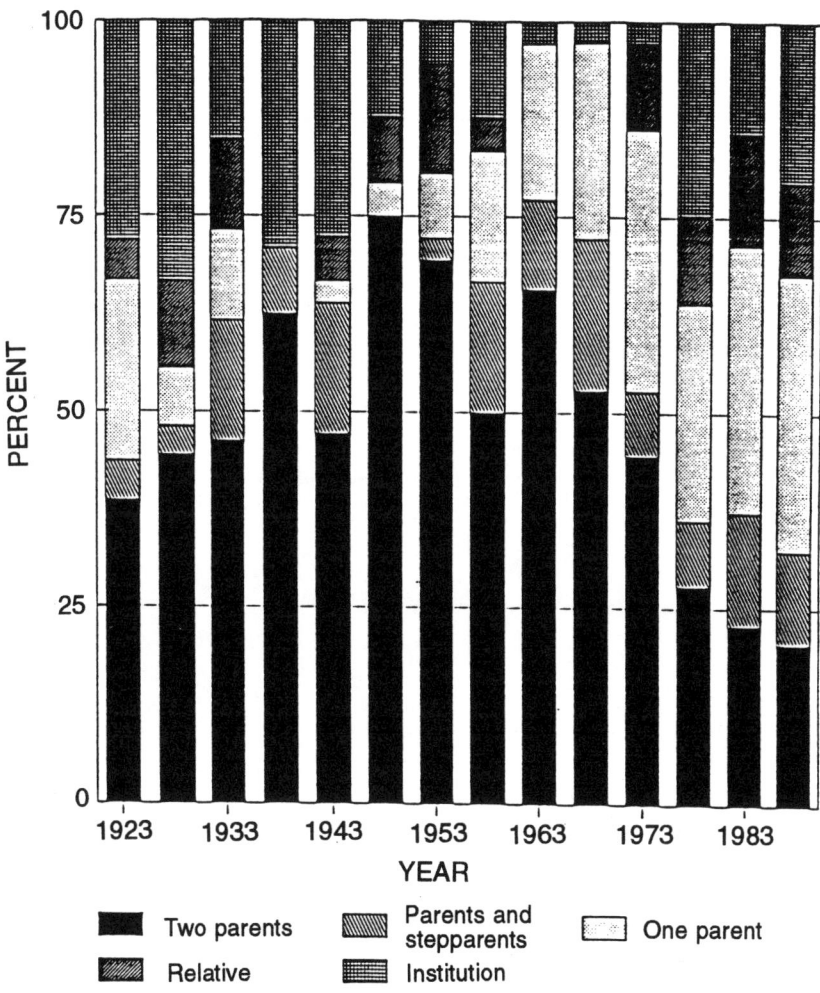

Figure 7.1. Bingham historical study demographics: child's current living arrangements.

were frequent problems. The school is the child's workplace and the site where stress from many sources is usually manifested. Figure 7.2 presents the trend lines for the top five children's presenting problems, and Figure 7.3 does so for the second five. The percentage of children presenting with academic and other school-related problems remained remarkably constant over the years, from about 26% in 1923 to about 24% in 1988. Parent-child relationship problems were almost as common as

Table 7.1
The Children's Top Ten Presenting Problems

Problem	Percentage Reporting
Academic, school learning problems	24.2
Parent-child relationship disturbance	22.4
Aggressive behavior	19.3
Peer problems	19.1
Anxious, nervous, obsessive, or phobic	16.9
Hyperactivity/hyperkinesis	14.5
Intelligence/cognitive deficit	14.3
Neglect, abuse	11.6
Temper tantrums	11.0
Stealing	10.1

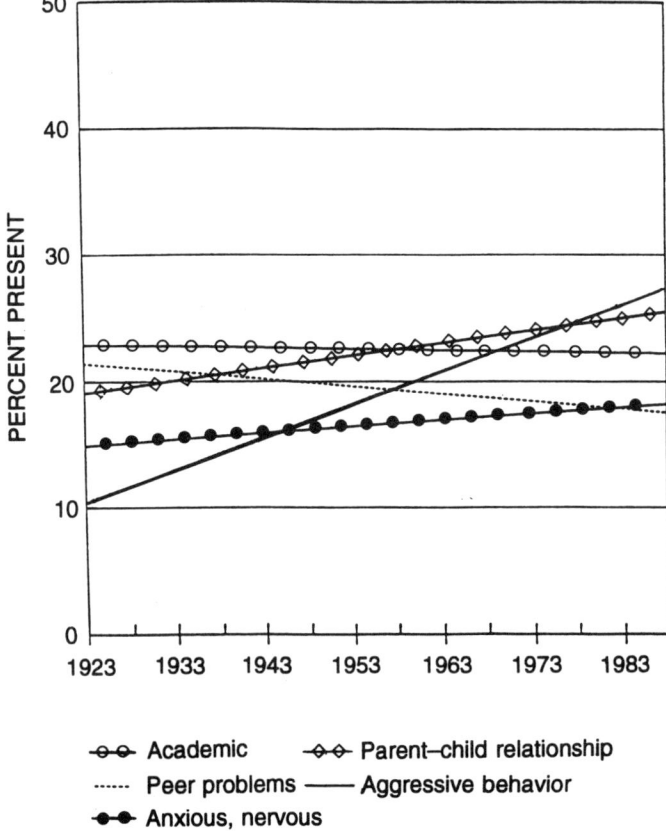

Figure 7.2. Bingham historical study trends of the top ten presenting problems (nos. 1–5).

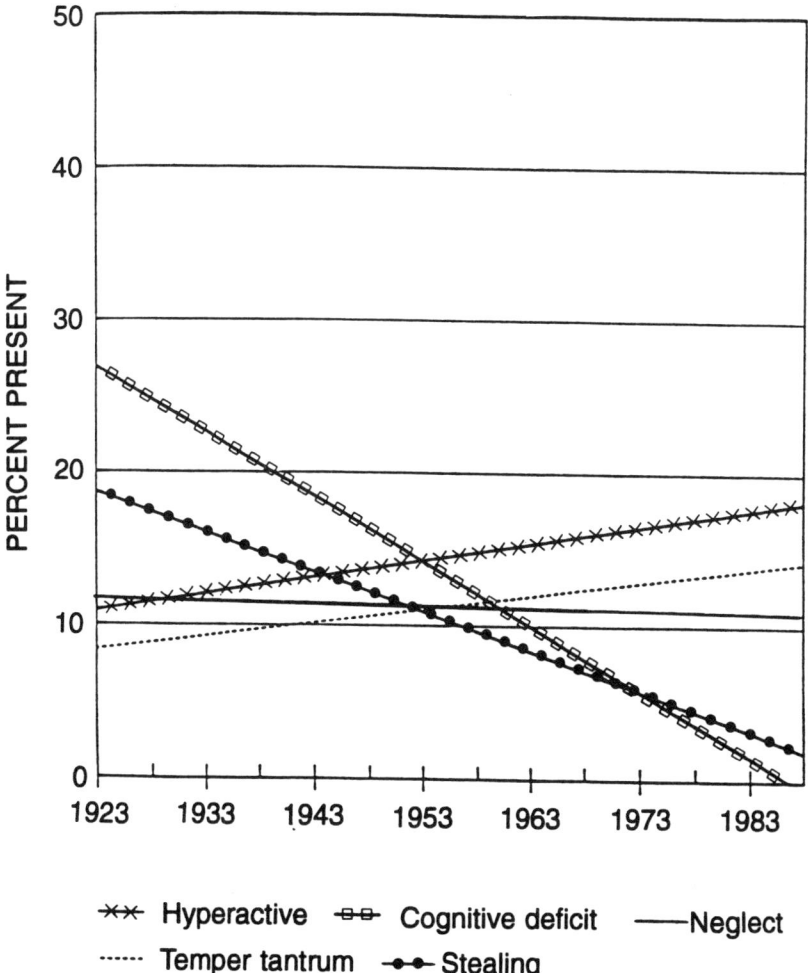

Figure 7.3. Bingham historical study trends of the top ten presenting problems (nos. 6–10).

academic/school problems but have increased somewhat, from about 19% in 1923 to 26% in 1988.

Other major changes over time were, first, the marked, almost steady increase in aggressive behavior (from about 10% of children in 1923 to 27% in 1988) and, second, the sharp declines in both cognitive deficits and stealing from the early 1920s until 1988, when they were only a few children's presenting problems. The decrease in children presenting cognitive deficits reflects the decline in the clinic's psychological testing for the schools as the school system developed its own programs. The decline in stealing as a presenting problem, however, probably reflects a culture change.

The constant 11% to 12% of children brought to the clinic over the years because of neglect is a tragic finding. We are concerned that it reflects no progress in enlightened child care and a possible decline in humanitarian sentiments during the past 10 to 15 years, when the Reagan "trickle-down" ethic pervaded our society and was paralleled by widespread greed and corruption in high places. As discussed in Chapter 1, the steady cutbacks in funding for such children's programs as Head Start and the Reagan administration's tragicomic definition of ketchup as a vegetable in order to slash money for funding children's school lunches exemplify the disregard of children's well-being that is associated with neglect and our nation's falling during the 1980s to 21st in the world in infant mortality.

Some of the changes in the children's presenting problems can be labeled signs of the times. They are mainly the increase in recent decades of the percentages of children presenting as depressed or with suicidal or other self-harming behavior. Although depression and suicidal/self-harming behavior were not among the children's overall top ten presenting problems, they have been the presenting problems for 10% to 15% of the children since about 1978. Also, the smaller but still steady increase in psychotic behavior, fire setting, and substance abuse as presenting problems since the mid-1950s, along with each one's being presenting problems for 4% to 7% of the children in the 1980s, depict the turmoil in our society. Is it possible that the irrationality and duplicity of such national behavior as the Watergate and Iran-Contra scandals have "trickled down" to become the children's presenting problem in the form of psychotic behaviors? Obviously, the drugs and arson on the streets of our cities during the past 15 years are conducive to drug abuse and fire setting becoming psychiatric problems for children.

Families' Problems

Table 7.2 presents the types and percentages of the children's family problems. Many have fluctuated in frequency since the 1920s; for example, there have been striking changes in the percentages of families reporting addictive behavior problems. Even though Prohibition was in effect in the 1920s, many families were reporting problems with alcohol. Problems related to alcohol and drugs declined during the 1930s and 1940s, but they have risen sharply since 1980.

Another recent trend is the marked increase in the percentages of families reporting mental illness, from less than 20% between 1923 and

THE HISTORICAL-CLINIC CHART STUDY

Table 7.2
Problems in the Children's Families

Problem	Percentage Reporting
Marital problems	18.7
Definite mental illness	16.9
Alcoholism	14.3
Financial problems	11.9
Probable mental illness	11.2
Recent serious physical illness	8.6
Unspecified family crisis	5.1
Recent death	4.4
Crime	3.7
Employment problems	3.5
Recent move (multiple)	3.5
Drug use/abuse	2.9
Gambling	2.0

1973 to 35% to 45% since then. It is possible that some of the recent increase is attributable to greater public awareness of mental illness and some changes in attitudes, including diminished stigma, greater recognition, and more reporting of mental illness than in the past. Inasmuch as ECA reports revealed that about 20% of the adults in the United States meet criteria for the diagnosis of a mental disorder, it appears that genetic and other biological influences, as well as the difficulty of living with a mentally ill parent, are combining with other stressors to influence the development of symptoms in the children.

The percentages of families reporting marital problems have fluctuated widely, from about 30% in the 1920s to a low of 10% or less in the 1930s and early 1940s, and then a sharp increase after World War II to about 30% in 1948. During the middle 1950s and early 1960s the proportion reporting marital problems was only about 10% to 15%, but by 1973 it had skyrocketed to almost 45%, and since then it has dropped rather steadily to about 11%. The decline in the percentage reporting marital problems during the depression and early World War II years is in accord with historians' and family scholars' views of the family becoming more cohesive during such times of great unrest. The large increase in marital problems reported in 1953 reflects the many problems of the postwar marriages. During the familistic 1950s and early 1960s, however, the percentage reporting marital problems dropped markedly, only to rise again following the turmoil of the late 1960s and early 1970s.

Unfortunately, the decline in the percentages reporting marital problems during the past 10 years reflects not a true decline in such problems but the sad fact that the percentage of the children living with two parents since 1978 has decreased considerably. During the 1980s, fewer than 25% of the children being seen at the clinic were living with two parents. As would be expected, there was a great increase in the percentage of children living with one parent or in institutions, situations in which there would not be reports of families' marital problems. Thus, the reports of the number and type of parents' marital problems reflect the historical events of the century and are poignant testimony to the influence of the wider society on the family, one of the major theses of our work.

We used curve-fitting techniques to fit trend lines to the data on family problems. As shown in Figure 7.4, the most meaningful trends in family problems over the years are the steadily increasing percentages of families reporting problems of mental illness, marital problems, and addictive behaviors (especially alcohol and drugs). The percentages reporting such specific family crises as deaths, moves, physical illness, and financial difficulties, as well as unspecified family crises, were relatively constant over the years. We wondered whether the increases in parental mental illness, marital problems, and the adults' addictive behaviors combined with the more constant crises of everyday family life could account for the apparent earlier onset and increased severity of children's emotional and behavioral problems observed in recent years.

Figure 7.5 shows that the percentage of the children's families reporting no family problems has declined from about 45% in 1958 to about only 7% to 8% in the 1980s, and concurrently, the percentages of families reporting problems increased during those years. But an even more sinister finding is that since 1973, the percentages reporting more than one family problem have risen greatly, from about 22% to almost 77%. Such data attest to the critical situation of the American family in the 1980s and have grave portents for the family in the near future.

CONCLUSIONS

The findings from the review of children's case reports since 1923 supply clinical support to the concerns about the stability and well-being of the American family throughout the twentieth century that were discussed in Chapters 1 and 3. Even though these cases are just the tip of the emotional distress–psychopathology–family unrest iceberg, the major changes in the children's presenting problems and living situations

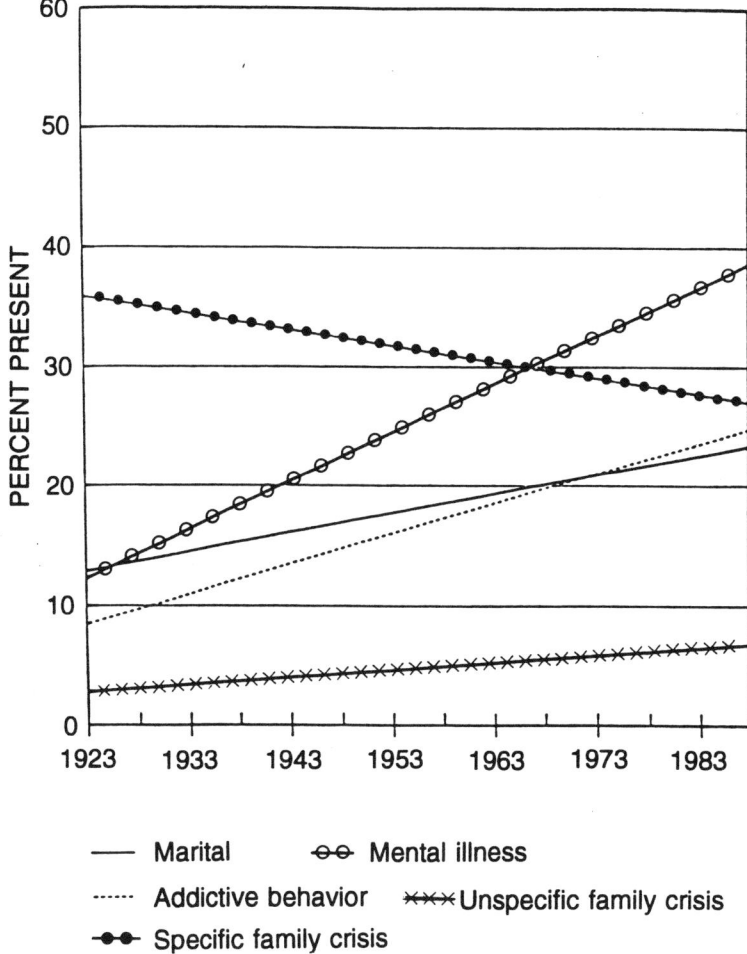

Figure 7.4. Bingham historical study family problems trends.

and in their families' problems illustrate the profound changes that have been taking place in the family in recent years. These include, but are by no means limited to, such prominent demographic changes as the decline in family size in recent decades and the extreme change in the marital status of children's biological parents. The decline in family size has occurred in most of Western society during this century and is associated with an increasingly higher standard of living, but the shrinkage in the percentage of children whose biological parents were married (to

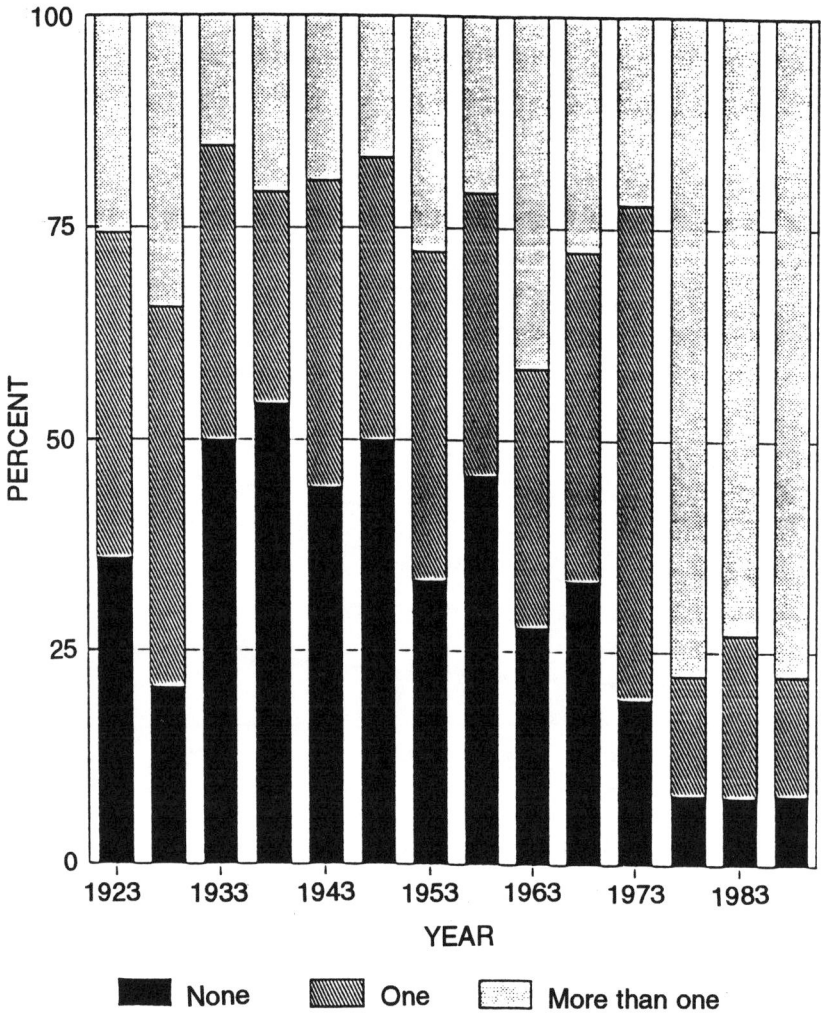

Figure 7.5. Bingham historical study family problem indicator.

only about 25% in 1990) represents an unfortunate trend that apparently began in the late 1960s. This trend is paralleled by the increased number of children of divorce and of children whose parents never married. Our clinical data can only reflect what is happening within a society and suggest trends, because many factors determine whether any patient (in this instance, a child patient) will seek or be brought for care and then be entered into the records. For every case seen in the clinic, there were many who never received care; but we can see that data collected over a long period of time (65 years in our study) probably are indicators of social change and, in this respect, have greater generalizability than some more time-limited and rigorously controlled studies.

The findings about the parents' marital status dictate questions. For example, to what extent is divorce associated with children's emotional distress, psychopathology, and need for mental health care? We cannot answer the question, and there may not yet be a definitive answer because such a question requires data from a large, longitudinal case-control study to be answered scientifically.

Perhaps a more profound, but related question concerns what life will be like for the large percentage of children whose parents never married. Recent reports indicate that about 25% of all births in the United States in 1990 were to unmarried mothers (Hill, 1991). Undoubtedly, many of these mothers were living with male partners who could serve as father figures or role models for the boys. Nevertheless, the possibility that the mothers were, are, and/or will be many of these children's only adult parental figure raises disturbing questions. The main question—whether children need to have two parents or parent figures—strikes at the roots of concepts of child and personality development that are the products of clinical observations and research since at least the 1890s and have been incorporated into standard textbooks of psychiatry, psychology, and child development. As mentioned in Chapter 3, Galdston (1958) feared that our society was becoming "matriarchive" and that its pathologies would be children's emotional distress, juvenile delinquency, and personality disorders. Even though most theories of personality development hold that a father figure is needed for the adequate development of the child's superego, no systematic research is yet available that can be used to determine the extent to which that tenet holds.

In the 1980s, most of the children seen in the clinic were living in one of five settings—institutions, with relatives, with one parent, with a parent and stepparent, or with two parents. We plan to examine associations between the children's problems and their parents' marital status and demographic characteristics on one hand and those different "living arrangements" on the other.

The analysis of children's presenting problems revealed a disturbing increase (almost a tripling) of the percentage of children with problems of aggressive behavior. Were the aggressive children mimicking what was happening in the wider society, or were they "protesting" the marked changes in the family and in the living arrangements for children that have been occurring and were found in our data? The increase in parent-child problems suggests that children were upset about the changes in their families. It is tempting to postulate that they were reacting to family instability and the discrepancies between their own situations and the traditional family that they see for hours each day on television. The children's symptoms of anxiety (many children have fears of their parents divorcing) and/or angrily exhibiting aggressive behavior could spark or increase the parent-child behavior problems. Already, schools in New York are conducting group therapy programs for children of divorce in the fifth and sixth grades.

The parents' marital problems depict the family troubles that have become so prominent and are now admitted by family scholars and researchers. The sharp increase in addictive behavior parallels individuals' apparently increasing needs for "escape" with the help of chemicals or by involvement with all-absorbing compulsive activities. The addictive behaviors, including gambling as well as drugs, are a tragic commentary on our society; ironically, many state-controlled lotteries were started in the 1980s.

The increase in children's depressive symptoms and suicidal behavior parallels the rise in depression and suicide in the young that we observed in the early 1970s and that has been tragically confirmed by continuing reports of high rates of depression in young adults (Shafii & Shafii, 1992). Cohort analyses reveal that those born after 1945 have had very high rates of depression; Klerman (1988) has postulated the existence of "agent blue"—a mixture of social and biological factors—to account for this phenomenon.

The percentages reporting probable or definite mental illness in the family have risen to about 40%. The public's changing attitudes, greater awareness of mental illness, lowered stigma regarding it, and more widely available services are probably largely responsible for the increase. We, however, are plagued with the nasty, recurring question of whether rapid social change produces a true increase in mental illness. Esquirol (1967) asked this question about France after the French Revolution and the Napoleonic Era. In the 1830s, he collected data on admissions to hospitals throughout France from the 1780s to the 1820s and found that most of the increases in admissions could be accounted for by expansions of and increases in facilities; however, he hedged and stated that the change in "morals" in France in the 1820s and 1830s was deleterious and might be a cause of increased mental illness. Apparently, Esquirol could not determine whether the increased facilities and services were in response to greater need, but that is a possibility. One hundred fifty years later, ECA data in America indicate that the prevalence rate of mental disorder is about 20% (Regier et al., 1988), and in Sweden, Hagnell, Lanke, Rorsman, and Ojesjo's (1982) follow-up of the Lundby study from 1947 to 1972 revealed an increased expectancy for mental illness over time. The increased number of families in our clinic sample that reported mental illness in recent years may be reflecting an increased incidence as well as prevalence of mental disorder and strongly indicates that there is a need for both prevention programs and expanded mental health services for children.

In conclusion, our historical-clinic study substantiated some of the concerns about the status and well-being of the family expressed by family scholars, other social scientists, and in recent years, the general public (see Chapters 1 and 3). Our findings show that children and families are in distress. Perhaps the most ominous finding is that, over the years, increasingly smaller percentages of the children's families reported no problems, and increasingly larger percentages reported that they were having not just a single family problem but multiple problems.

CHAPTER 8

Clinical Implications

> Families who turn to their physicians for help at times of crisis can also teach the physician much about the nature of life in families, the struggle to find both meaning and intimacy in the connectedness of human existence, and the remarkable human capacity for change and growth.
> —Lewis (1979, p. 89)

Although our studies have scientific and other limitations, some of the prominent findings have clinical significance. In many ways, they support impressions gleaned from practice and also are consistent with the results of epidemiological studies of individuals. Inasmuch as our studies included historical research reviews, a longitudinal epidemiological study of families, and historical-clinical case studies, they provide a backdrop that has both breadth and depth against which clinicians can compare their experiences and gain perspectives on their own practices.

THE EXTENT OF SYMPTOMATIC DISTRESS IN FAMILIES

For clinical purposes, the most striking finding was the extent of symptomatic distress in the random sample of families from the community. At Time 1, of the 43 families, 25 (58%) were symptomatic. In about half of them, only one person was symptomatic—usually a daughter or the wife—but in the 12 remaining families, two or more members were symptomatic. Of the 129 adults and children, 44 (34%) were symptomatic, representing almost 1.8 persons per family in the 25 symptomatic families.

Therefore, when seeing a patient with a disturbance of mood, thought, or behavior, the clinician always needs to inquire about the likely possibility that another family member(s) is symptomatic. Providing treatment for just one member of the family will be helpful but often difficult or insufficient because of other members' psychopathology. Also, it is necessary for the clinician to consider the effects of the symptomatic person on other family members and, likewise, the effects of the others on the patient.

As was discussed in Chapter 4, substantial evidence shows that a symptomatic family member often has deleterious influences on the others in the family. When the patient has an affective disorder, it is especially important to find ways to improve communication within the family, lessen negativism, and diminish face-to-face contact between family members. And when the family member has a chronic mental disorder, it is necessary to think specifically about "the family burden"—emotionally, socially, and financially—of mental disorder and to help the family find ways to lessen its severity.

CHANGE AND VARIABILITY IN SYMPTOMATOLOGY IN THE FAMILY

The change and variability that we observed in the families' symptom statuses over just a 15-month period of time add to the complexity of the clinician's task. From Time 1 to Time 3, there were changes in symptom status from asymptomatic to symptomatic or vice versa in 8 (23%) of the 34 families, and there was a change in the family member who was symptomatic in 3 (9%) of the families.

Such findings substantiate clinicians' concerns about the "ping-ponging" of symptomatology from one family member to another that has been observed in practice and now has been found in a random sample of nonpatient, nonvolunteer families from the community. Such changes are indicators of the need for therapy for the entire family unit—family therapy, not just therapy for individual members. Consequently, whenever possible, clinicians need to involve the whole family in therapy or, as an alternative, to help other family members obtain treatment from another clinician. When there are two or more clinicians working with a family, it is important for one to keep in close touch with the other in order to lessen the possibility of overidentification with the family member one is seeing, which can lead to the clinicians' working at cross purposes and to problems for all concerned.

IDENTIFICATION OF FAMILY MEMBERS AT RISK

The family members most likely to be symptomatic were the wives/mothers, sons, and daughters; only half as many husbands/fathers as wives/mothers were symptomatic. Such results are in accord with those of community studies of individuals: Repeatedly, more females than males report symptoms of mental disorder, especially of the anxiety disorders and depressions. Also, our findings are in agreement with recent ones showing that unusually large numbers of young persons have symptoms of emotional distress. Weissman (1991) emphasized that the age of onset of the affective disorders is earlier—in the low 20s—than it was in previous generations, and some new reports indicate that the median age of onset for the anxiety disorders is 15 years (Christie et al., 1988).

Our findings point to a singular aspect of the reports of young persons being at high risk for mental disorders. Large percentages of the young adult children in their parents' homes were at especially high risk. Thus, it behooves clinicians to focus questions about the emotional well-being of family members in their late teens and 20s and to ask specifically about symptoms and substance abuse.

We also uncovered some young children whose disturbed parents projected their concerns and symptomatology onto them. We need to be aware of such cases in which the problem is in the parent, not the child, and also to learn more about what happens to those children over time. Do they pay a price later on in life for carrying their parents' "troubles?" Wallerstein and Blakeslee (1989) described the plight of children of divorce, especially that of the "overburdened child" who was carrying most of the parent's (usually the mother's) problems. The clinician needs to inquire specifically about the emotional state of children of divorce and to discuss them at least briefly with the parents in order to raise their awareness so that they can take steps to prevent or lessen the difficulties (see Chapter 1).

FAMILY HISTORIES AND THE INTERGENERATIONAL CONTINUITY OF SYMPTOMATOLOGY

The necessity to think in terms of the family unit when seeing a patient is reinforced by findings from the family histories we obtained. Almost 40% of the families had relatives with a history of mental illness and/or substance abuse problems. In those with family histories of either mental disorder or substance use/abuse, 33% were symptomatic, but in those with family histories of both mental illness and substance use/abuse problems, 57% were symptomatic. This strong evidence of the intergenerational continuity of mental disorder, substance abuse problems, and comorbidity points to the necessity for clinicians in all fields to take careful family histories and to alert family members to their risk status and the need for treatment when symptoms first appear. Preventive measures must be found for the children in families in which there is or has been mental illness and/or substance abuse problems in two or more generations.

COMORBIDITY

The extent of comorbidity (32% of the symptomatic families had members with both symptoms of mental disorder and alcohol/drug abuse problems) supports clinicians' impressions about its pervasiveness. Inasmuch as comorbid conditions are notoriously treatment resistant, clinicians can use such findings to back up their recommendations for intensive treatment programs for the afflicted family member(s) and supportive programs, often self-help, for other family members.

TREATMENT-RESISTANT FAMILIES

Families with characteristics similar to those that did not complete the study—almost all of which were symptomatic—require special efforts on the part of their clinicians to ensure that they receive adequate treatment. The adult sons and daughters were the family members most likely to be symptomatic, the sons with alcohol and/or drug problems and the daughters with symptoms of emotional distress and phobias. The families that dropped out told us that the research took a great deal of time and that it was difficult to get the family members together. Also, they admitted that the family members had differing opinions about the advisability of continued participation. Such statements depict the divisiveness within those families, their secretiveness, and the unwillingness to change that is inherent in resistance. Consequently, therapists working with large, low-income families (and specifically those with older parents, who tend to have relatively low educational levels) should expect to encounter considerable resistance and will have to make special efforts to keep them in treatment.

The special efforts include the clinician's serving as a family advocate and also mobilizing assistance from agencies. Some information that we obtained from the families that did not continue in the study suggested that they feared that ongoing evaluations would surface even more troubles than were already apparent, including problems that they feared to confront. Therapists need to obtain knowledge about such family members' fears and to use appropriate approaches and techniques to keep the family in therapy, to save it from drowning in misery, and to sustain hope.

Such multiproblem (and often minority) families frequently are both educationally and economically deprived. They are well-known to social agencies, hospital emergency rooms, and mental health professionals. Usually, however, they seek help only when they are in crisis, and their care is fragmented both because of bureaucratic turf-guarding and because they have a "culture of poverty" present-time orientation. To middle-class therapists, they seem just to be going from one crisis to the next; however, studies indicate that such families are enmeshed in accelerating cycles of stressors and symptoms that perpetuate each other (Schwab et al., 1979). The therapist needs to acknowledge these facts about the poor and the battered and to find ways to keep the families engaged in treatment and rehabilitation programs, including self-help programs and support groups, for years. Ideally, one professional should be orchestrating their care.

FAMILY RISK FACTORS

The three most significant family risk factors were family structure (being in a single-parent family or having one or more adult children at home), low socioeconomic status (SES), and the negative impact of stressors. Of the 9 single-parent families, 8 (89%) were symptomatic, and of the 16 families with adult children at home, 12 (75%) were symptomatic. Moreover, 73% of the adult children were symptomatic. Some approaches that can benefit the single-parent family and the family with adult children are suggested later in this chapter.

The heads of the symptomatic households tended to be less educated and more often unemployed than the heads of the asymptomatic families. Perhaps most importantly, disproportionately more of the symptomatic families were in the two lower SES quartiles and had annual incomes under $20,400; also, they tended to have lower annual incomes than the median for the census tract in which they lived, and they had less disposable or discretionary money after they had paid their fixed monthly expenses.

The strong associations between employment and income on one hand and symptomatic status on the other indicate that the family unit is influenced by the events and forces in the community and wider society. Thus, it is important for the clinicians to view the family as a social unit and not as something that exists in isolation, as too often happens in both clinical practice and family studies. It is imperative for the clinician to think about whether the family needs material assistance and to inquire explicitly about financial distress. We were in a number of homes in which the empty cabinets in the kitchens and the barrenness of the rooms spoke sadly of the bitter realities of poverty. In such instances, the clinician can readily use his or her status to obtain some help for the family, and it is important for him or her to do so personally and immediately. In recent years, the senior author has not hesitated to stop in the middle of an assessment or therapy session to telephone a caseworker or an agency, in the presence of the patient or family, in order to arrange for temporary assistance. His willingness to take such immediate action lowered suspicion and doubt and fostered a positive transference that could be used to work effectively toward the desired therapeutic outcome.

FAMILY STRESS

Our findings revealed that there were a number of stress-related family problems that require the clinician's attention. The concept of stress themes that we developed supplied a more comprehensive view of the effects of stressors on the family than is shown just by a listing of the stressful life events (SLEs) that occurred. For example, the concept of a stress theme brings such SLEs as job loss, lowered income, and increased family arguments about finances together as a multifaceted adversity for the family that can lead to changes in members' roles and statuses and, eventually, to some degree of family disorganization. Consequently, it is wise for the clinician to think in terms of how related stressors affect the family and to make the appropriate shifts in therapy when additional stressors threaten to overwhelm the family's capacity to cope or even to function. Also, it is necessary for the clinician to keep in mind that the effects of stressors pile up exponentially.

That negative SLEs and stress themes were associated with a family's being symptomatic was to be expected. But our categorization of them revealed that the intrafamilial themes were much more likely to be associated with symptomatology than the other-relatives or friends stress themes. Finding that work and finances was by far the most common

CLINICAL IMPLICATIONS

intrafamilial stress theme underscores the importance of clinicians being cognizant of the influences of economic and other sociopolitical events on families and the stress within the family created by financial hardships.

We saw family members mentioning their achievements proudly. Too often clinicians do not surface patients' and families' accomplishments and make use of them in therapy where they can partially balance the adversities of life.

The reports of increased arguments by 20% of the symptomatic members signals serious difficulties in their marriages, as well as the likelihood that either the husband or wife or both are depressed. Paykel and his colleagues (1969) reported that spouses' reports of increased arguments often indicated that one or both were depressed. Weissman (1991) emphasized that a husband's or (especially) a wife's reporting that the couple was quarreling and not getting along well was a significant indicator of depression and that just asking about arguments and how well the couple was getting along was an excellent screening method for depression.

The surprising lack of agreement among family members about whether an SLE had occurred within the past 6 months points to the necessity for clinicians to obtain information about stressors from more than one family member whenever possible. As discussed by Stephenson et al. (1990), the wives/mothers reported 33% of the SLEs that had occurred, the husbands/fathers 20%, and the children 15% to 25%; the overlap (i.e., reports by two or more family members that a particular SLE occurred) amounted to only 40%. Also, our results showed that adolescent children's perceptions of what was happening to the family and within it were different than their parents' perceptions. Significant lack of agreement between the partners about the occurrence and effects of SLEs, about satisfactions, and about family values and goals are red lights that flash warnings of symptomatology and/or impending disruption of the family.

The discrepancies between the marital partners' reports about whether an SLE had occurred is a sector in which the therapist can intervene effectively, even early in assessment or treatment. Also, further probing can often reveal other marital differences and problems. In addition to the occurrence of the SLE, discussions need to focus on its differing effects on various family members. Often, the adolescents' stressors—other than very serious problems or striking achievements— are given little consideration, even in marital and family therapy. Many events that adults consider trivial are serious for a child (especially an adolescent) and need to be brought into therapy.

A glaring problem, and one about which we have heard many sharp complaints, is that "my doctor didn't even ask me about stress!" Our clinical experience with patients and families and our research with nonpatient families reveal that patients and family members want to be questioned directly about stress and its impact.

FAMILY ENVIRONMENT

Cohesion

One of the prominent clinical implications of the findings with regard to the Family Environment Scale (FES) is that low scores on the nine-item cohesion subscale often were associated with symptomatology, especially lowered mood, current emotional distress, and depressive symptomatology. Thus, asking a family member the nine cohesion items gives the clinician a quick, brief evaluation of the family and its members' well-being. These items, which can be phrased as true-false questions for interview purposes, are as follows:

1. Family members really help and support one another. (T)
2. We often seem to be killing time at home. (F)
3. We put a lot of energy into what we do at home. (T)
4. There is a feeling of unity and cohesion in our family. (T)
5. We rarely volunteer when something has to be done at home. (F)
6. Family members really back each other up. (T)
7. There is very little group spirit in our home. (F)
8. We really get along well with each other. (T)
9. There is plenty of time and attention for everyone in our family. (T)

Each "correct" response (noted in parentheses above) receives a score of 1. A score of 7 or more usually indicates a high level of cohesion, a score of 6 reflects mid-level cohesion, and a score of 5 or less is indicative of a low level of cohesion—and usually of symptomatology and family problems.

Our findings on low cohesion scores support those of other investigators (Beavers, Hampson, & Hulgus, 1985; Beavers & Voeller, 1983; Green et al., 1991a, b; Olson, McCubbin et al., 1983) about the importance of a reasonable level of cohesion for effective family functioning. Even a short index of cohesion can be a sensitive and reliable index of family well-being and of the "togetherness" that Bowen has described so eloquently (Kerr & Bowen, 1988).

Expressiveness and Communication

Families with symptoms of lowered mood and other indicators of depression often had relatively low scores on expressiveness as well as on cohesion. Low expressiveness scores are evidence of problems with communication that can be grievous and pervasive, especially in families with a depressed person. As was discussed in Chapter 4 in the review of research on depression in the family, a depressed person's language and intonations communicate negativism and often arouse critical or hostile feelings in others. Hinchliffe, Hooper, and Roberts (1978) warned clinicians not to rely on the quality of the communication between the depressed patient and the clinician as an indicator either of the quality of the patient's communication with the spouse or of his or her response to therapy. Hinchliffe's research showed that depressed persons communicated more effectively when talking with a therapist or "outsider" than when talking solely with the spouse.

DEPRESSION IN THE FAMILY AND SOCIAL SUPPORTS

Inasmuch as many investigators and clinicians have noted the controlling and negative influences exerted by a depressed family member on others in the family as well as the depressed person's withdrawal from social and other activities, it is usually helpful to widen the family circle by suggesting that members invite relatives or friends to visit frequently and that they visit relatives and friends as often as possible. Vaughn and Leff (1976) found that when a couple with a depressed spouse visited friends or relatives weekly or had a friend or relative stay with them 1 or 2 days every week, there was a reduction of negativism and critical/hostile behavior in the home and improved communication.

The clinician also needs to urge the family, not just the depressed member, to enlarge its activities by participating in religious services, attending community and other social functions, and increasing activities with others whenever possible. The increased activity reduces the usually negative face-to-face contact between spouses that leads to marital and family disharmony. Increased social activities and structure in daily life also improve the quality of daily communication.

Our results are in accord with other investigators' findings that such social supports as family, friends, clubs, and churches dilute or otherwise protect against the full impact of stressors, especially negative SLEs. In particular, participating in (not just belonging to or passively observing) community, organizational, and especially church activities is beneficial to the family with a depressed member. Clinically, we insist upon increased activity—physical, mental, social, and spiritual—for all patients with depression and their family members.

THE USE OF RESEARCH MEASURES IN CLINICAL PRACTICE

Certain approaches that we used in our research can be employed for therapeutic and other clinical purposes. The most immediate are the techniques to engage families for assessment and therapy. Some of the relatively nonthreatening ones to which families responded with interest and that they voluntarily said they both liked and found valuable include the following.

1. *Setting personal and family goals.* An efficient, nonthreatening way to engage a family is to begin by asking each member to write three goals for himself or herself as an individual and also three goals for the family for the next 12 months, and then to have the family members gather to discuss the family goals as a group. The most common goals for the forthcoming year reported by our families were health and fitness, career advancement or job-related achievements, other personal achievements, education or academic attainments, closeness and harmony, leisure and travel, financial security, and material acquisitions. It was useful to learn about individual family members' goals and, especially, to see whether their goals were idiosyncratic.

Meaningful points in question include whether the family members have mainly the same general goals or whether they are highly individualistic. Also, are the goals realistic or unrealistic? Deviant, or even bizarre? An unusual goal reported by a family member may be symptomatic of his or her illness and/or reflect individualism at the expense of family cohesion.

When discussing a goal with the family and a family member, it will be of clinical benefit to ascertain whether it appears likely that the goal will be attained. Is there strong hope that it will be reached? Also, what will it mean, and what will the family member(s) do, if the goal is unattainable? Despairing about reaching a goal or giving up on it may be symptomatic of depression or demoralization, or be an indicator of lack of family vitality.

2. *Using screening instruments.* Using such screening instruments as the 20-item Center for Epidemiologic Studies Depression Scale (CES-D;

Radloff, 1977), enables clinicians to obtain a simple but reliable evaluation of current distress, lowered mood, mild depression, and/or demoralization. Family members and patients report uniformly that it is easy to take. Also, family members find the 90-item, true-false Family Environment Scale (FES; Moos & Moos, 1981) meaningful. It can be completed in 15 to 20 minutes, and the results show areas of strength and agreement between family members as well as areas of weakness and divisiveness. The members' subscale scores reveal orientations and point to sectors requiring further evaluations and/or interventions. The discrepancy score is a measure of the level of agreement-disagreement between two members that we have found useful when working with a married pair. In practice, it is helpful to ask the couple about items on which they differ, develop discussions about differences, and emphasize areas of agreement and strength.

3. *Drawing the genogram.* The genogram is beginning to be widely used in therapy because it points out repetitive problem areas in two or three generations, as well as some of the family's more recent tensions. To gather information for the genogram, the clinician can ask each family member to give an individual written response to the question "Who is in your immediate family?" From the answers, the clinician can draw the family genogram on a clipboard or tablet for all to see and to discuss. In response to the question about the immediate family, some of our husbands or wives omitted the other spouse! Such omissions need to be evaluated; we found that a high percentage of these families were symptomatic. Also, a spouse's including members of his or her family of origin in the immediate family raises questions about how successfully the main tasks of the first stage of the family life cycle—those of loosening ties to the parental family and the formation of the new family—were or are being carried out. Our finding that there were so many omissions of persons whom one would expect to be in the immediate family, and the inclusion of others not expected to be in the family, signals the clinician that when a patient refers to or responds to questions about "the family," it is imperative to ascertain exactly about whom he or she is speaking.

It is also helpful to ask the family members about the family tree. If the discussions of the family tree and the genogram did nothing more than increase family members' views of themselves as having been influenced by and of belonging to three generations, it would nevertheless be a valuable therapeutic tool that deepens their sense of belonging and connectedness and increases their grasp of repetitive intergenerational problems.

VIDEOTAPES OF THE FAMILIES

The interviews with, and the videotaping of, the study families in their homes supplied more information and more meaningful "pictures" of the families than we usually obtain in office or clinic visits. The home interviews were welcomed by the families and were carried out much more easily than we anticipated, and the videotaping did not present difficulties. In addition to the yield of information about the family and the views of its dynamics that enhance the clinician's understanding, the videotapes can be therapeutically helpful. The family members' facial expressions and other nonverbal communications, as well as their words and silences, often reveal strengths (not just tensions and conflicts) that can be mobilized for therapy.

We encourage clinicians to make videotapes of one or more of their marital or family sessions. After the tape has been evaluated between sessions, it often can be used therapeutically when the clinician(s) and family members view it together. Also, sometimes it is helpful to give the tape to the families to review, but it is important for the clinician to determine first whether the family is "ready" for and can benefit from the tape. From watching the tape, family members can see how they appear to others, spot conflicts and defenses, consolidate gains in therapy, and gauge progress. Videotaping and/or viewing the tape, however, are not appropriate procedures for some patients and families; family members may be unpleasantly surprised at how they come across. Also, a paranoid patient's suspicions can be increased, and a borderline patient can become threatened or even develop "histrionics." The clinician may have little or no control over such situations. It is important for the clinician to keep in mind that families in need of therapy are usually those that do not know how they appear to and affect others. In particular, it can be unwise for a family to review a videotape when pathology dominated the session. But when used selectively or when the clinician and the family view a specific segment together for a defined reason, videotapes have therapeutic potential.

HOME VISITS

As a result of our research, we think that only home visits can give the clinician a comprehensive view of the family and its conflicts, troubles, resources, and strengths. At home, families often are able to present their strengths more effectively than in the clinician's office and, in subsequent sessions, the clinician can use those strengths for therapeutic purposes.

THE PROBLEMS OF POVERTY

The problems of poverty felt by the many working poor as well as by the unemployed began to be recognized in 1990 as the cold war wound down and a prolonged recession was beginning. Families' financial problems need to be assessed explicitly by clinicians. Clinicians will be seeing more families with financial problems in view of the structural changes in the American economy that are occurring—specifically, the "Latinization" of United States, recently described by Halberstam (1991) as the result of a shrinking middle class and a widening income gap between rich and poor families. Both adults and children will be anxious and depressed about family finances, and the parents will be concerned about their children's future well-being. Also, family violence increases during recessions. Therefore, asking families directly about their income and expenditures can have clinical utility.

Finding that the family has a budget usually indicates planning and cohesion, family strengths that can be used in treatment and are associated with favorable outcomes. Conversely, the lack of such forethought and organization may reflect lack of cohesion, demoralization, or anomie, or simply a lack of resources. We were surprised to find that almost all the families we interviewed were willing to share the details of their finances with us, and we urge clinicians to include questions about finances and budgets in their assessment and treatment of couples and families. It is wise for the clinician to recall, as was discussed in Chapter 4, that the first systematic family research was Le Play's (Silver, 1982) mid-nineteenth-century investigations, in which the family budget turned out to be the basic research tool. In his work it provided significant information about the community and quality of life in the environment as well as about family well-being.

Although both parents may be working, many are employed in lower-paying service jobs and are compelled to work long hours (sometimes each parent at more than one job) to maintain the family. The long hours at work reduce family time and thus are associated with problems with the children as well as between the parents. Our low-income families had to spend a disproportionately large amount of their income on such fixed expenses as utilities and gasoline and had few dollars for the many extras that are pushed by advertising as necessities in our consumer-driven society.

A study such as ours of both the adults and the children in the community reveals the plight of families in poverty, usually multiproblem families. Frequently two or more members are symptomatic, and their emotional distress encompasses a wide range of affective symptoms, alcohol and/or drug problems, and too often, neglected physical illnesses. In addition to the number and complexity of problems and symptoms in these families, the adults and children have added disadvantages—the conditions of poverty, chronic illness, limited resources for coping, and often a fragile social support system whose members may be burdens because they are having just as many problems.

The clinician will need to obtain assistance from medical and social agencies to help multiproblem families with their parent-child conflicts, feelings of deprivation, chronic fatigue from overwork and family tensions, stressors that accompany worry and overwork, concurrent physical and emotional symptomatology, and often alcoholism. Unfortunately, the number of multiproblem families, many of which have children at home, is increasing greatly. Obviously, the children are vulnerable; they suffer from the pinch of poverty and consequent feelings of anxiety and inferiority. Some persons raised in multiproblem families do remarkably well in adult life, however, although even when successful most of them feel that they were scarred, and some have psychosomatic disorders as the price of upward mobility.

CHILDREN

Subclinical Cases

Our results revealed that there were many children and adolescents in the community who were in mild to moderate emotional distress and/or whose behaviors were only somewhat disturbing. Many were subclinical cases whose difficulties usually go unrecognized and untreated or are dismissed as transitory and relatively insignificant. Generally, children with anxiety, phobic, and depressive symptoms, as well as those who are withdrawn and "schizoid," suffer in silence. Only a rare child or adolescent spontaneously asks for help, although a few more children refer themselves than in the past. Some young children with obsessive-compulsive disorder (OCD) ask for help with their "bad thoughts." By and large, however, the young persons brought for psychiatric services are those with oppositional, conduct, or attention-deficit disorders, those whose behavior problems disturb others in the school or neighborhood, and/or those who are troublesome to their parents.

Thus, the findings on the children point to the necessity to get information about them from multiple sources. Our evaluations of the children's reports indicated that many of them were symptomatic but that their mothers were not aware of their distress (as evidenced by the mothers' limited reports of child symptomatology), possibly as a result of so many parents working long hours outside the home.

Another clinical implication of our research is that clinicians can use diagnostic instruments, such as the Child Depression Inventory (CDI; Kovacs, 1983, 1985), easily in their assessments of children. Children and adolescents are familiar with questionnaires from school and are willing to complete self-report inventories. The results identify subclinical cases as well as children in severe distress. When clinicians are treating adults and/or disturbed children, it is important to inquire about the emotional as well as physical health of all the children in the family in order to identify those who are subclinical cases.

When possible, child mental health specialists need to work with teachers and personnel in institutions serving children to increase their ability to identify and refer the distressed child who is not yet causing obvious difficulties. When children who are 2 or more years behind in reading are screened, all kinds of pathologies—physical, emotional, social, and developmental—are often found, and early intervention can be initiated. Screening and early treatment can prevent chronicity and stunted emotional development, as well as more severe illness.

Intergenerational Boundaries

When working with disturbed children and their families, often the greatest assistance the clinician can provide is his or her emphasis on the importance of the parental coalition and of definite boundaries between the parents and children. Pathology grows in the webs that entangle enmeshed families. Although the opposite extreme (detachment and distance) has its own set of problems, it is vitally necessary to see that families establish and maintain boundaries. Firm intergenerational boundaries prevent parent–child alliances that can perpetuate psychopathology in the family by diffusing it or by shifting the focus away from the marital or other problems that may be the central issues. Parent–child alliances also result, too often, in the child becoming the family's "identified patient" whose problems are the focus of attention and a distraction from repetitive marital and other conflicts that usually have been handed down to the parents from their families of origin. Our research with families in the community showed that boundaries and structure were strongly related to health.

Unfortunately, some degree of a parent–child coalition is almost inevitable in single-parent families when there is a child of about 10 years of age. The often lonely, disappointed parent, especially a mother, will find herself "leaning" on a child who can listen to complaints or help share the family chores and burdens. Wallerstein (1989) described the plight of the "overburdened" child as one of the most serious problems facing children of divorce. In view of the huge increase in the number of single-parent families, the clinician will find it necessary to devote considerable time and effort to alerting the parents to the danger of a coalition with a child and recommending that single parents join support groups and develop a number of activities to extend their social networks and interests.

Adult Children

The problems of adult children in the home appeared in our research when we began interviewing in 1983. Since then, there has been an increasing trend for adult children, even those in their early 20s, not to leave home and for adult children to return home if they lose work, cannot find a job, or are divorced. The parents were concerned about these adult children, many of whom were still caught up largely with their own maturational problems. Their presence in the home often leads to divisiveness and conflict.

The trends toward "extended youth" and return to the sanctuarial parental home are likely to continue throughout the 1990s. Therefore, clinicians need to learn about the special problems produced by the changes in family composition and structure resulting from the return of adult children. Our finding that 73% of the adult children were symptomatic, and that their families were the most likely of all to be symptomatic, indicates that many will need treatment.

Two important questions that have complex clinical implications concern the extent to which social (especially economic) and cultural factors are responsible for the increased number of adult children in the home in recent years, and whether such adult children are vulnerable persons who have not yet resolved the developmental tasks of early adulthood (and, in a sense, are returning home to do so). Perhaps, as is seen in so many clinical situations, both social/cultural factors and personal problems with identity and maturation are responsible. At a more profound level, however, the social and cultural processes carry the basic responsibility, inasmuch as their influences on family life and values determine many aspects of personality development and the character of the young. Thus, families with adult children present special challenges to clinicians.

Often, the clinician's initial task is to obtain clarification. When the adult child's problems appear to be preponderantly sociocultural (e.g., economic rather than maturational), the clinician can direct efforts toward advising the person to obtain the additional education and/or training that will enlarge his or her qualifications and skills and increase opportunities for employment. But when the latter condition—a delay in maturation or in resolving essential developmental tasks—is the chief problem, psychotherapy and/or family therapy may be needed, not as a substitute for education or training but to enhance it.

When the clinician learns that there are adult children in the home, it is wise to ask the parents about their concerns regarding the adult child and advise them, first, that it is necessary for all the family members to establish the ground rules for their daily life together, and second, that it is essential for them to maintain their own parental identities. The parents' reinforcing their intergenerational boundaries can prevent tensions and quarrels stemming from the change in the composition of the family after the adult child returns home. Sometimes it is helpful for the clinician to schedule discussions with the adult children and the parents. Such discussions need to focus on all the family members' household obligations and responsibilities, the necessity to have mutual respect and firm boundaries, and, especially, the adult children's and parents' expectations of each other. In addition, it is important to have the adult children present their plans and specific goals.

Trends in Children's and Families' Problems

Demographic Changes

Some of the prominent findings from our 1923–1988 historical-clinic chart reviews supply guidance to clinicians working with children, couples, or families. There is a recent upward trend in the number of young girls needing treatment, especially those in early adolescence. In light of the lower age of menarche, increased alcohol and drug use, and greater sexual activity than in the past, we expect that the trend for larger numbers of young girls to be in treatment will continue and also that there will be an increase in both their "acting-in" and "acting-out" disorders. For example, a 40-year-old high school teacher sought therapy because of job stress and associated marital tensions that threatened to explode because her husband "was drinking again." The stress stemmed from "my difficulty keeping order with a group of young teenage girls with raging hormones and drinking problems." Her outlook for the young girls was grim.

An increasing number of black children and families have been seeking treatment since the 1960s. It appears that some of the overlooked mental health problems of black children in their segregated communities are finally being surfaced. Also, the development of a wider black middle class and of positive black role models has probably resulted in greater awareness of their children's problems and insistence on their receiving mental health care.

The large increase in the number of single-parent families is probably the greatest demographic change that we observed. It raises concern about children not having a father figure and difficulties with their superego development and character formation. Such changes and concerns indicate that clinicians need to find ways to help families forge a link with existing support systems to foster the health, education, and welfare of these children from early in life—the single parent needs support, not condemnation. The changes in the composition and structure of the family that are occurring are a signal to clinicians that they need to enlarge and vary their therapeutic approaches to children and their families, and to help plan primary and secondary prevention strategies.

Children's Aggression, Depression, and Suicidality

The increase in the number of children presenting with aggressive behavior and/or depression and suicidal thoughts and behaviors is deeply disturbing, both as a societal trend and as an indicator of grave personal distress. The parallel increases in aggressive behaviors and depressive symptoms confirm theorists' and clinicians' views that they are two sides of the same coin. One changes place with the other, and the consequences are tragic—aggression toward others as homicide or other violence and/or toward the self as risk-taking and/or suicidal behaviors.

When there is a problem with aggressive behavior or with suicidal ideation, threats, or behaviors, it is imperative that the family remove firearms from the home and keep medications that could be used for suicidal purposes in places where children and adolescents do not have access to them. There are no easy ways to treat aggression in childhood and adolescence. It occurs most often in children suffering from oppositional or conduct disorders but also is manifested by psychotic or brain-damaged children. Approaches that have been used include individual, family, and group therapies; institutional care; and pharmacological agents, either alone or in combination with other treatments. Although a number of children have responded to one or more of these treatment approaches, there is always the fear that the aggressive child will become an adult with an antisocial personality or other severe character pathology. But when a child whose behavior becomes aggressive receives intensive treatment promptly, often he or she is helped considerably, especially when the aggressivity is symptomatic of lack of care or of frustration about learning and is not yet "fixed."

The treatment of depression in children now often includes both pharmacotherapy and psychotherapy for the child, as well as family therapy when possible. One of the main problems for the clinician will be the prevention of relapse. The early age of onset of depression usually is associated with a high relapse rate, and in many cases, there is a history of affective disorders in parents and grandparents. The intergenerational continuity needs to be recognized, and preventive measures need to be extended to all the family members.

Trends in Parents' Problems

The increased reports of marital conflicts in recent years augur poorly for marriage and the future of the family. Clinicians need to inform quarreling parents that divorce is no sure cure; 60% of divorced persons' second marriages end in divorce, and those who quarrel in their first marriage tend to do so in their second marriage (Smith, 1990). When there are children in the family, we recommend significant efforts to save the marriage. Increased spousal arguments are an indicator of major depression and, as our review of the literature on depression and the family summarized, continued marital conflict often is evidence of chronic or recurrent depression. Consequently, when a clinician is seeing a child whose parents are quarreling, the clinician needs to be alert to the high probability that one or both of the parents are depressed. Treatment of the parents' depression can benefit the child and his or her siblings considerably. Many studies show that a depressed parent, especially a depressed mother, has a deleterious effect on children in the home. Investigators have found that depressed mothers have difficulty caring for their children and are unable to give them warmth and affection. In addition to treating the mother, it is important to diminish the amount of daily mother-child face-to-face contact. Young children will benefit by being placed in day care part of each day, and school-age children need extended peer-group and other activities to lessen contact with the mother and reduce the negative messages and discouraging sentiments that a depressed person cannot help sending to others who are near him or her.

The increasing number of parents reporting addictive behaviors is a worrisome finding. The entire family is affected by a parent's drinking, smoking, and gambling, and the children are influenced both directly and indirectly. They often regard the parents' behaviors as sanctioning their own experiments with risk-taking behaviors. Sometimes the children identify with the parents, or there is reaction formation and a strong denunciation of alcohol, tobacco, and/or gambling.

The reports of parents' increased addictive behaviors are especially disturbing when we see the increasing use of alcohol by children who are only seventh or eighth graders, the lowering of the average age of girls' initial sexual experiences to about age 15, the marked increase in unwed mothers, and teenagers' almost epidemic drug problems. The findings from our historical chart survey point to the importance of clinicians' taking comprehensive alcohol, drug, smoking, and gambling histories on all the family members and dealing with those behaviors as effectively as possible by offering intensive treatment, making appropriate referrals, and, especially, turning to support groups.

INDIVIDUALISM VERSUS FAMILISM

Inasmuch as companionship and togetherness were the most highly valued goals of our random sample of families from the community, the clinician working with couples and families needs to put this subject under the microscope. The clinician and the family members can begin by looking at family members' personal and family goals. This scrutiny calls for more than just detecting inconsistencies or deficiencies; it requires analysis of the strengths as well as the weaknesses that appear and discussions of approaches that are likely to be helpful.

The clinician can surface the tensions of individualism versus familism by using those terms explicitly and describing their significance for the family in question. It helps to recall Bowen's emphasis on autonomy and togetherness as basic human drives and the critical importance of finding and maintaining a meaningful balance between them (Kerr & Bowen, 1988). At the appropriate time, the clinician can comment that a number of influences at various levels are affecting the conflict inherent in the polarization of individualism and familism and that those influences need to be recognized and their effects evaluated. The various interacting levels and their influences are as follows:

1. The *sociocultural* level, with its emphasis on consumption and accumulation that is resulting in the now widely held view of the 1980s as the decade of greed and that, implicitly as well as explicitly, tilts strongly toward the pole of individualism and away from the family. Also, the polarity of individualism has been strengthened by the strident antifamilism of prominent political leaders who scapegoat the family for society's ills (see Chapter 1).
2. The *familial* level, particularly the intergenerational continuity of family problems, mental illness, and divorce (Elias, 1991). Bowen's concepts of the development of mental illness over a number of generations, the repetition of family problems and triangles from one generation to the next, and depression "running in the family" all attest to the significance of intergenerational influences (Kerr & Bowen, 1988). It appears that many intergenerational influences are destabilizing the family and promoting individualism. It is likely that those influences will continue during the 1990s and the next few decades inasmuch as the older generations now contain many divorced persons and many who are living in a variety of types of families and stepfamilies. As always, the younger generation tends much more often to do what the older generation does or did than to adhere or listen to the latter's precepts and admonitions.
3. At the *individual* level, the influences include the many strong personal strivings for individuality revealed, for example, by the growing emphasis on personal development, the narcissism attributed to young adults in the United States in the 1980s and early 1990s, and even the vogue of self-psychology.

SUPPORTIVE FAMILY THERAPY

In view of the complexity of the family as a group, some type of family rather than individual therapy often is helpful even when only one member is suffering from emotional distress. We think that supportive, insight-oriented family therapy is a fruitful approach, especially when it is directed toward identifying stressors, clarifying communication, explicating selected psychodynamic processes, lowering defensiveness, working with the distrust that can pervade the family, promoting mutual support, and mobilizing resources. Generally, symptomatic families need to increase their church and social activities and thereby reduce negative face-to-face interactions. Work with the clergy and joining self-help groups can be especially beneficial.

While carrying out our research, analyzing the data, and preparing this book, we repeatedly (and often spontaneously) began to talk about the need for psychiatrists and other mental health professionals to become, when possible, family psychiatrists, family psychologists, family social workers, or other family mental health specialists. We were thinking not just of the desirability of professionals having a family orientation, but of the need to penetrate the barriers raised by specialization and to work with and follow families over the years by observing their transitions, being available at times of crises, and "quarterbacking" them through the family maze and/or both the social and mental health system to obtain material and human assistance when necessary.

CHAPTER 9

Summary and Conclusions

> On the psychological side, the thoughts, feelings and impulses that centre round the family belong to the most intimate and fundamental part of man's spiritual nature.
> —Flügel (1921, pp. 241–242)

INTRODUCTION: CONCERNS AND QUESTIONS

The crises in marriage and the family that became so prominent on the American scene in the 1980s was accompanied by reports from the nationwide Epidemiologic Catchment Area (ECA) studies that about one of every five adults in the United States had a disorder of mood, thought, and/or behavior that met criteria for the diagnosis of a mental disorder (Freedman, 1984). Also, an Institute of Medicine (IOM) report (1990) indicated that at least 12% of all children and adolescents had definite mental disorders and that the percentage was probably closer to 20% in the inner city and/or among those living in poverty. The pitiable condition of many children was evidenced by horrible facts—for example, that the United States ranked 21st in the world in infant mortality and 56th (after Albania) in immunizations. But such facts cannot adequately portray the misery of the millions of children who go to bed hungry and/or are sick and in need of care. There is some hope, however, that instead of indulging in the immature defense mechanisms of denial, projection (blaming others), and immediate gratification, policymakers and leaders will be guided by concern for the public and their social consciences will awaken and they will decree that the 1990s will be the "decade of the child."

These problems of families, adults, and children were matched by the breakdown of community life, the deterioration of the once proud cities of America, and fragmentation of the social structure. According to Yankelovich (1991), the United States went on a holiday in the 1980s, but by the end of the decade the vacation was over and the bills were coming due. The metaphor was appropriate: That vacation, which was accompanied by presidential assurances that everything was in good shape, led to massive national and personal indebtedness, political and economic excesses, widespread greed and corruption in the marketplace, family turmoil (with divorce at an all-time high), and a decline in the nation's social and medical well-being. The structural deterioration of the great cities of America includes their being dirty, odoriferous, and looking in places as if they had been ravaged by war. They are filled with beggars, violent gangs, the mentally ill (often publicly hallucinating), and the homeless, who huddle on newspapers on sidewalk grates or lie together for warmth like stacks of cordwood. The worsening social health also is evidenced by the increasing numbers of adults and children living in poverty, child neglect and juvenile delinquency, pervasive violence with child and spouse abuse, and the rising crime rate. The worsening physical health includes the high infant mortality rate, increasing homicide and accident rates among those aged 15 to 24, the spread of the AIDS epidemic, and even the return of "conquered" diseases such as tuberculosis (which had not been a major health problem for almost four decades).

Those widespread pathologies have been accompanied by a rising tide of antifamilism that is led by the increasing approval of divorce and of conspicuous consumption by the nation's elite, especially its political and financial leaders. In addition to the high divorce rate, other indicators of the antifamilistic trend are the postponement of marriage and the later age of first marriage, the changing structure of the family (with, for example, the legal recognition of the "domestic partners" living arrangement), the increasing number of single-parent families, publicly accepted cohabitation without marriage, the recent (and shocking) Census Bureau report that almost 25% of the 3.9 million women who had babies in 1990 were not married and that "more than half of all births to 18- and 19-year-olds in the last 5 years were out of wedlock" (B. Hill, 1991, p. 3).

Two prominent questions stand out against this somber background. First, do the activities at the societal and community level influence the functioning and well-being of the family and its members at other levels? Second, how and to what extent is the family's well-being related to individual members' physical and emotional health?

SUMMARY AND CONCLUSIONS

Any answer to the first question must be tentative. The question is fundamental, but its scale is so vast that the only data that can be used to formulate opinions about it are those from historical studies of societies and their cultures that lend themselves to inference and analogy. Although the question about the influences of society, the family, and the individual on each other has puzzled the great rulers, historians, and philosophers through the ages, as well as social and behavioral scientists during the past two centuries, the need to obtain knowledge about it has become urgent. Those influences appear to be gaining epidemic force, as they are transmitted in seconds from world capitals and studios via the media and telephone to homes and individuals. Also, Western society has been transformed in this century by the brutalities of two world wars, the horrors of nuclear weapons, the atrocities of totalitarian regimes, and the follies of the cold war that, as Graubard (1992) recently noted, "coarsened the American political system—made it less moral . . . less ready to address fundamental social problems. Institutional damage has been severe" (p. A23).

Thus, as the century ends, we are seeing rapid political and economic changes of such magnitude that they amaze historians and even veteran news commentators. Margaret Mead (1970) insisted that the rapidity of change, not change itself (which has always been present), was the current major source of stress in Western society. It is likely that the last part of the stressful, brutal twentieth century will be seen as the beginning of the postmodern era, just as the sixteenth century marked the beginning of the modern era. With these thoughts in mind, we conducted extensive studies in social history, cultural anthropology, sociology, and the history of the family.

Since at least the time of Herodotus, the "father of history," the character of a society and the nature of its culture have been associated with its marital customs, family structure and relations, and type of education for the young. Zimmerman (1947) emphasized that the cycles of history have been paralleled by changes in family type. When the government was weak, for example, the large trustee family tended to be the main family type. Family or clan law and customs prevailed, as in Homeric Greece and even in the mountainous regions of Appalachia a few decades ago. But when a government was strong and it prized the family, there was an equilibrium between it and the dominant domestic family type, which had its own beliefs and customs and directed its energies toward traditional family functions—the stabilization of the adults' personalities and the rearing of the children. The domestic family is responsive to governmental authority but bears the responsibility for socializing the young and for transmitting the cultural legacy.

Increasing power of government and a decline in traditional values, however, have been associated with Zimmerman's anomic family, which is small, lacks cohesion, and is individualistically oriented. The anomic family's weaknesses go hand in hand with the central government's assuming many family functions. The anomic family became the dominant type in ancient Greece in the fourth century B.C. following the internecine Peloponnesian War and was prominent in the Roman Empire during its last decadent centuries (about A.D. 200 to 476). The anomic family type also began to be identifiable in Western society in the late nineteenth century. In the 1860s, Le Play (Silver, 1982), who termed such families "unstable," conceptualized them as a disintegrating type that benefited neither the society to which they belonged nor, in the long run, the family members. Since at least the 1960s, the anomic family has been the dominant type in the United States, and many of its features, especially divorce and excessive individualism, are evidence of family instability (and, possibly, pathology).

Thus, in contrast to the popular evolutionary views of the family espoused by Westermarck, Burgess, and many other family scholars, history shows that societies and their cultures grow and decline in organic (if not cyclic) fashion over time. Likewise, families change in type with the changes taking place in the wider society. The neglect of history and the tendency to see the family as an isolated institution—relatively uninfluenced by the character and vitality of the central government—probably led such prominent family sociologists as Burgess and Locke (1945), Ogburn and Nimkoff (1955), and Parsons and Bales (1955) to view the changes in the family in the early to middle decades of the twentieth century as evidence not of family disorganization but of an appropriate transition "from institution to companionship" (Burgess & Locke, 1945).

Changes in the family in this century are marked by the frequency of divorce—one half of all marriages now end in divorce, including 60% of divorced persons' second marriages—and the ascendancy of individualism, the concurrent decline of familism, and a corresponding increase in the authority of the state. This increased authority has been accompanied by the Reagan-Bush administrations' blaming, if not scapegoating, of the family for the social ills that mar America. Barbara Bush (Radcliffe & Dionne, 1992) declared that the country's problems were not produced by the government but were attributable to values: "We're doing a really lousy job as parents." Blaming the family for the nation's social ills absolves the leaders of the government of responsibility for social problems even while they are increasing their regulation of family

SUMMARY AND CONCLUSIONS 357

functions and setting examples of irresponsibility that filter down to influence the young. Thus, in the United States since the 1960s (and especially in the 1980s), the national government has become stronger and its antifamilism has contributed to the disorganization and weakening of the family, which is becoming fragile and perhaps unappealing.

The second question concerns how and to what extent are the changes in the family associated with its members' marital problems and behavioral disorders? The emotional and relationship problems presented by children of divorce, the plight of the large number of children now living in poverty, the high rates of mental disorders in the separated and divorced, and the younger age of onset of the depressive disorders add to the seriousness of the ECA finding that about 20% of all adult Americans have a diagnosable mental disorder (Freedman, 1984).

Weissman (1991) recently reported that the peak age of onset of depression is now in the early 20s; 12% of cases appear before age 15 and 22% to 23% by age 20. The lower age of onset has ominous implications; a maxim of epidemiology is that when the age of onset of any chronic or recurring illness decreases, there will be an increased prevalence of that condition in the future. Cohort studies (e.g., Klerman, 1988; Klerman, Lavori, Rice, et al., 1985) are verifying our report (Schwab, Warheit, & Holzer, 1973) of high rates of depressive symptoms among teenagers and young adults. Weissman (1990) concluded that there were "higher rates in more recent birth cohorts and an earlier age of onset . . . with an increase in the rates of depression for all ages but particularly . . . an increase in the teenage and early adult years" (pp. 9-10). Some of the multiple biological and psychosocial factors responsible are changes in the family structure and especially drugs and divorce.

The association between family disruption and distress on one hand and depression on the other, which has been described by the great writers and has been a melancholic theme in song, is supported by many reports of higher rates of depression in the separated and divorced than the married. As noted earlier, Weissman (1991) reported that just asking how a patient was getting along with his or her spouse was a good screening question for depression. Of those who replied that they were not getting along well and were quarreling, 14.9% of males and 45.3% of females were found to have major depression.

Thus, evidence indicates that there are significant relationships between the family, the vitality and character of the society, and the well-being of the family members. History reveals parallels between the strength and integrity of the government at one level and the soundness of the family at another level. And data-based evidence shows that although the causal sequences have not been established, healthy and competent families usually are composed of healthy and emotionally stable persons, whereas mental illness "runs" in other families.

OUR STUDIES

We carried out three different types of studies to evaluate the increasing concerns about the family in this century and the associations between the family and mental disorder. We wanted to look at the interactions and sequences involved among stressful life events (SLEs), the family environment, family functioning, and the presence and development of symptoms of emotional distress and mental disorder in family members. The first study consisted mainly of a comprehensive review of the literature on the family in Western society, including a survey of research on the family and mental disorder. The second was a pilot longitudinal epidemiological study of a random sample of families in the Louisville area. The third was a historical-clinical chart review of almost 500 cases between 1973 and 1988 from our child guidance clinic that was designed to complement both the historical studies and the epidemiological research.

We devoted special attention to the history of the family in an attempt to enlarge our perspective on the many changes in the family in this century. Our specific aims were, first, to learn about associations between societies and their cultures and evaluate possible relationships between them and the family on one hand and mental disorder on the other; and second, to identify the roots of the modern nuclear family to see if knowledge about its past could increase understanding of the problems families are encountering in the 1990s and be used to prevent mental disorder.

The History of the Family

We found that the modern nuclear family has three major roots—the legacy of antiquity from ancient Greece and Rome, its Judeo-Christian heritage, and its enduring Anglo-Saxon traditions. Most historians, however, have overlooked or have given little attention to the Egyptian family, which antedates that of the Old Testament by about 1,500 years. From the Pharaonic texts of about 2500 B.C. and other sources, evidence reveals that the family during Egypt's long history (from about 3000 B.C. to Alexander's conquest in 323 B.C. and Roman occupation by Caesar in 50 B.C.) often was a strong institution and that its vitality fluctuated with the cycles of governmental stability and decadence. Marriage customs in ancient Egypt were firmly established, the status of women was high, and there were laws referable to divorce, family property settlements, and even infanticide. Breasted's (1933) intensive studies indicated that the "dawn of conscience" and of social responsibility came when the sentiments binding the family together began to be extended to the community. The maxims of Amenhotep, which emphasized marital and other family obligations, preceded the Mosaic commandments by about 1,000 years. Durant (1935) pointed out that much of the culture transmitted to us from ancient Greece and Rome was taken from the Egyptians.

The modern family's legacy from classical Greece and ancient Rome was mainly their emphasis on marriage as a sacred ceremony and the importance of the family as a religious institution. Also, many of our marriage ceremonies and the function of the home as a basic economic unit have been passed down to us in relatively unchanged form. The Judaic heritage of the modern family consisted primarily of its transformation from a maternal kinship system to a strong patriarchal family unit. Christianity introduced reforms in Mediterranean societies 2,000 years ago by requiring monogamy, elevating the status of women, and making marriage a sacrament. Thus, it bound the family to religious as well as social foundations. The Reformation included a revival of Old Testament views and values, especially the vise-like authority of the father, the loosening of which in this century has been associated with family instability. The Anglo-Saxon traditions of monogamy, individualism, and self-sufficiency supported the emergence of the nuclear family and capitalism in the eleventh and twelfth centuries and, even earlier, the recognition of the married union as based on the mutual desire of the bride and groom rather than a parental arrangement.

The historical review sharpened our appreciation of the interrelationships of the society, the family, and the individual. We were surprised to learn that, contrary to many twentieth century sociologists' opinions, the modern nuclear family has been in existence in England since about the eleventh or twelfth centuries. Its rise to become the dominant family type in western Europe and the United States, particularly among Anglo-Saxon groups, is associated with capitalism and individualism, but a cause and effect relationship (and even the sequence) is unclear. Some family scholars and researchers have maintained that the rise of capitalism led to the emergence of the nuclear family as the dominant family type; however, considerable new evidence indicates that the nuclear family as we know it was responsible for the rise of capitalism in the twelfth and thirteenth centuries, or that the nuclear family and capitalism arose together at about the same time and abetted each other's development. Thus, the supposedly strong influence of the Industrial Revolution on the development of the modern nuclear family has been largely discredited, although it changed family life (often adversely).

The review of the history of the family also showed that it has had resilience and durability, even though it has been affected by social and cultural events and processes. The Greek family that Thucydides praised early in the Peloponnesian War was satirized by Aristophanes only 50 to 60 years later as being ineffectual, if not ridiculous, and the Roman family changed significantly during the second century B.C. after women began to run the state during the Punic Wars. In the United States, changes in the family began after the Civil War. The black family emerged as a unit, women's roles started to change, and industrialization and urbanization began to transform the character of American life. Increasing numbers of women started working in the sweatshops and industries in the cities and, later, in the factories in the notorious mill towns of the South. By the 1880s, desertion and divorce were increasing, and the first family organizations were formed. During the early years of this century, concern about the family mounted following the economic panic of 1893, the closing of the frontier in 1896, and continuing urbanization.

The "century of concern" started with these developments and became manifest with the appearance of serial monogamy and growing tensions between individualism and familism. Family scholars saw that the institutional foundations of the family had been weakened by Darwinism and concepts of evolution, increasing secularism, and the rapid social change accelerated by inventions and early technologies. Many of the changes in the family were considered to be appropriately modern, but by the late 1960s, glaring pathologies had surfaced. By the 1980s, individualism and familism were divisively polarized.

In this century, the American family has been changed further by Western society's wars. Wars loosened family cohesion, relaxed mores, and changed roles within the family. Divorce rates climbed after both world wars and never returned to prewar levels. Probably most importantly, as Burgess and Locke (1960) noted, the main effect of the wars on the family was to hasten changes already taking place.

Family Research

Research on the family and its functions, well-being, and illness had a slow start. It began as a consequence of the changes in the social order, especially the emergence of the middle class in western Europe and the changes in institutions precipitated by the French Revolution. It was stimulated by the urbanization and other social developments accompanying the Industrial Revolution and by the rise of the social sciences. Le Play's studies of European families' budgets in the 1850s and 1860s showed that different family types were associated with levels of societal vitality. For example, the stem family, in which the oldest son inherited the family property and the other children were given various monetary allotments and expected to go out into the world, was the common type in thriving societies. In contrast, the unstable family was becoming the common type in the new urbanized and bureaucratized societies. Although Le Play supplied an effective method for studying families, there was little research during the rest of the nineteenth century except for fruitless studies and debates about the origin of the family, mainly about whether early families were matriarchal or patriarchal. But, early in this century, cultural anthropologists became interested in the new psychoanalytic theory and began to evaluate associations between groups' customs, child-rearing practices, and personality types, usually in families in the South Seas or among Indian groups in North America.

About the turn of the century, some surveys of families living in poverty were conducted in England. The most famous were Charles Booth's (1892) studies of the London poor and Rowntree's (1903) study of York. They showed that about 25% to 30% of families in those large cities were so poor that their health was compromised by deprivation. Jack London's (1904) *People of the Abyss* is a grim, haunting portrayal of that misery. At about the same time, some of Kraepelin's associates carried out pedigree studies of psychiatric patients' families to determine whether mental disorders were heritable. They found that mental disorders were more common in patients' families than in those of nonpatient controls and thus launched the research that is now being conducted to isolate genes responsible for specific mental illnesses, especially bipolar disorder or schizophrenia.

The rising divorce rate after World War I prompted early studies of marital happiness, success, or adjustment. Studies in the 1920s and 1930s showed generally that selected young middle- and upper-middle-class urban dwellers' degree of marital satisfaction was related to the partners' mental health. Also, in the 1930s, researchers looked at the effects of the Great Depression on the family, and in the 1940s at the effects of World War II. By 1950, family scholars agreed that family research had been retarded, in part because it was considered unethical to invade the privacy of the family. The rising divorce rate during and after World War II, however, focused attention on family stress and coping. Sociologists began to formulate conceptual models of family functioning, and in psychiatry, Ackerman developed methods for family studies in an attempt to construct a family typology that would have clinical significance.

During the past 20 years, major family studies have been aimed toward assessing the family life cycle and intergenerational influences on health and well-being; evaluating stress and the family; and, currently, developing models and instruments to evaluate family functioning and/or competence. The ongoing longitudinal studies of families after the birth of the first or another child show promise, especially those being conducted by Lewis and his colleagues (1988) and by Belsky and his associates (1983, 1985, 1988). Longitudinal studies have potential for supplying data that contribute to knowledge about family functioning and the members' health as transitions and other stressors influence the family over its life cycle. Unfortunately, there have been few controlled studies of divorce and marital disruption, even though this has been one of the greatest family problems in the last decades of the century.

The Family and Mental Disorder

After World War II, psychiatrists and behavioral scientists began to study the possible etiological role of the family in the development of schizophrenia. Although Bateson and his colleagues' (1956) highly touted double bind was found not to be specific for schizophrenia, studies led to the development of such concepts as Bowen's (1959) multigenerational influences and triangling, Jackson's (1957) family homeostasis and the "identified patient," Lidz, Fleck, and Cornelison's (1965) narcissistic and "paranoidal parents," and Wynne and his colleagues' (1976) pseudomutuality and communication deviance. Family members' mental disorders were found to be associated with family dysfunctions, but there were no specific associations between a particular disorder and family dysfunction. Family research shifted to studies of biological factors and schizophrenia, especially after Rosenthal and Kety's (1968) Danish adoptees study showed that schizophreniform illnesses were more common in patients' biological than adoptive parents.

Until recently, there was much less research on the family and the affective disorders, especially major depression, than on the family and schizophrenia. Repeated clinical, case-control, and family studies, however, have found that depression is associated with a disturbed, negative family environment. The depressed person's irritability and withdrawal, along with the communication problems accompanying depression, can dominate the family environment. A depressed mother's interactions have a deleterious effect on young children in the home, and depression is associated with marital arguments and discord.

SUMMARY AND CONCLUSIONS

The review of the literature showed that mental disorders tend to run in families and are associated with stressful life events (SLEs), an adverse home environment, and disturbances in family functioning, but the sequences involved have not been untangled. Also, possible causal family dysfunctions have not been identified. Both clinical experience and such research as that of Penrose (1944) and Kreitman (1962) have shown that mental disorder in a family member can have a deleterious effect on other family members. There is a need for large-scale longitudinal epidemiological studies of the family and mental disorder that evaluate the antecedents of mental disorder as well as its effects.

The Pilot Epidemiological Study

Our second approach, therefore, was to carry out a pilot epidemiological study of a random sample of families in their homes at three times over a 15-month period to develop and test methods for large-scale studies. Most research on the family, stress, and/or mental disorder has been on highly selected groups, mainly patients' families or middle- and/or upper-middle-class volunteer families, and most of the research has been cross-sectional (i.e., families were studied at only one time). Our major aim was to conduct a pilot study to ascertain whether the stressful life events–family functioning–onset of symptoms sequence could be disentangled and not subject to the chicken-egg question that is a valid criticism of the results of much cross-sectional research.

An epidemiological approach was necessary because the problems facing families required studies of social and cultural processes, communities, and groups of families over time. Inasmuch as a mentally ill family member changes the interactions, environment, and functioning within the family, it is necessary to study and follow families in which there is no emotional symptomatology. Only comprehensive longitudinal efforts can evaluate the reciprocal influences of the three systems—the society, the family, and the individual—and explicate possible causes and sequences involved in relation to mental illness.

Another reason for beginning with a pilot epidemiological study was that investigators working in psychiatric genetics and in biological psychiatry needed baseline data from large-scale studies of mental disorder in families against which they could compare their results. Also, epidemiological studies of families complement the extensive pedigree research being carried out in an attempt to isolate genetic defects for particular mental illnesses.

Still another reason to conduct an epidemiological study of even a small random sample of families was that psychiatric epidemiology had reached a plateau with the successful completion of the ECA studies during the 1980s. A necessary step in psychiatric epidemiology required the development of concepts and methods and the testing and refining of procedures that would enable investigators to conduct longitudinal epidemiological studies of families representative of the general population. To the best of our knowledge, such studies had not been done, and methods for such research were not available. We had the opportunity to adopt and adapt the instruments and methods used in the ECA studies of individuals to family studies. One of our major objectives, therefore, was to raise the epidemiological unit, both conceptually and methodologically, from the level of the individual to that of the family.

Concepts and Methods

To carry out our pilot feasibility study, we obtained a true random sample of 43 families from the greater Louisville area. We trained interviewers, developed the interview schedules, and interviewed all the adults and children individually in their homes at three times—at baseline, 6 months later, and then after 9 more months. The age-appropriate interviews were designed to elicit information about (a) the family members' sociodemographic characteristics and personal and health histories: (b) the occurrence of SLEs and their impact on the family; (c) the characteristics and quality of the family environment; (d) marital and family satisfaction or dissatisfaction; and (e) both the presence and onset of symptoms of mental disorder and physical illness. Some of the instruments we used were the Center for Epidemiologic Studies Depression Scale (CES-D; Radloff, 1977), the Diagnostic Interview Schedule (DIS; Robins et al., 1979), the Short Michigan Alcoholism Screening Test (SMAST; Selzer et al., 1975), the Diagnostic Interview Schedule for Children (DISC; Costello, Edelbrock, & Dulcan, 1985), the Child Behavior Checklist (CBCL; Achenbach & Edelbrock, 1983), and the Denver Developmental Screening Test (DDST; Frankenburg et al., 1975). In addition to interviews of the family members, we made videotapes of each family as a group in their homes while the members were carrying out a specified task.

To relate what was happening in the wider society and the community to the information that we obtained from the family members, we studied the current events impinging on the Louisville area, previous community surveys, and the 1970 and 1980 census data. We looked at social indicators and census tract data for the tracts in which each of our families lived, and the we compared the families' incomes and other

SUMMARY AND CONCLUSIONS

social facts and characteristics with data on the census tracts in which they lived.

As the conceptual basis for our work, we selected general living systems theory elaborated by James G. Miller (1978) from von Bertalanffy's (1966) *General Systems Theory*. We considered Miller's general living systems theory to be appropriate because it specifies interacting hierarchical levels such as the individual, the group (family), and the society, and also the subsystems at each level. We reviewed definitions of the family and operationalized a definition that would have utility at a time when family structure and relationships were changing rapidly. We defined the family as two or more persons who live in a circumscribed dwelling that has definite boundaries (e.g., a house, apartment, or mobile home), who interact, and who are bound together in some way (legal, affectional, etc.). We found that the definition had utility and also that it had certain limitations; in particular, it did not include any members of the extended family who lived outside the designated household area, even though, in some instances, one or more such members might have influenced what was happening to a family. There is a need for epidemiological studies of larger family units and extended families.

Some of our findings compounded the problem of defining the family. Even in the same household, we received varied answers to the question "Who do you think is in your immediate family?" In view of the extent of family disruption and of the newer types of family living arrangements, it is not possible to anticipate the composition and structure of the family unit or the cohabiting group of the future, even in the next generation or two. Perhaps, as Hagestad (1986) has suggested, the grandmother-mother-daughter vertical axis may become the most stable social unit, rather than the horizontally oriented nuclear family to which many, especially in the middle class, have been accustomed.

General living systems theory provided the conceptual basis that we needed. It kept our attention directed toward the community and the society as well as the family. The census tract data showed, for example, that the symptomatic families tended to have somewhat lower annual incomes than the median income for the census tracts in which they lived, whereas the asymptomatic families tended to have somewhat higher annual incomes than the median.

An early problem was that there was no agreement about the definition or concept of family functioning. Also, the instruments for measuring family functioning are still in various stages of development. Inasmuch as one of the chief aims of our feasibility study was to develop and test instruments and procedures for assessing family function, we designed a general living systems model of family functioning mainly from the family videotapes. We constructed the Bell and Schwab (1985) Family Systems Assessment Scale, which addresses the functioning of each of the 19 subsystems conceptualized according to general living systems theory. We will report a description of the family functioning model, the scale, and the results of our use of it in the second volume in this project.

Sampling, Recruitment, and Attrition

Some of the procedures were easier to carry out than we anticipated, and some were more difficult. The city-county directories used to establish the sample frame were adequate. Comparisons of the sociodemographic characteristics of our 43 families with data from the 1980 census indicated that the sample was representative of the Louisville community. Recruitment of families for research has been a problem since the 1950s; when we first contacted the families, we gave them copies of local officials' endorsements of the research to dispel suspicion about what we were "really" looking for. We learned from experience: We recruited only 35% of the first 51 families contacted, but 49% of the remaining 52 families. Although the participation rate was only 42%, a much smaller percentage than we have obtained in our epidemiological studies of individuals, it compares favorably with other researchers' participation rates, even with mainly middle-class volunteer or clinic families that often belonged to a certain church (Hinchliffe et al., 1978; Olson et al., 1983). We wondered whether reimbursing family members for the time they gave to the study would have increased participation but are doubtful that it would have done so. Probably it would have helped to keep teenagers interested, and it would have been a nice incentive for families living in poverty.

Recruiting depended mainly on reaching the decision maker in the family. Repeatedly the interviewers were able to enlist the person first contacted (usually the wife/mother), but after the family discussed participation, they often informed us that it would not be possible for them to participate for a variety of reasons. When a family agreed, they signed the informed consent form and we scheduled the first interview.

We worried about attrition and did our utmost to keep it low; consequently, it was not severe. The first interview session was critical because families that dropped out did so soon after the first interview: 7 (16%) dropped out of the study and 2 (5%) others moved away, but 34 (79%) families continued for the entire 15-month period.

To maintain the families' interest in the study, we sent them holiday greeting cards and kept in touch with them regularly. When we read in the newspaper about a family's activity (e.g., graduation from a school), we sent cards; also, the same interviewers continued to work with the same families. The families responded favorably to the interviewers' interest. At the end of the study, many told us they had participated because they wanted to help others. We admired the extent of altruism that we observed. Contrary to our fears, most of the families reported that participating in the study had been helpful; it had made them think about their family interactions and the high priority that needed to be given to family well-being.

Field Procedures and Interviews

We had little difficulty obtaining information. Almost all of the families disclosed their budgets, including their income and expenditures, but only 26 (60%) of the 43 families agreed to be videotaped. They worried more about the confidentiality of the videotapes than about information given to the interviewers. We scheduled appointments for family interviews and videotaping at times convenient to the families. Videotaping in the homes was technically easier than we had anticipated inasmuch as the video camera could be used with ordinary lighting. Interviewing the families in their homes was both feasible and desirable; we urge other investigators to study families in the home whenever possible.

We had a major problem balancing the amount of information we wanted to obtain with family members' interest in the study and their fatigue threshold. Some topics that we wished we had covered more completely are the family histories and the number, type, and quality of relationships (marital, parental, sibling, with the extended family, with those at work or in school, and within the community). The need to examine such a broad group of relationships is heightened by the rapidity and variability of the changes taking place in the family and other personal relationships. Also, we wished that we had been able to obtain a more complete history of family milestones, the life course, and the children's development, but we just could not pack all of these items into the 1½ hour interview. We concluded that interview schedules for epidemiological studies of families needed to be carefully designed and limited because it is more important to get some information at frequent intervals than a great deal at one time only. Also, lengthy interviews at the beginning increase the probability that the family or some members will drop out and that valuable information about what happens over time will be lost. It would be valuable to have families keep diaries of important events and family milestones, and we would attempt to do so in another study.

After a training period, the interviewers were able to use the Diagnostic Interview Schedule (DIS) effectively. We were pleased that we could make symptom counts and thus rate family members for symptom status on the DIS, not just diagnoses. The DIS probes also yielded satisfactory information about the nature of the symptoms reported; however, the relatively early version of the DIS that we used was too detailed. An epidemiological family study needs to focus on the common manifestations of emotional distress (symptoms of various anxiety disorders and affective disorders) rather than on such relatively rare illnesses as schizophrenia.

Asking family members (first individually, and then as a group) to set goals for themselves and for the family supplied significant information about family interactions and members' values and orientations, especially on the individualism versus familism issue. In addition, observing them at a goal-setting task gave us insights into the family's decision-making process and the amount and quality of communication between them. It was not, however, a comprehensive approach to studying family functioning.

During the course of the study, the interviewers began to suffer from fatigue and/or disinterest. Inasmuch as the home interviews were scheduled at times convenient for the family, burnout was bound to develop. We learned that having the interviewers attend weekly meetings of the entire research team heightened their interest in the study and invigorated them. During those meetings, we asked them to present interesting or troublesome situations.

Data Management and Analyses

We were able to use the commercial software package SIR for management and organization of the data on 75 adults and 54 children at three periods of time. It is an integrated database management system that is easy to learn, available on a variety of mainframe and personal computers, and interfaces with such statistical packages as the Statistical Package for the Social Sciences (SPSS). SIR handles both variable-length records and hierarchically structured data sets. For our analyses, we used the statistical procedures in SPSS, including chi-square, analysis of variance, cluster analyses, discriminant function analyses, and logistical regression. We demonstrated that discriminant function analysis and logistical regressions could predict symptom status, even though the analyses were limited by the small size of the sample.

Although we have studied SLEs in patient groups and in random samples of the general population for about 20 years, we were somewhat

SUMMARY AND CONCLUSIONS

dissatisfied with the SLE information that we obtained from family members. To experiment and to develop methods as needed, at Time 2 we gave the SLE inventory to the family as a group while they were being videotaped. Fewer SLEs were reported than we anticipated; we think that various family members did not report certain events because of the lack of confidentiality. Consequently, at Time 3 we returned to the method we had used at Time 1, asking each family member about SLEs during the confidential individual interview.

To evaluate family stress, we took the information from the level of the individual (i.e., each family member's responses to the SLE inventory and to questions about who was affected and why the event had occurred) and, as a panel, grouped related events and their effects into stress themes that we rated for each family. For example, a stress theme that involved work might include such SLEs as a family member's being laid off from a job and obtaining a new job at a lower wage, resulting in less family income, another member starting work, and reduced expenditures for the children's education.

We placed the themes in three major categories: intrafamilial (involving only the members of the household); other relatives (involving family members not living in the household); and friends. We rated the stress themes in each category as to whether they were positive or negative, included ratings of the theme's impact on the family, and gave them scores that ranged from +4 to −4.

We now think that to gain in-depth information about stress and an understanding of its effect upon a family, it is necessary to supplement the SLE inventory for adults and adolescents with measures that evaluate chronic stressors, particularly the "hassles" of everyday life and the stressors related to marriage, work or school, finances, parent-child relationships, and the neighborhood. Also, there is a need to devise instruments that will assess the families' habitual patterns of reacting to stressors and their social supports. Ilfeld (1977) found that chronic stressors scores explained much more of the variance in respondents' depression scores than did their sociodemographic characteristics. More recently, Gary and his colleagues (1989) found that the everyday "hassles"—especially chronic financial and marital difficulties—were strongly associated with high depression scores in black males.

Results

Extent of Symptomatology. The results of the epidemiological study were surprising. We did not know what to anticipate; to the best of our knowledge, it was the first such study of a sample of families from the general population that had been carried out in the United States. Although no family member met full DIS criteria for the diagnosis of a mental disorder at Time 1, during the course of the study, 3 members in different families did so. At Time 1, however, 25 (58%) of the families met the criteria we established for being symptomatic (see Chapter 5); thus, we had evidence of significant distress in the community. In 13 (52%) of those 25 families, only one member was symptomatic, but the other 12 (48%) were multisymptomatic—two members in 6 (24%) of the families, and three or more members in the other 6 (24%). In those 25 families, 44 members were symptomatic. Members most likely to be symptomatic were adult daughters (100%), followed by adult sons (90%), young daughters (60%), and mothers (50%); those least likely were fathers (38%) and young sons (29%). The adult daughters tended to be symptomatic on current emotional distress, the adult sons for alcohol and/or drug problems, the mothers on the affective measures (CES-D and depression) and panic, and the fathers for depression. The CES-D, which measured dysphoria during the past week, was the symptom measure most often positive in the family members (13%). The others were depression symptoms on the DIS (11%), drug problems (10%), alcohol problems (6%), panic symptoms (6%), and phobic symptoms (4%).

Many of the symptomatic individuals were subclinical cases. Their being uncovered by a study such as ours is one of the "uses of epidemiology" (Morris, 1964). Identifying such cases before they reach full intensity has implications for the prevention of more serious illness. Unfortunately, very few symptomatic family members were receiving care; only 4 families had members who received mental health care during the past year.

After the first wave of interviews, 2 (5%) of the 43 families moved away, and 7 (16%) dropped out of the study. A disproportionately high number, 8 (89%) of these 9 families, were symptomatic. They tended to be single-parent, poor, often black families that had multiple problems and a great deal of symptomatology. Almost all of them had young and/or adult children at home, most of whom were symptomatic—the adult sons with alcohol or drug problems, and the adult daughters with depression symptoms, panic, and/or phobias. Although the families pleaded that the study took too much time, it appeared that the interviews were surfacing troubling problems that had been avoided because there were no solutions in sight. When such families are enlisted in studies, researchers need to make special efforts to retain them, and when they are in treatment, therapists need to take special steps to understand their burdens, provide concrete help with crises, and work through their resistance to keep them in therapy over time.

SUMMARY AND CONCLUSIONS

Change and Variability in Symptomatology and Family Composition Over Time. The second most important result was that even though our study was conducted only three times over a 15-month period, there was substantial variability in the family symptomatic status and family composition from one time to the next.[1] The 34 families that completed the study constituted a panel for Time 1–Time 3 comparisons. At time 1, in all 34 families, 26 (25%) members in 17 (50%) families were symptomatic; of those 17 families, 11 had only one symptomatic member, but in the other 6 families, two or more members were symptomatic. As in the dropout families, the adult sons and daughters were the members most often symptomatic, the sons for alcohol and drug problems and the daughters for current affective distress and phobias. The symptomatic and asymptomatic families differed in that the symptomatic families were somewhat larger, more often contained adult children (few of whom were employed), and had heads who were older and had less education and lower incomes.

At Time 3, we found less symptomatology than at Time 1. Of the 34 families, 19 (19%) members in 15 (44%) families were symptomatic. In 12 (80%) of the 15 families, only one member was symptomatic, but in the remaining 3 (20%) families, two or more members were symptomatic. At Time 3, as at Time 1, the sons and daughters were most often symptomatic, and the fathers the least often. And, as at Time 1, the symptomatic males tended to report alcohol and drug abuse problems and the females depressive symptoms. Finding less symptomatology at reinterviews (the regression toward the mean) has been reported often in epidemiological studies, especially when the interviews were only months or about a year apart. The recent ECA report of the second-wave interviews (1 year after the initial surveys) noted that the respondents reported fewer symptoms (Eaton et al., 1989).

The symptom patterns that tended not to change from Time 1 to Time 3 were the affective symptoms on the CES-D and the depressive symptoms list. Also, those symptoms of dysphoria were the ones that "developed" over a 15-month period, whereas panic and phobic symptoms and some of the alcohol and drug problems tended to clear up.

We divided the 34 families into four subgroups according to their symptomatic status at both interviews. Only 14 (41%) of the 34 families were asymptomatic at both Time 1 and Time 3; 8 (24%) changed in

[1] Inasmuch as one of our main purposes was to develop methods and carry out a feasibility study, we used the Time 2 interviews to test innovative and alternative approaches and procedures. Thus, as explained in Chapter 5, the Time 2 data were less complete and not comparable either to the Time 1 or to the Time 3 data (which were obtained by using most of the Time 1 procedures again).

symptom status, and the remaining 12 (35%) were symptomatic at both times. About two thirds of the families that were asymptomatic at both times were "older" families (couples in their mid-50s or early 60s), but three had children under age 15 at home, and two others had adult children at home.

Of the 8 (24%) families that changed in symptomatic status over the 15 months, 3 changed from being asymptomatic to symptomatic; thus, the 15-month incidence rate for developing symptoms was 9%. One was an elderly couple in which the husband developed symptoms of depression. Another was a couple with two children (ages 11 and 2) in which the mother became symptomatic on the CES-D and reported depressive symptoms at Time 3; her father had recently died, and she was having a grief reaction. The third was a young couple who had a new baby; the mother was symptomatic on the CES-D at Time 3 and had symptoms of depression, probably a post-partum syndrome.

The 5 other families that changed were symptomatic at Time 1 but asymptomatic at Time 3; thus, the 15-month family remission rate was 15%. At Time 1, in 3 of those families, the mother was symptomatic for panic; in the fourth, the father was phobic; and in the fifth, an adult daughter (who was about to leave home for college) was symptomatic on the CES-D. In all of the families, the parents were in early middle age and had children under age 16 at home. Generally, they were "functioning" families that had reasonable financial and extended family "resources."

Unfortunately, we also identified chronicity: 12 (35%) families were symptomatic at both Time 1 and Time 3. In 5 families, there were children under age 16 at home; in another 6, the parents were older, and most had adult children still living at home. Features that characterized these families were the persistence and multiplicity of symptomatology in the same family members over time. In 9 (75%) of the 12 families, there was at least one family member who was symptomatic at both Time 1 and Time 3, often on multiple measures. In the 34 families interviewed at both times, the family members most likely to be symptomatic at one or both times were the adult sons (60%), followed by the young daughters (50%), the adult daughters (43%), and the mothers (30%). Fathers and young sons had the lowest percentages with symptomatology (23% and 19%, respectively).

Family composition as well as symptom status was dynamic and variable. Members moved in and out of the families, even during the 15 months of the study. In the 34 families, there were five major changes; three persons entered families (two were born and one returned home), and two left to marry. Such a flow of family members affects family

SUMMARY AND CONCLUSIONS

interactions and points to the necessity to continue family studies over a significant period of time. We now think that an epidemiological family study should include interviews over at least 5 years with brief reports at 4- to 6-month intervals in order to evaluate changes that accompany the growth of the children and the family members' transitions. Also, probably 5 years is the minimum period of time in which to identify the patterns of family life and health that are stable and those that are variable during that part of the life course. Inasmuch as the family is a dynamic complex system, we suggest that family therapists need to assess continually the changing composition as well as interactions within the family.

Family Risk Factors. The three major family risk factors were structure (belonging to a single-parent family or having adult children at home), low socioeconomic status (SES), and stress. At time 1, 8 (89%) of the 9 single-parent families in the study were symptomatic, in contrast to 17 (50%) of the 34 families with two parents. The many problems of single-parent families include their usually being the bitter fruits of a parent leaving the family (through separation, divorce, or desertion) or, increasingly, of unmarried women having children and thus heading families. Single-parent families usually are headed by the mother who carries the total parenting burden. In those families, symptoms surface when the parent-child boundaries break down and members become entangled in each other's distress. Too often, financial difficulties, if not outright poverty, compound the grim everyday problems of living.

The risks associated with having adult children at home can be serious. At Time 1, 12 (75%) of the 16 families with adult children at home were symptomatic, and 73% of the adult children were symptomatic (usually with alcohol and/or drug problems). Also, often other members in those families were symptomatic; they tended to be the mothers, many of whom were in affective distress. The adult children seemed to be producing distortions in the family structure that possibly caused or at least were associated with the symptomatology in other family members.

Low SES, reflecting low educational, occupational, and income levels, has both direct and mediating affects that are deleterious. The association between low SES and high mental illness rates is the most consistent finding in psychiatric epidemiology. Our families that were headed by fathers and mothers with less than high school educations and/or by heads who were unemployed or had only part-time employment, along with the families with annual incomes of $12,000 (1983 dollars) or less, were significantly more likely to be symptomatic than the better educated, the employed, and those with higher annual family incomes.

In the first systematic family research, Frederic Le Play, in the 1850s and 1860s, related the adequacy of "family budgets" to family stability. Our symptomatic families had lower monthly incomes than the asymptomatic, but their living expenses were about the same. The symptomatic families spent a higher percentage of their income on food, utilities, and gasoline, but a lower percentage on child care than the asymptomatic. Such findings are consistent with those described by Le Play and reflect the validity of his "family budget" method for studying family well-being.

In Chapters 1 and 3, we discussed the devastating effects of poverty on the family; it is common in single-parent families and is the factor responsible for many of their problems. Its direct effects on children in the United States are recounted in harrowing descriptions of distress. Seeing such children and their tired, usually depressed mothers in health clinics arouses grave misgivings about the character of our society and its values, especially the attacks on welfare by national leaders. Nationally, the poverty rate has increased greatly. Gwen Ifill (1992) reported that "declining incomes forced 2 million more people below the Federal poverty line—$10,419 for a family of three . . . [yet] 40 states cut or froze benefits to families with children" (p. 1). She reported a statement by Robert Borosage from the Institute for Policy Studies: "People are feeling a compassion fatigue. . . . They're tired of the homeless, tired of poor people" (p. 1). And the poor are becoming invisible. An advisor to Senator Tom Harkin (D-Iowa) pointed out "nobody's speaking for poor people" (p. 1).

Paul Krugman (1990) cited tax data compiled by the Congressional Budget Office showing that "the top 1% got 60% of the gain in the '80s boom" (Nasar, 1992, p. A1). From 1977 to 1989, the average pretax income for families in the top 1% rose from $377,000 per year to almost $560,000. Nasar pointed out that the great reduction of tax rates (down from a 90% top rate during the Kennedy presidency), along with high incomes for executives, accounted for the massive distribution of income upward to the wealthy. The typical American family, however, from 1977 to 1989 had only a 4% rise in family income to $36,000 per year, "and the bottom 40% of families had actual declines in income" (Nasar, 1992, p. A1). Some of our results revealed the symptomatology often associated with the declining family incomes of so many in America in the 1980s. If the widening of the gap in family income between those at the top and the bottom of the social ladder continues, the "Brazilification" of the USA will have occurred. The large, poverty-stricken lower social class groups will become a permanent underclass that is impaired by physical and mental symptomatology and limited by little education, drugs, and other afflictions and handicaps. The intergenerational continuity of distress and disadvantage will cloud the American dream and besmirch the "land of opportunity."

The concept and development of stress themes and their ratings enabled us to relate family-level stress and its type to the presence or absence of symptomatology. The symptomatic group's mean intrafamilial stress theme score was -1.8, significantly different from the asymptomatic group's positive score of 0.6. The most common intrafamilial negative stress themes were work and finances, minor law violations, and hospitalizations; the main positive theme was a personal achievement. The two groups' other-relatives and friends stress theme scores differed only slightly; the symptomatic group's mean scores were -0.8 and -1.0, respectively, and the asymptomatic group's were -0.1 and -1.2, respectively. The most common negative other-relatives stress themes were work and finances and hospitalization; again, the main positive theme was a personal achievement. The friends themes were all negative (e.g., the death of a friend, or a friend moving away).

Stressors and their effects on the family cannot be evaluated as discrete or isolated phenomena. The nature of the stressor and the magnitude of its effects are influenced by families' coping abilities and resources. Also, the significance of SLEs for individuals and families depends on previous experiences with stressors, as well as psychodynamic and other factors. In future studies we will ask subjects to rate the significance of stressors for themselves, other family members, and the family as a whole.

The results of our family research supported those from studies of individuals, especially the associations between lower SES, increased number of negative life events, and symptoms of distress. Also, the highly stressed symptomatic families had lower social support ratings (i.e., little participation in churches, clubs, and other organizations and activities) than those that were asymptomatic. We did not obtain data on social supports over the 15 months, because we thought that it was too short a period of time to yield meaningful results. But it would be important in a larger study to evaluate changes in social supports over at least a few years, and especially to determine the sequential relationship between stressors, social supports, and the onset of symptoms. The major questions are as follows: (a) Does the lack of participation in social support systems contribute to or result from stressors and symptoms? (b) Does the lack of participation in such social support systems as church and club activities contribute directly to symptom status or, indirectly, by not helping to buffer the effects of stressors? (c) Specifically, is being embedded in a social support system, in itself, protective? Repeated studies show that married men are in better physical and mental health than the unmarried. But in their study of SLEs, social supports, and both physical and mental health in black adults, D. R. Brown and Gary (1987) reported that black females in poor physical health had more social supports than those in better physical health because the physically ill had developed friendships and also turned to their family members and to the church. Only longitudinal studies can supply answers to the questions about the influences of SLEs, chronic stressors, and social supports on symptoms.

Family Life Cycle and Stress. We modified the more conventional classifications of the stages of the family life cycle because they lacked an adult-children-at-home stage and because we had a relatively small number of families. Our five stage classification included the beginning of the family, young children at home (oldest child 12 years), adolescents at home (oldest child 18 years), adult children at home, and an aging couple alone. We had only a few first-stage families, but about ten in each of the other four stages. There were significant differences in stress theme levels and symptomatology between families in different stages. The mean intrafamilial stress theme score was positive for those in the first and second stages, but negative for the third-, fourth- and fifth-stage families. The other-relatives and friends stress theme scores were all negative and, as to be expected, were more negative for those in the older than the younger stages. The percentages of symptomatic second-, third-, and fourth-stage families (about 73%) were significantly larger than the percentage (18%) in the last stage.

Studies generally have reported that stress and symptomatology are prominent features of life during the adolescent family stage, when teenagers are testing limits and parents are having their own midlife strains. Our finding such a high level of stress and symptomatology in the fourth stage, when many parents were in their 50s, may be indicative of problems stemming from the continued presence or return of adult children to the parental home.

We carried out an analysis for covariance (ANCOVA) to determine the effects of both Time 1 and Time 3 symptoms status on the Time 3 intrafamilial stress theme ratings. The Time 1 intrafamilial stress theme rating was the significant predictor of the Time 3 ratings. This finding has grave implications for families that are hammered by SLEs; unfortunately, their stressors continue to occur and to exert deleterious influences. Our findings, however, raise questions about the variable effects of SLEs. In studies of individuals and in clinical work we have seen different individuals in the same or different families react variably to similar SLEs. Their reactions bring to mind the old saw that one person's

SUMMARY AND CONCLUSIONS

trash is another person's treasure, and also W. I. Thomas's (1923) profound "definition of the situation."

Family Environment. We obtained a great deal of information about the family environment by using the Family Environment Scale (FES; Moos & Moos, 1976, 1981). We and others have reported that the norms for Louisville were different from those Moos and Moos (1983) reported for samples of Bay Area populations on which the scores were standardized. Louisville respondents had significantly higher mean cohesion, moral-religious emphasis, and organization subscale scores and significantly lower mean conflict, intellectual-cultural orientation, active-recreational orientation, and control subscale scores than the California norms. Therefore, the norms need to be evaluated for use with other populations.

The FES subscale scores revealed significant differences between the symptomatic and asymptomatic families. The symptomatic families had significantly lower mean cohesion and expressiveness subscale scores, slightly higher conflict scores, and a tendency toward lower independence, intellectual-cultural orientation, and active recreational-orientation subscale scores, and they also had higher family incongruence scores than the asymptomatic families. The FES subscale scores of subjects positive on just a single measure of psychopathology (e.g., the CES-D, depression symptoms, drug problems, or the children's symptom status) were different from those who did not have that particular type of symptomatic distress, suggesting that they had different family environments. For example, families with members having high scores on the CES-D (which assesses emotional distress during the preceding week) had significantly lower cohesion, expressiveness, and moral-religious emphasis subscale scores and a higher family incongruence score than those with low CES-D scores. Also, families with depressive symptoms had significantly lower mean cohesion and expressiveness scores and a higher mean incongruence score than those without depressive symptoms.

Such findings from a community sample support the reports by clinicians and other investigators of the disturbing effects of depressive symptoms on family functioning. When depressive symptoms are prominent, the bonds holding the adults together are strained, and difficulties are compounded by the communication problems intrinsic to depression (as reflected by such families' low expressiveness scores). These families were divisive as well as negative and incommunicative, and various members held differing views of the family environment (as evidenced by relatively high family incongruence scores).

The seven families with drug problems had significantly low cohesion and intellectual-cultural orientation scores and a significantly high mean conflict score—the highest of any group in the study. Such findings point to the devastation of the family and its turmoil when members, usually adult sons who returned home, had drug problems.

Families with symptomatic children differed significantly from those without symptomatic children by having a lower mean independence subscale score; also, their mean incongruity scores tended to be higher than those of asymptomatic families. We wondered whether they were low on the independence subscale because they were enmeshed families; many of the adults in those families had symptoms of depression, however, and it is possible that their negativism and despair were manifested by the low independence scores.

We think that we would have obtained even more significant differences in the various groups' FES subscale scores if we had used a larger and/or less heterogeneous sample. Nevertheless, we were able to use the FES subscale scores to evaluate the various dyads in the families and also, in discriminant function and logistical regression analyses, to predict whether a given family would be either asymptomatic or symptomatic both at Time 1 and at Time 3.

The evaluation of the dyads' FES subscale scores in the families with children enabled us to look at the family structure and boundaries from the "inside." The mother-daughter dyad's mean score reflected their similar attitudes and values, but as would be anticipated, the sibling-sibling mean score reflected the sharp differences between those two family members. We were concerned because the husband-wife mean dyad score showed almost as much difference between the partners as the sibling-sibling mean score did for the young family members. This lack of husband-wife concordance is a troubling finding in families that, in many ways, were a representative cross-section of families in much of America and had many healthful and other positive characteristics. We think that determining dyad scores on the various subscales has a potential for deepening investigators' and clinicians' understanding of family structure and relationships.

Predictors of Symptomatic Status. We used the Time 1 FES subscale and family incongruence scores in discriminant function analyses and logistical regressions to determine how well they predicted Time 1 and Time 3 symptom status. The discriminant function analyses correctly classified 67.4% of the families' Time 1 symptom status, except for the 17 families with young children; these families were classified into symptomatic and asymptomatic groups with 100% accuracy on the basis of eight mean

SUMMARY AND CONCLUSIONS

FES subscale scores. Depression symptom status was correctly classified in 86.1% of the families. Low cohesion subscale scores generally were the most powerful predictors of overall symptomatology, of high CES-D scores, or of depressive symptoms. High conflict subscale scores were predictors of drug problems, and low independence scores were the best predictors of child psychopathology.

The logistical regressions correctly classified 63% to 84% of the families on overall symptom status, their CES-D scores, depressive symptomatology, drug problems, or child symptom status. The mean cohesion score was a powerful predictor of symptom status, high CES-D scores, or depressive symptoms. As the discriminant function analyses had shown, high conflict subscale scores were predictors of drug problems, and low independence scores were predictors of child symptomatology. Both the discriminant function analyses and the logistical regressions correctly classified higher percentages of the asymptomatic families than the symptomatic ones, possibly because the asymptomatic group was larger. The discriminant function analyses classified higher percentages of the families correctly than the logistical regressions but used more variables and thus were the less parsimonious of the two methods.

We then used the Time 1 FES subscale and family incongruence scores in discriminant function analyses and logistical regressions to see how accurately they predicted family symptom status 15 months later at Time 3. For the discriminant function analyses, a linear combination of six Time 1 subscale scores correctly classified 82% of the families as either symptomatic or asymptomatic. With logistical regressions, the Time 1 cohesion subscale scores alone correctly predicted 62% of the families' Time 3 symptomatic status.

Thus, our results indicated that families' subscale scores, particularly on cohesion, were both associated with symptomatology and predictive of symptom status 15 months later at better than an 80% level of accuracy. We regarded these associations between the quality of the family environment and family well-being, or even specific types of symptoms and problems, as having importance, especially the associations between low cohesion scores and depressive symptoms, between high conflict scores and drug problems, and between low independence scores and the children being symptomatic.

To evaluate further associations between FES scores and symptom status, we conducted separate analyses of covariance with FES scores and both Time 1 and Time 3 symptom status. The Time 1 FES subscale and incongruence scores were more powerful predictors of the Time 3 FES subscale and incongruence scores than symptom status. These results suggest not just that the quality of the family environment is associated with symptomatology, but that it did not change much over the 15 months. This resistance to change is a sector toward which family therapists can direct their efforts and is one that needs further research.

Genograms, Family Structure, and Symptom Status. The genograms developed by Bowen and his colleagues were informative and added some valuable findings (McGoldrick & Gerson, 1985). Genograms constructed from family members' responses to the question "Who do you think is in your immediate family?" classified them into five types. Type I consisted of the 21% of the families in which all the family members agreed about the composition of the family. Type II (47% of the families) consisted of all the members of the household plus the inclusion by a spouse of one or more of his or her relatives. Type III (23% of the families) contained those in which one spouse omitted the other as part of the immediate family but included persons outside the family. Type IV (5%) consisted of a small miscellaneous group, and Type V (another 5%) consisted of those with only one adult respondent. A significantly lower percentage, 22%, of the Type I (consensus) families was symptomatic than the 68% of the Type II–Type V families.

We urge researchers to use genograms in their family studies. They gave us a graphic picture of the structure of the family, revealed cohesion or a lack thereof, and pointed to the probable influences of those outside the household on the family. Such findings raise questions that have clinical significance and generate hypotheses for further study. Does the omission of a spouse, for example, signify failure or incomplete resolution of the task of the first stage of the family life cycle (e.g., separation from one's family of origin and the formation of a new "attached" family), or does it depict the lack of bonds indicative of low cohesion? Or does it emphasize the undue influence of those outside the household or of outsiders being burdens that add to family stress?

Family and Sexual Satisfaction. Our evaluation of marital satisfaction consisted mainly of each spouse's ratings of his or her marital satisfaction, comparisons with the previous year, and perceptions of the other spouse's views. Almost 90% of the husbands and wives rated their marriages as excellent or good, and about 60% to 70% of them agreed on various measures of satisfaction. The main finding was that more couples who disagreed about their level of marital satisfaction tended to be symptomatic than those who agreed. Also, wives who reported that the marriage had a deleterious effect on their mental health tended to be symptomatic. Generally, the reports about satisfaction were skewed toward harmony to a degree that is not consistent with the many reported relationship problems in modern America. About 75% of the couples agreed that their sexual relationship was important; in response to questions about their own and their partner's sexual satisfaction, 80% to 90% reported satisfaction. The only association with symptomatology was that disproportionately more of the couples that disagreed about levels of sexual satisfaction and frequency of intercourse were symptomatic than those that agreed.

We think that self-report of marital and sexual satisfaction provides only a crude measure of these important but somewhat nebulous aspects of marriage. Perhaps "intimate" data are not usually revealed fully to interviewers except in clinical settings. We recommend repeating questions about marital and sexual satisfaction on reinterviews in the hope that the respondents will then have sufficient confidence in the interviewers to confide in them. We found that the critical finding was not the level of reported satisfaction but, specifically, the extent of agreement between the spouses about their own and their spouses' levels of satisfaction. It is an indicator of interpersonal sensitivity and also cohesion.

Likes and Dislikes About Marriage and the Family, Goals, and Household and Family Responsibilities. To reach into the intricacies of their marital relationships, we asked the spouses about their likes and dislikes about their marriages and their personal and family goals for the forthcoming year. Companionship and togetherness were what the couples liked best; the husbands reported raising a family as their second "like," and the wives reported security. Most reported that there was nothing they disliked, but when pressed, the husbands reported responsibilities, and the wives, household chores.

The most frequently listed family goals were "health and fitness" and "closeness and harmony." We also asked each family member to judge the probability that each goal would be attained and, if it were, to what he or she would attribute the attainment. About 85% of family members were optimistic about the goals being reached. Between 50% and 60% attributed attainment to the efforts of the family as a unit, but 30% to 40% emphasized that each member's individual efforts would be the most important determinant. About 15% to 20% gave considerable weight to chance, fate, or circumstances beyond control. The questions about attributions were designed to supply data about locus of control and the emphasis given either individualism or familism. We concluded that a significant percentage, possibly as many as 40% to 45% of our family members, were "individualists."

To determine the extent to which our families subscribed to traditional sex roles and a gender-stereotyped division of labor, we asked about which family members assumed responsibilities for household chores, home upkeep, and child care. Generally, there was a traditional division of labor, but there also was a significant degree of sharing, especially of child care. The results were generally in accord with Hochschild's (1989) findings, discussed in Chapter 1.

There were no associations between symptom status and family goals, optimism about attaining them, or the attributions. Also, symptom status was not related to whether the household and child care responsibilities followed traditional gender-stereotyped roles or were shared.

Young Children. At Time 1, 20 of our 43 families had a combined 34 children under age 16 at home, but 2 children in 2 families did not participate; our analyses were therefore based on 32 children in 18 families. They were representative of the general population, and we had no teenage or elderly parents. Almost all of the children had unremarkable developmental histories. Also, the parents reported generally that the children had normal relationships with their siblings, behaved reasonably well with the parents, played well by themselves, and did at least reasonably well in school.

The parents generally agreed about their expectations of their children and the values they wished to instill in the latter. The extent of that agreement should be a healthful determinant of the children's development. The mothers were the disciplinarians, but the fathers were stricter. There was parental accord about what was punishable behavior, and both parents mentioned similar punishments. Approximately half of the parents, however, disagreed about discipline; such disagreement, seen often in clinical work with disturbed families, suggests that the children experienced some inconsistencies about rules. But we found no associations between agreement and disagreement on expectations, values, and discipline and families' symptomatic status.

The fathers reported being much more dissatisfied than the mothers with the amount of time they spent with their children. Such reports are not surprising in view of the emphasis in recent years on the importance of fathers devoting time to their children. The mothers reported doing many more different things with their children than did the fathers, but many of the parent-child activities varied in accord with traditional male/female parental roles. Overall, the families were doing what ordinary families do together.

The findings suggested a good outlook for these children in the future, but some caution is indicated because of parental inconsistencies, especially the relative lack of agreement about punishment. Parental variability and disagreement about punishment handicap the growing child's psychosexual development. For the child, anxiety stems from uncertainty about whether and how he or she will be punished, and risk taking is stimulated by inconsistencies in the home. The unpredictability of punishment also impairs superego development by arousing the child's fantasies of rage, which can become self-punitive and potentially destructive to self and others. Also, we wondered whether the extent of such disagreement in a nonclinical population such as ours might be representative of a new trend that was accompanying the many changes in the family taking place since the 1960s. If so, it could have major implications for children's personality development, superego formation, and character as adults. The ramifications include effects on the family of the future and, eventually, society.

At Time 1, 10 (33%) of the children in 8 (44%) of the 18 families with children were symptomatic. In clinical settings, finding that more than one child in the family is symptomatic is not unusual; also, in some of the families both a child and another family member were symptomatic. Of the 18 families with young children, 13 (72%) were symptomatic, in contrast to 12 (52%) of the 23 families without young children. In 5 (39%) of the 13 families, other family members as well as young children were symptomatic; in another 3 (23%), only the young children were symptomatic; and in the remaining 5 (39%), other family members were symptomatic and the young children were asymptomatic. In some families there was a shift of symptoms from one family member to another from Time 1 to Time 3; it appeared that having one symptomatic member was needed in order to maintain homeostasis, even though the equilibrium was uneasy.

Analysis of the children's symptomatic status at Time 1 revealed that 5 (16%) in 3 families were symptomatic on the Achenbach Child Behavior Checklist (CBCL). In contrast, the child psychiatrist's rating of the children's reports on the Diagnostic Interview for Children (DISC) indicated that 7 (22%) showed psychopathology. Of the 10 (33%) children symptomatic on at least one of the two measures, 2 were symptomatic on both the CBCL and DISC ratings; 3 were symptomatic only on the CBCL, and 5 had only DISC ratings of psychopathology. The disagreement between the mothers' reports on the CBCL and the ratings of the children's reports on the DISC is in accord with clinical experience and researchers' strong recommendations that to identify mental disorder in children, information is needed from at least two (if not all three) conventional sources—the parents, the child, and the latter's schoolteacher. Information about the child from these sources is complementary and helpful for assessment and treatment planning.

A disproportionately large percentage of the adults and children in the families that did not continue in the study were symptomatic compared to those who continued. In the 3 families with 7 young children that either dropped out or moved away after Time 1, 4 (57%) children were symptomatic, 2 (29%) only on the CBCL and 2 (29%) only on the DISC ratings. In the 15 families with 25 young children that completed the study, however, 6 (24%) children in 5 (33%) families were symptomatic on one or both of the child measures; 3 (12%) children were symptomatic on the CBCL and 5 (21%) had DISC ratings of psychopathology, but only 2 were symptomatic on both measures.

At Time 3, 6 (24%) children in 4 (27%) of the families with children were symptomatic; some were symptomatic at both times, and some only at Time 3. Of the 6 symptomatic children, 3 were symptomatic on the CBCL, and 5 had DISC ratings of psychopathology (2 were symptomatic on both measures). At Time 3, as at Time 1, their symptomatology consisted mainly of the "mixed neurotic" symptoms of anxiety, various phobias, and some depression, not severe behavioral or conduct disturbances. More boys than girls were symptomatic, as is usually the case in clinical situations.

Finding such a high percentage of symptomatic children in a community sample is consistent with researchers' and agencies' reports that there are many children with unrecognized and untreated psychopathology in the community, and it is also in accord with the data presented in the recent Institute of Medicine (1990) report. Probably an even more distressing finding was that about 40% of the symptomatic children's families also contained older children or parents who were symptomatic. It points to the intergenerational continuity of emotional distress and mental disorder and also suggests that the family environment is conducive to the development of symptomatology. Although we could not determine many sequential relationships in just a 15-month study, some of our data indicate that the family environment was relatively stable over that period of time and showed less variability and fluctuations than did symptomatology. If that preliminary finding can be replicated, it has both fortunate and unfortunate implications. Those living in healthful family environments will tend to be healthy families, whereas those in family environments characterized by lack of cohesion, problems with expressiveness, conflict, and disparate views of the home situation will tend to continue to have emotional distress. Therefore, our findings that so many of the children were symptomatic is another indicator signifying that the American family is in need of help and that there is danger that the next generation will be composed of large numbers of disturbed young people.

Adult Children. As discussed in Chapter 6, we were surprised in 1983 to find that a relatively large number (16, or 37%) of our families contained adult children who either had not left their parental homes or had returned home after job loss or divorce. These adult children changed the structure of the family and often appeared to be a concern to their parents, especially older parents who had lived as a dyad for a number of years and had accustomed patterns of living. At Time 1, a high percentage (73%) of these young adults were symptomatic.

We divided the 22 participating young adults into three subgroups: preparing for the future (those aged 16 to 22, most of whom were students), extended youth (those aged 21 to 25), and returnees (those aged 24 to 38, who had once left home but now had returned to live with their parents). We were very surprised to find that 67% to 78% of the individuals in each of the three subgroups were symptomatic. Generally, the symptomatic persons in the preparing subgroup were females with affective distress who had high scores on the CES-D and depressive symptoms. The symptomatic in the extended-youth group also were mainly females, many of whom were affectively symptomatic. The returnees, however, were mainly males, many of whom had alcohol and drug problems.

The tendency for such young adults as those in the extended-youth stage to stay at home was reinforced by the adversities and harshness of life in the United States in the 1980s, a tone noted by then-Vice President Bush in 1988 when he called for a "kinder and gentler" America. Economic and other sociocultural forces, the emphasis on consumption, and a lack of meaningful jobs have led to the "twentysomethings" having diminished expectations and negative (if not cynical) sentiments. More of them are young men than young women; unmarried young men appear to be having significant difficulties living alone.

The returnees were usually men who came back home not to care for aging parents but to find a sanctuary where they could have many of their dependency needs satisfied and live more narcissistically than when working or having responsibilities for spouses and children. The high percentage of them with alcohol and/or drug problems, sometimes accompanied by comorbid mental disorders, raises the possibility that emotional instability may have been the significant factor that led to their lack of success on their own and the need to return to the parental home. But demographers (Glick, 1988) report that economic conditions generally have been the major determinants of when young adults leave their parents' homes. In view of the continued recession of the early 1990s and the structural changes in the American economy, it is likely that many families in the ensuing decade will contain adult children. Family members will be compelled to adjust to a family composition and structure that had belonged to the America of yesteryear.

When there are adult children in the home, it is critically important to surface the parents' and adult children's expectations of each other. Many of the parents worry about these adult children. Clarifying responsibilities and goals can provide some of the structure needed in such situations where there is a tendency for the boundaries essential for domestic stability and harmony to break down.

There is need for special studies of families with adult children in the home and also of adult children's children. The information from such studies should increase our understanding of adaptation to varying family structures and of intergenerational patterns of mental health and illness.

The Historical-Clinic Chart Study

Our third major approach was to carry out a historical-clinical study by analyzing a random sample of 455 records from our Bingham Child Guidance Clinic from 1923 to 1988. We gathered data on the children's sociodemographic characteristics, their presenting problems, their families' problems, and their living situations from samples of the charts at 5-year intervals, beginning in 1923. We were interested in changes in the children's and their families' problems over time and in ascertaining whether different sociocultural epochs were associated with particular types of problems. Thus, this third approach was designed to furnish clinical data that would complement the reviews of the history of the family in this century and the results of the epidemiological study.

The analysis of the clinic charts revealed that the percentages of children presenting with certain problems (especially aggressive behaviors) increased over time, whereas others, (e.g., academic problems) were relatively constant. Although some fluctuations were associated with changes in the staffing or the service philosophy of the clinic, year-to-year fluctuations also could be attributed to changing family attitudes toward mental illness, the community selecting the behaviors that were designated as illness, and/or economic and other outside factors that impinged on families.

The major changes from the 1920s to the 1980s in the children's presenting symptoms were increases in aggressive behavior, difficulties in the parent-child relationships, and anxiety and nervousness. We speculated that the increase in aggressive behavior and in parent-child problems could be related to the changes in the family structure that the charts showed had occurred during the "century of concern." In 1983, when we were first interviewing in the community, the clinic was tending to see older children and smaller families than in preceding decades. Most importantly though, in recent years only a small percentage (27%) of the children's biological parents were married; about 33% were divorced, and the rest were never married. In 1988, only 23% of the children were living with two parents, about 10% were living with a parent and a stepparent, 27% were living with a single parent, 20% were with grandparents or other relatives, and the remaining 20% were in various institutions, mainly foster homes. We worried whether the absence of two parents was associated with the emotional distress and aggressive behavior that was being seen.

Reports of children's depressive symptoms and suicidal thoughts and behaviors were especially prominent in the late 1970s and early 1980s. During those years, depression and suicide were increasing greatly in adolescents and young adults throughout the United States. Unfortunately, depression is no longer a rare mental disorder in children, and the mean age for the onset of the affective disorders has been dropping for several decades. Researchers agree that the marked increase in the frequency of depression is the result of multiple biological and social factors, especially family instability.

Concern about the multiple factors producing such mental disorders as depression is compounded by our finding that increasing percentages of the clinic families have been reporting the history or presence of mental illness in a family member in recent years. These increases, along with the extent of family disruption and changes in the family structure (evidenced by the divorce rate and the many single-parent and stepfamilies), are a combination of influences that have deleterious effects on the children. Such factors are responsible in large part for the data in the recent Institute of Medicine (1990) report showing that 12% of children in the United States (20% in inner cities and among the poor and disadvantaged) have diagnosable mental disorders.

An especially serious finding was the large increase in recent years of multiple family problems in addition to the children's presenting problems. These family problems often included an increase in the percentage of parents with problems stemming from addictive behaviors (e.g., alcohol, drugs, and gambling). Also, there has been a strong trend toward increased reports of marital problems. Thus, many of the findings from our historical-clinical chart study substantiate the concerns about the status and well-being of the American family expressed by family scholars throughout this century.

CONCLUSIONS

T. S. Eliot (1936) asked, "Where is the wisdom we have lost in knowledge? Where is the knowledge we have lost in information?" (p. 147). When we look at the mass of data and the many findings from our three major approaches to the study of the family, we need to select a handful that we think are important.

First, history shows that the status and well-being of the family are both inevitably and inextricably linked to the vitality and stability of the society and the state. Studies that do not account for political and other cultural influences are bound to yield only fragmentary results. Currently, the antifamilism in the United States that is trumpeted by many of the nation's political and financial leaders is contributing to the family turmoil that too often results in marital disruption, divorce, and the many problems of the children of divorce.

Second, our epidemiological longitudinal study of a random sample of 43 families from the general population showed that there was at least one emotionally distressed, symptomatic member in more than half of them. The symptomatology was strongly associated with living in a single-parent family, being poor, and/or exposure to stressors. Moreover, a family member who was symptomatic when interviewed in the home the first time often was not the member who was symptomatic when the family was reinterviewed 15 months later, and the type of symptomatology (e.g., depressive symptoms or drug problems) sometimes changed from one interview to the next. Thus, we think that results of studies and even clinical evaluations at just one point in time are limited. Only longitudinal studies or a series of clinical evaluations can hope to capture the variable shifts in symptoms, composition, and interactions of such a complex group as the family.

Third, the quality of family environment, as reflected by the Family Environment Scale (FES) subscale scores on cohesion, expressiveness, conflict, and independence, is strongly associated with symptomatology and is predictive of symptom status over at least a 15-month period. Our Time 1 FES subscale scores classified families as being either symptom-

SUMMARY AND CONCLUSIONS

atic or asymptomatic 15 months later at better than an 80% level of accuracy. Also, the analyses indicated that the quality of the family environment changed relatively little over the 15 months. Thus, the quality of life in the home is of decisive importance for the mental health or illness of the family members.

Fourth, the plight of the young children and the many symptoms and problems of the adult children (those in the stage of extended youth, as well as the returnees) merit special attention. More than one fourth of the children under age 16 were symptomatic, as were three fourths of the adult children, and often parents as well. The extensive psychopathology in these families bodes poorly for the well-being of those who are aging, as well as for those who will be coming of age by the end of the century. Those findings also sound a note of alarm about the intergenerational continuity of mental disorder and the cycles of disadvantage (Rutter & Madge, 1976), which can be never-ending (especially when they are propelled by poverty). Our extensive literature reviews and the results of our studies indicate that the health of children in America is not good and probably declined during the 1980s, an era when many in the nation got richer and when poverty was strongly associated with children's deteriorating health (Bane & Ellwood, 1989).

The problems of adult children in the home were evidenced by our finding that they were the family members who were most likely to be symptomatic. Although both sociocultural and personal (i.e., mental health) factors are associated with adult sons and daughters, mainly sons, staying at home in adulthood, economic forces seem to be the major determinants of this trend that started early in the 1980s and is continuing. Nevertheless, we found that most of these adult children at home were still attempting to master the developmental tasks of late adolescence and early adulthood and many of them showed self-centered, if not somewhat regressive, narcissistic tendencies. We concluded sadly that just being a young child or an adult child in the United States at this time in history is a risk factor for mental illness!

We began our studies with thoughts about the "century of concern" regarding the stability of the American family since the late 1880s. The findings from our in-depth review of clinical studies over the years substantiated many of the concerns that had been expressed by such family scholars as Willystine Goodsell in 1915, Pitrim Sorokin in the 1930s and 1940s, and Carle Zimmerman from 1935 to the early 1970s. Our data showed that the percentage of clinic children living with two parents had dropped sharply, to a frightening low of about 30% in 1988. Children's problems with aggressive behavior were rare until about 1960 but have jumped dramatically during the last two decades, as have children's cases of depression and suicidal thoughts and actions. These tragedies are paralleled by a sharp increase in recent years in parents' addictive behaviors, marital conflicts, and family histories of mental illness.

Thus, the children's and their parents' increasing problems are marching in step with our society's problems (crime, violence, institutional decay, corruption in the marketplace, and massive indebtedness), which appear to have trickled down from the presidencies and Congresses of the 1980s that deregulated business and weaponry (when profitable), as well as their own actions. There is a frightening parallel between political leaders refusing to control the sale of handguns and other weapons of destruction at home and abroad and the increase in children's aggressive behaviors, the risk-taking behaviors that we observe almost daily in our clinics, and the flood of reports about increased sexual abuse of children (Owens, 1992). Washington, D.C., is the murder capital of the world (more Americans were killed in Washington in 1991 than in the Persian Gulf War), and teenagers are conducting executions, for example, in New Haven, Connecticut. Meanwhile, we see the starving children in Somalia and are bound to be appalled by the realization that American weaponry supplied to that country has kept food from being distributed to its inhabitants, just as our weapons at home have made our streets unsafe.

When we ask what the results of our extensive literature reviews, pilot epidemiological study, and analyses of clinical records mean, we conclude that the family in the United States in the early 1990s is in serious difficulty. The balance between individualism and familism has been tilted precariously toward excessive individualism. Support for the family has been bludgeoned from above (from the top levels of our society and government) and eroded from below (from individuals' pursuits of gain and gratification). The projective nature of our society in the late 1980s and early 1990s is an additional unfortunate development that handicaps efforts to restabilize the family, the institution that for millennia has satisfied adults' and children's needs for intimacy and nurturance, provided for survival of the group and the development of the young, and ensured the continuity of the cultural legacy. The massive indulgence intrinsic to blaming others—Japan for the problems of the American automobile industry, Colombia for the drugs on the streets of our cities, and banks for "bounced" checks—is a disavowal of personal and collective responsibility that injures family life and stability. The other great barrier to restabilization of the family is the widening gap between the rich and the poor and the debilitating effects of such disparity on individuals and families.

As the 1990s began, it appeared that a number of forces were strengthening the family. The divorce rate started dropping slowly in the late 1980s; the fear of AIDS reduced so-called casual sex; economic considerations and the problems of divorce tempered hasty decisions to marry (as evidenced by the late age of first marriages); and there was a general revulsion against the excesses of the 1980s. The fate of the family in this decade, which Zimmerman (1972 a, b) saw as being critical for its future, depends on whether those forces can surmount individual and group abandonment of responsibility and the increasing stratification of our society.

Although the findings from our studies point to pathologies and problems, we learned that the family is a unit that has both resilience and other qualities ensuring that it will endure. We were especially gratified by the altruism that we observed firsthand in the families that we interviewed in their homes. Repeatedly they told us that they had participated in the study to learn more about themselves and, especially, to help others. That spirit, which in many ways is the heart of family life, is one of the qualities most likely to strengthen the family in its struggle for survival.

References

ABC News (August 27, 1992). *Prime time live* [Television broadcast].
Abraham, K. (1968). Notes on the psychoanalytical investigation and treatment of manic-depressive insanity and allied conditions. In *Selected papers of Karl Abraham*. London: Hogarth Press. (Original work published 1912).
Achenbach, J. M., & Edelbrock, C. S. (1983). *Manual for the child behavior checklist and revised child behavior profile*. Burlington, VT: Queen City Printers.
Ackerman, N. (1937). The family as a social and emotional unit. *Bulletin of the Kansas Mental Hygiene Society*.
Ackerman, N. (1957). An orientation to psychiatric research on the family. *Marriage and Family Living, 19*(1), 68–74.
Ackerman, N., & Behrens, M. L. (1956). A study of family diagnosis. *American Journal of Orthopsychiatry, 26*, 66.
Ackerman, N. W., & Behrens, M. L. (1974). Family diagnosis and clinical process. In S. Arieti & G. Caplan (Eds.), *American handbook of psychiatry, vol. 2* (2nd ed., pp. 37–50). New York: Basic Books.
Adams, B. N. (1971). *The American family: A social interpretation*. Chicago: Markham.
Adams, B. N. (1988). Fifty years of family research: What does it mean? *Journal of Marriage and the Family, 50*, 5–17.
Adler, A. (1964). *Problems of neurosis*. New York: Harper and Row.
Aichhorn, A. (1935). *Wayward youth*. New York: Viking.
Alanen, Y. O. (1980). In search of the interactional origin of schizophrenia. In C. K. Hofling and J. M. Lewis (Eds.), *The family: Evaluation and treatment*. New York: Brunner-Mazel.
Alarcon, R. D. (1976). Drug and psychotherapy interactions in depression. *American Journal of Psychiatry, 133*(5), 502–508.
Alexander, F. (1927). *Psychoanalyse der gesamtpersönlichkeit; neun Vorlesungen über die Anwendung von Freud's ichteorie auf die neurosenlehre*. Vienna: Internationaler Psychoanalytischer Verlag.
American Psychological Association. (1991, March 19). *News bulletin*. Washington, DC: Author.
American Psychiatric Association. (1987). *Diagnostic and statistical manual of mental disorders* (rev. 3rd ed.). Washington, DC: Author.
Angell, R. C. (1936). *The family encounters the depression*. Gloucester, MA: Charles Scribner & Sons.

Aries, P. (1962). *Centuries of childhood: A social history of family life* (R. Baldick, Trans.). New York: Knopf.
Aries, P. (1977). The family and the city. *Daedalus, 106*(2), 227–235.
Arieti, S. (1959). Schizophrenia: Symptomatology and mechanisms. In S. Arieti (Ed.), *American handbook of psychiatry, vol. 1* (1st ed.). New York: Basic Books.
Aristophanes (1917). The trial of Euripides. In E. Rhys (Ed.), *Everyman's Library*, (Vol. II). New York: E. P. Dutton.
Aristophanes (1987). *Lysistrata*. Oxford: Clarendon Press.
Aristotle (1952). Politics, vol. 2. In R. M. Hutchins (Ed.), *Great books of the Western world, vol. 9*. Chicago, IL: Encyclopaedia Britannica.
Asbury, H. (1938). *The French quarter: An informal history of the New Orleans underworld*. New York: Garden City.
Astell, M. (1970). *Some reflections upon marriage*. New York: Source Book.
Bachofen, J. J. (1954). *Mutterecht und urreligion*. Stuttgardt: A. Kroner.
Bahr, S. J. (Ed.). (1991). *Family research: A sixty year review, 1930–1990, vol. 1*. New York: Lexington.
Bane, M. J., & Ellwood, D. T. (1989). One fifth of the nation's children: Why are they poor? *Science, 245,* 1047–1053.
Bartlett, D. L., & Steele, J. B. (1992). *America: What Went Wrong?* Kansas City, MO: Andrews and McMeel.
Bateson, G., Jackson, D., Haley, J., & Weaklend, J. (1956). Toward a theory of schizophrenia. *Behavioral Science, 1*(4), 251–264.
Beavers, W. R., & Hampson, R. B. (1990). *Successful families: Assessment and intervention*. New York: W. W. Norton.
Beavers, W. R., Hampson, R. B., & Hulges, Y. F. (1985). Commentary: The Beavers systems approach to family assessment. *Family Process, 24,* 398–405.
Beavers, W. R., & Voeller, M. N. (1983). Family models: Comparing and contrasting the Olson Circumplex Model with the Beavers Systems Model. *Family Process, 22,* 85–98.
Bell, D. (1980). *The winding passage: Essays and sociological journeys 1960–1980*. Cambridge, MA: ABT Books.
Bell, R. A., Goldsmith, H. F., Lin, E., Hirzel, R. K., & Sobel, S. (Eds.). *Social indicators for human service systems*. Louisville, KY: Department of Psychiatry and Behavioral Sciences.
Bell, R. A., & Schwab, J. J. (1985). *Bell and Schwab Family Systems Assessment Scale*. Unpublished manuscript, University of Louisville, Department of Psychiatry, Louisville, KY.
Bell, N. W., & Spiegel, J. P. (1966). Social psychiatry: Vagaries of a term. *Archives of General Psychiatry, 14,* 337–345.
Bell, R. A., & Sundel, M. (1975). *The Louisville metropolitan health and family life study*. Unpublished manuscript.
Bellah, R., Madsen, R., Sullivan, W. M., Swidler, A., & Tipton, S. M. (1985). *Habits of the heart: Individualism and commitment in American life*. Berkeley: University of California Press.
Belsky, J. (1985). Experimenting with the family in the newborn period. *Child Development, 56,* 409.
Belsky, J., Rovine, M., & Fish, M. (1989). The developing family system. In M. Gunnar (Ed.), *Systems and development, Minnesota symposium on child psychology, vol. 22*. Hillsdale, NJ: Erlbaum.
Belsky, J., Spanier, G. B., & Rovine, M. (1983). Stability and change in marriage across the transition to parenthood. *Journal of Marriage and the Family, 45*(3), 567–577.
Benedict, R. (1934). *Patterns of Culture*. Boston: Houghton Mifflin.

REFERENCES

Berardo, F. M. (1990). Trends and directions in family research in the 1980s. *Journal of Marriage and the Family, 52*, 809–817.

Bernard, J. (1933). The distribution of success in marriage. *American Journal of Sociology, 39*, 194–203.

Berry, W. (1992, April 26). The fall of community, the ruins of sex. *Louisville Courier Journal*, pp. D1, 4.

Bertalanffy, L. von (1966). General systems theory and psychiatry. In S. Arieti (Ed.), *American handbook of psychiatry* (pp. 705–721). New York: Basic Books.

Bishop, D. S. (1986). Psychosocial issues in stroke rehabilitation. In M.E. Brandstater & J. V. Basmajian (Eds.), *Stroke rehabilitation*. Baltimore, MD: Williams & Wilkins.

Bloch, M. (1962). *Feudal Society* (vols. 1 & 2, 2nd ed.) (L. A. Manyon, Trans.).

Blumberg, S. R., & Hokanson, J. E. (1983). The effects of another person's response style on interpersonal behavior in depression. *Journal of Abnormal Psychology, 92*(2), 196–209.

Boake, C., & Salmon, P. G. (1981, October 22). Demographic correlates and factor structure of the Family Environment Scale. *Journal of Clinical Psychology, 39*(1), 95–100.

Bohannon, P. (Ed.). (1970). *Divorce and after*. Garden City, NY: Doubleday.

Booth, C. (1892). *Life and labour of the people in London* (vol. 1). London: Macmillan.

Bosanquet, H. (1906). *The family*. New York: Macmillan.

Bowen, M. (1988). Epilogue: An odyssey toward science. In M. E. Kerr and M. Bowen (Eds.), *Family evaluation*. New York: W. W. Norton.

Bowlby, J. (1965). *Child care and the growth of love*. Baltimore: Penguin.

Brecht, B. (1961). Mother courage and her children. In E. Bentley (Ed.), *Seven Plays*. New York: Grove Press.

Breasted, J. H. (1933). *The dawn of conscience*. New York: Charles Scribner's Sons.

Breuer, J., & Freud, S. (1895). *Studien über hysterie*. Vienna: Deuticke.

Briffault, R. (1927). *The mothers*. New York: Macmillan.

Broder, D. (1992, May 6). The GOP's Big Lie. *Louisville Courier Journal*, p. A12.

Broderick, C. B. (1971). Beyond the five conceptual frameworks: A decade of development in family theory. In C. B. Broderick (Ed.), *A decade of family research and action 1960–1969* (pp. 3–24). Minneapolis, MN: National Council on Family Relations.

Brown, D. R., & Gary, L. R. (1987, Winter). Stressful life events, social support networks, and the physical and mental health of urban black adults. *Journal of Human Stress*, 165–174.

Brown, G. W., Harris, T., et al. (1975). Social class and psychiatric disturbance among women in an urban population. *Sociology, 9*, 225–254.

Brown, G. W., & Harris, T. (1978). *Social origins of depression: A study of psychiatric disorder in women*. New York: Free Press.

Bruhn, J. G., Chandler, B., & Miller, M. C. (1966). Social aspects of coronary heart disease in two adjacent ethnically different communities. *American Journal Public Health, 57*, 1493–1506.

Budge, E. A. W. (1969). *The gods of Egyptians, or studies in Egyptian mythology*. New York: Dover.

Bullock, R. C., Siegel, R., Weissman, M., & Paykel, E. S. (1972). The weeping wife: Marital relations of depressed women. *Journal of Marriage and the Family, 34*, 488–495.

Burgess, E. W. (Ed.). (1926). *The urban community: Selected papers from the proceedings of the American Sociological Society 1925*. Chicago: University of Chicago Press.

Burgess, E. W. (Ed.). (1929). *Personality and the social group*. Chicago: University of Chicago Press.

Burgess, E. W., & Cottrell, L. S., Jr. (1939). *Predicting success or failure in marriage*. New York: Prentice-Hall.

Burgess, E. W., & Locke, H. J. (1945). *The family: From institution to companionship.* New York: American.

Burgess, E. W., & Locke, H. J. (1960). *The family: From institution to companionship* (2nd ed.). New York: American.

Bush, B. (1992, August 20). Barbara Bush lauds virtues of family life. *Louisville Courier Journal,* p. A13.

Burrows, G. M. (1828). *Commentaries on the causes, forms, symptoms, and treatment, moral and medical, of insanity.* London: T. G. Underwood.

Byington, M. F. (1910). *Homestead: The households of a mill town.* Philadelphia: Russell Sage Foundation.

Calhoun, A. W. (1917–1919). *A social history of the American family,* vols. 1, 2, & 3. Cleveland: Arthur H. Clark.

Carstairs, G. M. (1969). A land of lotus eaters? *American Journal of Psychiatry, 125,* 130–134.

Caton, L. M. (1990). *Homeless in America.* New York: Oxford University Press.

Christensen, H. T. (Ed.). (1964). *Handbook of marriage and the family.* Chicago: Rand McNally.

Christie, K. A., Burke, J. D., Regier, D. A., Raie, D. S., Boyd, J. H., & Locke, B. Z. (1988). Epidemiologic evidence of early onset of mental disorder and higher risk of drug abuse in young adults. *American Journal of Psychiatry, 145,* 971–975.

Churchhill, W. S. (1956). *A history of the English-speaking peoples: The birth of Britain.* New York: Dodd, Mead.

Clowes, W. L. (1970). *Black America: A study of the ex-slave and his later master.* Westport, CT: Negro Universities Press. (Original work published 1891.)

Coats, D. (1991). America's youth: A crisis of character. *Imprimis, 20*(9).

Coleman, R. E., & Miller, A. G. (1975). The relationship between depression and marital maladjustment in a clinic population: A multitrait-multimethod study. *Journal of Consulting and Clinical Psychology, 43*(5), 647–651.

Collins, R. (1985). *Sociology of marriage and the family: Gender, love, and property.* Chicago: Nelson Hall.

Conference Board. (1985). *Corporation and families: Changing practices and perspectives.* Report No. 868. New York: Author.

Connelly, J. (1989, August 28). The CEO's second wife. *Fortune,* 52–66.

Croce, B. (1960). *History. Its theory and practice.* New York: Russell & Russell.

Costello, A. J., Edelbrock, C., Dulcan, M. K., et al. (1984). *Development and testing of the NIMH Diagnostic Interview Schedule for Children in a clinic population.* Final Report (Contract #RFP-DB-81-0027). Rockville, MD. Center for Epidemiologic Studies, National Institute of Mental health.

Coupland, D. (1991). *Generation X: Tales for an accelerated culture.* New York: St. Martin's Press.

Cox, H. G. (1969). *The feast of fools: A theological essay on festivity and fantasy.* Cambridge: Harvard University Press.

Coyne, J. C. (1990). Interpersonal processes in depression. In G. I. Keitner (Ed.), *Depression and families: Impact and treatment.* Washington, DC: American Psychiatric Press.

Cutler, J. E. (1916). Durable monogamous wedlock. *American Journal of Sociology, 22*(2), 226–250.

Davis, K. B. (1929). *Factors in the sex life of twenty-two hundred women.* New York: Harper & Brothers Publishers.

de Coulanges, F. (1901). *The ancient city: A study on the religion, laws and institutions of Greece and Rome* (11th ed.). Boston: Lothrop, Lee and Shepard.

REFERENCES

de Maulde, R. (1911). *The women of the Renaissance, vols. 1 & 2.*
De Parle, J. (1991, December 19). The welfare attack. *Louisville Courier Journal*, p. A11.
de Tocqueville, A. (1945). In F. Bowen (Ed.), *Democracy in America, vol. 1.* New York: Random House.
Defoe, D. (1748). *A tour through the whole island of Great Britain, vol. III* (pp. 137–139).
Demers, R. G., & Davis, L. S. (1971). The influence of prophylactic lithium treatment on the marital adjustment of manic-depressives and their spouses. *Comprehensive Psychiatry, 12*, 348.
Demos, V. (1990). Black family studies in the "Journal of Marriage and the Family" and the issue of distortion: A trend analysis. *Journal of Marriage and the Family, 52*, 603–612.
Dickens, C. (1958). *Hard times.* New York: Harper and Row.
Dickinson, R. L. (1931). Medical analysis of a thousand marriages. *Journal of the American Medical Association, 97*(8), 529–535.
Dicks, H. V. (1967). *Marital tensions: Clinical studies towards a psychological theory of interaction.* London: Routledge & Kegan Paul.
Doane, J., West, K. L., Goldstein, M. J., Rodnick, E. H., & Jones, J. E. (1981). Parental communication deviance and affective style. *Archives of General Psychiatry, 38*(6), 679–685.
Du Bois, W. E. B. (1908). *The Negro American family.* New York: Negro Universities Press.
Dugdale, R. L. (1910). *The Jukes: A study in crime, pauperism, disease, and heredity.* New York: Putnam.
Durant, W. (1927). *Philosophy and the social problem.* London: George Allen & Unwin.
Durant, W. (1935). *Our Oriental heritage: Part 1. The story of civilization.* New York: Simon & Schuster.
Durkheim, E. (1951). *Suicide, a study in sociology* (J. A. Spaulding & G. Simpson, Trans.). New York: Free Press.
Eaton, W. W., Kramer, M., Anthony, J. C., Dryman, A., Shapiro, S., & Locke, B. Z. (1989). The incidence of specific DIS/SMM-III mental disorders: Data from the NIMH Epidemiologic Catchment Area program. *Acta Psychiatric Scandinavia, 79*, 163–178.
Eaton, Y. (1991, July 21). Family ties. *Louisville Courier Journal*, pp. H1–H6.
Egeland, J., & Hostetter, A. (1983). Amish study I: Affective disorders among the Amish, 1976–1980. *American Journal of Psychiatry, 140*, 56–61.
Egeland, J. A., Gerhard, D. S., Pauls, D. L., Sussex, J. N., Kidd, K. K., Allen, C. R., Hostetter, A. M., & Housman, D. E. (1987). Bipolar affective disorders linked to DNA markers on chromosome 11. *Nature, 325*(6107), 783–787.
Ehrenreich, B. (1989). *Fear of falling: The inner life of the middle class.* New York: Pantheon.
Elder, G. H., Jr. (1974). *Children of the Great Depression: Social change in life experience.* Chicago: University of Chicago Press.
Elder, G. H., Jr., & Rockwell, R. C. (1979). Economic depression and postwar opportunity in men's lives: A study of life patterns and health. In R. G. Simmons (Ed.), *Research in community and mental health: An annual compilation of research, vol. 1* (pp. 249–302). Greenwich, CT: Jai Press.
Elias, M. (1991, May 14). Divorce is likelier for kids of divorce. *USA Today*, p. D1.
Ellenberger, H. F. (1970). *The discovery of the unconscious: The history and evolution of dynamic psychiatry.* New York: Basic Books.
Eliot, T. S. (1936). Choruses from "The Rock." *T. S. Eliot selected poems.* New York: Harcourt, Brace & World.
Eliot, T. S. (1971). *The complete poems and plays, 1909–1950.* New York: Harcourt, Brace & World.

Ellis, H. (1903). *Analysis of the sexual impulse: Love and pain, the sexual impulse in women*. Philadelphia: F. A. Davis.

Ellwood, C. A. (1910). *Sociology and modern sociology problems*. New York: American.

Engel, G. L. (1977). The need for a new medical model: A challenge for biomedicine. *Science, 196*(4286), 129–136.

Engels, F. (1972). *The origin of the family, private property and the state*. New York: Pathfinder.

Epstein, N. B., Bishop, D. S., & Baldwin, L. M. (1984). McMaster Model of Family Functioning: A view of the normal family. In *Family studies review yearbook* (pp. 75–101). Beverly Hills, CA: Sage.

Erikson, E. H. (1950). *Childhood and society*. New York: Norton.

Erikson, E. H. (1959). Identity and the life cycle. In *Selected papers*. New York: International Universities Press.

Esquirol, J. E. (1967). A treatise on insanity [1845]. In C. E. Goshen (Ed.), *Documentary history of psychiatry: A source book on historical principles* (p. 346). New York: Philosophical Library.

Euripides. (1952). The Trojan women. In R. M. Hutchins (Ed.), *Great books of the western world* (vol. 5). Chicago, IL: Encyclopaedia Britannica.

Eysenck, H. J. (Ed.). (1960). *Handbook of abnormal psychology: An experimental approach*. New York: Basic Books.

Fairbairn, W. R. D. (1954). *Object-relations theory of the personality*. New York: Basic Books.

Falloon, I. R. H., Boyd, J. L., & McGill, C. W. (1984). *Family care of schizophrenia*. New York: Guilford Press.

Feldman, L. B. (1976). Depression and marital interaction. *Family Process, 15*, 389–395.

Fenichel, O. (1945). *The psychoanalytic theory of neurosis*. New York: W. W. Norton.

Fleck, S. (1980). The family and psychiatry. In A. M. Freedman & H. I. Kaplan (Eds.), *The comprehensive textbook of psychiatry* (3rd ed., pp. 513–530). Baltimore: William & Wilkins.

Flügel, J. C. (1921). *The psycho-analytic study of the family*. London: International Psycho-Analytical Press.

Footlick, J. K. (1990, Winter/Spring). What happened to the family? *Newsweek*, 14–23.

Forster, E. M. (1908). *Howards end*. London: Edward Arnold.

Frankenburg, W. K., Dodds, J. B., Fandal, A. W., et al. (1975). *Denver developmental screening test reference manual* (rev. ed.). Boulder: University of Colorado Medical Center.

Frazier, E. F. (1966). *The Negro family in the United States* (rev. ed.). Chicago: University of Chicago Press.

Freedman, D. X. (1984). Psychiatric epidemiology counts. *Archives of General Psychiatry, 41*(10), 931–933.

French, M. (1985). *Beyond power: On women, men, and morals*. New York: Summit.

Freud, S. (1927). *Totem and taboo*. New York: New Republic.

Freud, S. (1930). *Civilization and its discontents*. New York: J. Cape & H. Smith.

Freud, S. (1939). *Moses and monotheism* (K. Jones, Trans.). New York: Vintage Books.

Freud, S. (1955). In J. Strachey (Ed.), *The interpretation of dreams*. New York: Basic Books.

Friedenberg, E. Z. (1964). *The vanishing adolescent*. Boston: Beacon.

Fromm-Reichmann, F. (1958). Basic problems in the psychotherapy of schizophrenia. *Psychiatry, 21*, 1.

Furstenberg, F., & Spanier, G. (1984). *Recycling the family*. Beverly Hills, CA: Sage.

Galdston, I. (1958). The American family in crisis. *Mental Hygiene, 42*, 229–236.

Gary, L. R., Brown, D. R., Milburn, N. G., Ahmed, F., & Booth, J. (1989). *Depression in black American adults: Findings from the Norfolk Area Health Study*. Washington, DC: Mental Health Research and Development Center, Howard University.

Gershon, E. S., & Guroff, J. J. (1984). Information from relatives. Diagnosis of affective disorders. *Archives of General Psychiatry, 41*, 173–180.

REFERENCES

Gershon, E., Hamovit, J., Guroff, J., Dibble, E., Leckman, J., Sceery, W., Targum, S., Nurnberger, J., Jr., Goldin, L., & Bunney, W., Jr. (1982). A family study of schizoaffective, bipolar I, bipolar II, unipolar, and normal control probands. *Archives of General Psychiatry, 39,* 1157–1167.
Gershon, E. S., Hamovit, J. H., Guroff, J. J., & Nurnberger, J. I. (1987). Birth-cohort changes in manic and depressive disorders in relatives of bipolar and schizoaffective patients. *Archives of General Psychiatry, 44,* 314–319.
Gibbs, N. (1989, April 24). How America has run out of time. *Time,* 58–67.
Gies, F., & Gies, J. (1987). *Marriage and the family in the middle ages.* New York: Harper and Row.
Glick, P. C. (1947). The family cycle. *American Sociological Review, 12,* 164–174.
Glick, P. C. (1988). Fifty years of family demography: A record of social change. *Journal of Marriage and the Family, 50,* 861–873.
Goddard, H. H. (1973). *The Kallikak family.* New York: Arno.
Goldberg, E. M., & Morrison, S. L. (1963). Schizophrenia and social class. *British Journal of Psychiatry, 109,* 785–802.
Goldenberg, I., & Goldenberg, H. (1980). *Family therapy: An overview.* Monterey, CA: Wadsworth.
Goldsmith, O. (1909). *The deserted village.* New York: Dodd, Mead.
Goldstein, M. J. (1985). Family factors that antedate the onset of schizophrenia and related disorders: The results of a fifteen year prospective longitudinal study. *Acta Psychiatrica Scandinavica, 319*(71), 7–18.
Goldstein, M. J., Judd, L. L., Rodnick, E. H., Alkire, A., & Gould, E. (1968). A method for studying social influence and coping patterns within families of disturbed adolescents. *Journal of Nervous and Mental Disease, 147*(3), 233–251.
Goode, W. J. (1964). *The Family.* Englewood Cliffs, NJ: Prentice-Hall.
Goodman, E. (1989, August 1). Sharing home chores. *Boston Globe,* p. 10.
Goodsell, W. (1915). *A history of the family as a social and educational institution.* New York: Macmillan.
Goodsell, W. (1934). *A history of the family as a social and educational institution* (2nd ed.). New York: Macmillan.
Graubard, S. (1992). *Mr. Bush's war: Its moral and political consequences.* New York: Hill and Wang.
Green, R. G., Harris, R. N., Jr., Forter, J. A., & Robinson, M. (1991a). Evaluating FACES III and the circumplex model: 2,440 families. *Family Process, 30*(1), 55–73.
Green, R. G., Harris, R. N., Forter, J. A., & Robinson, M. (1991b). The wives data and FACES IV: Making things appear simple. *Family Process, 30,* 79–83.
Grinker, R. R., & Spiegel, J. (1945). *Men under stress.* Philadelphia: Blakiston.
Group for the Advancement of Psychiatry Committee on the Family. (1954). *Integration and conflict in family behavior.* GAP Report #27. New York: Author.
Group for the Advancement of Psychiatry Committee on the Family. (1970). *The field of family therapy.* GAP Report #78, vol. 7. New York: Author.
Grover, K. J., Paff-Berger, L. A., Russell, C. S., & Schumm, W. R. (1984). The Kansas Marital Satisfaction Scale: A further brief analysis. *Psychological Reports, 54,* 629–630.
Groves, E. R., & Ogburn, W. F. (1928). *American marriage and family relationships.* New York: Henry Holt.
Guidubaldi, J., & Perry, J. (1985). Divorce and mental health sequelae for children: A two-year follow-up of a nationwide sample. *Journal of the American Academy of Child Psychiatry, 24*(5), 531–537.
Gurin, G., Veroff, J., & Feld, S. (1960). *Americans view their mental health: A nationwide interview survey.* Monograph Series, No. 4. Washington, DC: Joint Committee on Mental Illness and Health.

Hagestad, G. (1986). The aging society as a context for family life. *Daedalus, 115,* 119–139.
Hagnell, O., & Kreitman, N. (1974). Mental illness in married pairs in a total population. *British Journal of Psychiatry, 125,* 293–302.
Hagnell, O., Lanke, J., Rorsman, B., & Ojesjo, L. (1982). Are we entering a new age of melancholy? Depressive illnesses in a prospective epidemiological study over 25 years: The Lundby Study, Sweden. *Psychological Medicine, 12,* 279–289.
Halberstam, D. (1991). *The next century.* New York: Morrow.
Hamilton, G. V. (1929). *A research in marriage.* New York: Medical Research Press.
Hampson, R. B., Beavers, W. R., & Hulgus, Y. F. (1988). Commentary: Comparing the Beavers and circumplex models of family functioning. *Family Process, 27,* 85–92.
Hampson, R. B., Beavers, W. R., & Hulgus, Y. (1990). Cross-ethnic family differences: Interactional assessments of white, black, and Mexican-American families. *Journal of Marital and Family Therapy, 16*(3), 307–319.
Hareven, T. K. (1977). Family time and historical time. *Daedalus, 106,* 57–70.
Harrington, M. (1963). *The other America: Poverty in the United States.* Baltimore, MD: Penguin.
Harris, M. (1968). *The rise of anthropological theory: A history of theories of culture.* New York: Crowell.
Hell, D. (1982). The spouses of depressive and schizophrenic patients: A controlled study. *Archiv Psychiatrie Nervenkrank, 232*(2), 167–178.
Henderson, S. (1981). Social relationships, adversity, and neurosis: An analysis of prospective observations. *British Journal of Psychiatry, 13,* 391–398.
Henry, J. (1963). *Culture against man.* New York: Random House.
Hewlett, S. A. (1991, Sept. 1). A neglected generation. *Louisville Courier Journal,* p. D1.
Hewlett, S. A. (1990). *When the bough breaks: The cost of neglecting our children.* New York: Basic Books.
Hill, B. (1991, December 7). *Louisville Courier Journal,* p. 3.
Hill, R. (1949). *Families under stress: Adjustment to the crises of war separation and reunion.* New York: Harper.
Hill, R. (1958). The sociology of marriage and family behavior, 1945–1946: A trend report and bibliography. *Current Sociology, 7,* 1–98.
Hill, R. (1970). *Family development in three generations: A longitudinal study of changing family patterns of planning and achievement.* Cambridge, MA: Schenkman.
Hill, R., & Hansen, D. A. (1960, November). The identification of conceptual frameworks utilized in family study. *Marriage and Family Living,* 299–311.
Hill, R., & Rodgers, R. H. (1964). The developmental approach. In H. T. Christensen (Ed.), *Handbook of marriage and the family.* Chicago: Rand McNally and Co.
Hinchliffe, M. K., Hooper, D., & Roberts, F. J. (1978). *The melancholy marriage: Depression in marriage and psychosocial approaches to therapy.* New York: John Wiley.
Hinchliffe, M. K., Hooper, D., Roberts, F. J., et al. (1975). A study of interaction between depressed patients and their spouses. *British Journal of Psychiatry, 126,* 164–172.
Hinchliffe, M. K., Vaughn, P. W., Hooper, D., et al. (1978). The melancholy marriage: An inquiry into the interaction of depression: III. Responsiveness. *British Journal of Psychiatry, 51,* 1–13.
Hippocrates. (1952). On airs, waters and places. In R. M. Hutchins (Ed.), *Great books of the Western world.* Chicago, IL: Encyclopaedia Britannica.
Hirshfeld, R. M. A. (1981). Situational depression: Validity of the concept. *British Journal of Psychiatry, 139,* 297–305.
Hirshfeld, R. M. A., Klerman, G. L., Clayton, P. J., & Keller, M. B. (1983). Personality and depression: Empirical findings. *Archives of General Psychiatry, 40,* 993–998.

REFERENCES

Hochschild, A. (1989). *The second shift.* New York: Viking.
Hofling, C. K. & Lewis, J. M. (Eds.). (1980). *The family evaluation and treatment.* New York: Brunner/Mazel.
Hogarty, G. E., Anderson, C. M., Reiss, D. J., Kornblith, S. J., Greenwald, D. P., Javna, C. D., & Madonia, M. J. (1986). Family psychoeducation, social skills training, and maintenance: Chemotherapy in the aftercare treatment of schizophrenia. *Archives of General Psychiatry, 43,* 633–642.
Hokanson, J. E., Sacco, W. P., Blumberg, S. R., & Landrum, G. C. (1980). Interpersonal behavior in depressive individuals in a mixed-motive game. *Journal of Abnormal Psychiatry, 89*(3), 320–322.
Holman, T. B., & Burr, W. (1980). Beyond the beyond: The growth of family theories in the 1970s. *Journal of Marriage and the Family, 42,* 729–741.
Holzer, C. E., Shea, B. M., Swanson, J. W., Leaf, P. J., Myers, J. K., George, L., & Bednarski, P. (1986). The increased risk for specific psychiatric disorders among persons of low socioeconomic status. *American Journal of Social Psychiatry, 4,* 259–271.
Hooley, J. M. (1990). Expressed emotion: A review of the critical literature. In G. I. Keitner (Ed.), *Depression and families: Impact and treatment.* Washington: American Psychiatric Press.
Howard, G. E. (1904). *A history of matrimonial institutions: Chiefly in England* (3 vols.). Chicago, IL: University of Chicago Press.
Hudson, W. (1982). *The clinical measurement package: A field manual.* Homewood, IL: Dorsey Press.
Ifill, G. (1992, January 19). Whose welfare? *New York Times,* sec. 4.
Ilfeld, F. W. (1977). Current social stressors and symptoms of depression. *American Journal of Psychiatry, 134*(2), 161–166.
Information please almanac atlas and yearbook 1990 (43rd ed.). (1990). Boston: Houghton Mifflin Company.
Institute of Medicine. (1990). *Research on children and adolescents with mental, behavioral and developmental disorders* (DHAS Pub. No. ADM-90-1659). ADAMHA.
Jackson, D. (1957). The question of family homeostasis. *Psychiatric Quarterly Supplement, 31,* 79–90.
Jarvis, E. (1971). *Insanity and idiocy in Massachusetts: Report of the Commission on Lunacy, 1855.* Cambridge, MA: Harvard University Press.
Jaspers, K. (1963). *General psychopathology* (J. Hoenig & M. W. Hamilton, Trans.). Chicago: University of Chicago Press. (Original work published 1923)
Jellinek, M.S., & Slovik, L. S. (1981, September 3). Divorce impact on children. *New England Journal of Medicine,* 557–560.
Jennings, M. (1990, November 13). Students' replies on sex, suicide, alcohol alarm education chief. *Louisville Courier Journal.*
Johnson, J. (1990, October). Cases old, cases new, cases treated, cases blue: Incidence, chronicity, and attributable risk in ECA. In J. J. Schwab (Chair), *Epidemiology and Social Psychiatry.* Symposium conducted at the meeting of the 12th World Congress of Social Psychiatry, Washington, DC.
Kanter, J., Lamb, H. R., & Loeper, C. (1987). Expressed emotion in families: A critical review. *Hospital and Community Psychiatry, 38*(4), 374–380.
Kantor, D., & Lehr, W. (1975). *Inside the family: Toward a theory of family process.* San Francisco: Jossey-Bass.
Kantrowitz, B., & Wingert, P. (1990, Winter/Spring). Step by step. *Newsweek,* 24–37.
Kaplan, H. I., Freedman, A. M., & Saddock, B. J. (Eds.). (1980). *Comprehensive textbook of psychiatry/III* (vol. 1). Baltimore, MD: Williams & Wilkins.

Kardiner, A., & Ovesey, L. (1962). *The mark of oppression*. New York: World.
Keen, J., & Harney, J. (1992, May 21). Words spark passion, but few answers. *USA Today*, pp. 1–2.
Keitner, G. I. (Ed.). (1990). *Depression and families: Impact and treatment*. Washington: American Psychiatric Press.
Kendler, K. S., McGuire, M., Gruenberg, A. M., O'Hare, A., Spellman, M., & Walsh, D. (in press). The Roscommon family study: 1. Methods, diagnosis of probands and risk of schizophrenia in relatives. *Archives of General Psychiatry*.
Kennedy, J. F., & Keeney, V. T. (1987). Group psychotherapy with grandparents rearing their emotionally disturbed grandchildren. *Group, 11*(1), 15–25.
Kennedy, J. F., & Keeney, V. T. (1988). The extended family revisited: Grandparents rearing grandchildren. *Child Psychiatry and Human Development, 19*(1), 26–35.
Kerr, M. E., & Bowen, M. (1988). *Family evaluation: An approach based on Bowen theory*. New York: W. W. Norton.
Kety, S. S., Rosenthal, D., Wender, P. H., & Schulsinger, F. (1968). The types and prevalence of mental illness in the biological and adoptive families of adopted schizophrenics. In D. Rosenthal & S. S. Kety (Eds.), *The transmission of schizophrenia*. Oxford, England: Pergamon.
Kinnaird, K. L., & Gerrard, M. (1986). Premarital sexual behavior and attitudes toward marriage among young women as a function of their mothers' marital status. *Journal of Marriage and the Family, 48*, 757–765.
Kinsey, A. C., Pomeroy, W. B., & Martin, C. E. (1948). *Sexual behavior in the human male*. Philadelphia: W. B. Saunders.
Kinsey, A. C., Pomeroy, W. B., Martin, C. E., & Gebhard, P. H. (1953). *Sexual behavior in the human female*. Philadelphia: W. B. Saunders.
Klein, J. (1992, June 18). Whose values? *Newsweek*, pp. 19–22.
Klein, M. (1932). *The psychoanalysis of children*. London: Hayworth.
Klerman, G. L. (1988). The current age of youthful melancholia: Evidence for increase in depression among adolescents and young adults. *British Journal of Psychiatry, 152*, 4–14.
Kolata, G. (1992, June 21). More children are employed, often perilously. *New York Times*, pp. 1, 18.
Koller, J. (1950). In E. Strömgren (Ed.), *Proceedings of the Congrés International de Psychiatrie Paris VI, Psychiatrie Sociale*. Paris: Hermann.
Komarovsky, M., & Waller, W. (1945). Studies of the family. *American Journal of Sociology, 50*, 433–451.
Koos, E. L. (1946). *Families in trouble*. New York: King's Crown.
Kozol, J. (1988). *Rachel and her children*. New York: Crown.
Kozol, J. (1990, Winter/Spring). The new untouchables. *Newsweek*, 48–53.
Kozol, J. (1991). *Savage inequalities: Children in America's schools*. New York: Crown.
Krause, N. (1983). Conflicting sex-role expectation, housework dissatisfaction, and depressive symptoms among full-time housewives. *Sex Roles, 9*(11):1115–1125.
Kreitman, N. (1962). Mental disorder in married couples. *Journal of Mental Science, 108*, 438–446.
Kreitman, N. (1964). The patient's spouse. *British Journal of Psychiatry, 110*, 159–173.
Kreitman, N. (1968). Married couples admitted to mental hospital. *British Journal of Psychiatry, 114*, 699–718.
Kreitman, N., Collins, J., Nelson, B., & Troop, J. (1971). Neurosis and marital interaction: IV. Manifest psychological interaction. *British Journal of Psychiatry, 119*, 243–252.
Kris, Ernst. (1952). *Psychiatric explorations in art*. New York: International Universities Press.
Krugman, P. (1990). *The age of diminished expectations: U.S. economic policy in the 1990s*. Cambridge: MIT Press.

Landsberg, M. (1992, June 29). New laws ban stalking. *Louisville Courier-Journal* p. A3.
Lasch, C. (1975). *Haven in a heartless world: The family besieged*. New York: Basic Books.
Leff, J., & Vaughn, C. (1980). The interaction of life events and relatives' expressed emotion in schizophrenia and depressive neurosis. *British Journal of Psychiatry, 136,* 146.
Leff, J., & Vaughn, C. (1987). Expressed emotion [Letter to the Editor]. *Hospital and Community Psychiatry, 38*(10), 1117–1118.
Leighton, D. C., Harding, J. S., Macklin, D. G., MacMillan, A. M., & Leighton, A. H. (1963). *The character of danger: The Stirling County study.* New York: Basic Books.
Levinson, D. J. (1978). *The seasons of a man's life.* New York: Knopf.
Levi-Strauss, C. (1985). *The view from afar* (J. Neugroschel & P. Hoss, Trans.). New York: Basic Books.
Lewin, K. (1951). Field theory in social science. In D. Cartwright (Ed.), *Social science: Selected theoretical papers.* New York: Harper and Row.
Lewis, J. (1988). The transition to parenthood: 1. The rating of prenatal marital competence. *Family Process, 27,* 149–165.
Lewis, J. M. (1979). The family of the patient. In J. Usdin & J. M. Lewis (Eds.), *Psychiatry in general medical practice* (p. 89). New York: McGraw Hill.
Lewis, J. M. (1989). *The birth of the family: An empirical inquiry.* New York: Brunner/Mazel.
Lewis, J. M., Beavers, W. R., Gossett, J. T., & Phillips, V. A. (1976). *No single thread: Psychological health in family systems.* New York: Brunner/Mazel.
Lewis, J. M., & Looney, J. G. (1983). *The long struggle: Well-functioning working-class black families.* New York: Brunner/Mazel.
Lidz, R., & Lidz, T. (1949). The family environment of schizophrenic patients. *American Journal of Psychiatry, 106,* 332–345.
Lidz, T. (1974). The family: The developmental setting, In S. Arieti (Ed.), *American handbook of psychiatry* (vol. 1, 2nd ed., pp. 252–263). New York: Basic Books.
Lidz, T. (1980). The family and the development. In C. K. Hofling & J. M. Lewis (Eds.), *The family: Evaluation and treatment.* New York: Brunner/Mazel.
Lidz, T., Fleck, S., & Cornelison, A. (1965). *Schizophrenia and the family.* New York: Universities Press.
London, J. (1904). *People of the abyss.* New York: Nelson.
Loomis, C. P., & Hamilton, C. H. (1936). Family life cycle analysis. *Social Forces, 15*(1), 225–231.
Lorch, D. (1991, May 12). Where day is night. *New York Times,* pp. 32–35.
Lucretius (1952). On the nature of things. In R. M. Hutchins (Ed.), *Great books of the Western world* (H. A. J. Munro, Trans.). Chicago, IL: Encyclopaedia Britannica.
Lupton, K. (1979). *Mungo Park the African traveler.* Oxford: Oxford University Press.
MacDonald, M. (1981). *Mystical bedlam: Madness, anxiety, and healing in 17th-century England.* Cambridge: Cambridge University Press.
MacFarlane, A. (1978). *The origins of English individualism.* New York: Cambridge University Press.
MacFarlane, A. (1986). *Marriage and love in England: Modes of reproduction 1300–1840.* New York: Basil Blackwell.
Mackay, C. (1932). *Extraordinary popular delusions and the madness of crowds.* New York: L. C. Page.
MacLean, P. D., Ogston, K., & Grauer, L. (1973). A behavioural approach to the treatment of depression. *Journal of Behaviour Therapy and Experimental Psychiatry, 4,* 323–330.
Maine, H. (1861). *Ancient law.* London: J. Murray.
Malinowski, B. (1927). *Sex and repression in savage society.* London: Routledge and Kegan Paul.
Marcus, S. (1966). *The other Victorians: A study of sexuality and pornography in medieval nineteenth-century England.* New York: Basic Books.

Martindale, D. (1960). *The nature and types of sociological theory.* Boston: Houghton Mifflin.
Matheny, A. P., Jr., & Dolan, A. B. (1980). A twin study of personality and temperament during middle childhood. *Journal of Research in Personality, 14,* 224.
Marx, K. (1952). Das kapital. In R. M. Hutchins (Ed.), *Great books of the Western world.* Chicago, IL: Encyclopaedia Britannica.
Masters, W., & Johnson, V. (1966). *Human sexual response.* Boston: Little, Brown.
May, R., Angel, E., & Ellenberger, H. F. (Eds.). (1958). *Existence: A new dimension in psychiatry and psychology.* New York: Basic Books.
McGoldrick, M., & Gerson, R. (1985). *Genograms in family assessment.* New York: W. W. Norton.
McLaren, E. F. (1992). A transcultural paradox. In E. Sorel (Ed.), *Social psychiatry in the later twentieth century.* Selected Proceedings XII World Congress of Social Psychiatry, Washington, DC, 1990. New York: Legas Press.
McLennan, J. F. (1865). *Primitive marriage.* Edinburgh: Adam and Charles Black.
Mead, M. (1928). *Coming of age in Samoa.* New York: Morrow.
Mead, M. (1930). *Growing up in New Guinea.* New York: Blue Ribbon.
Mead, M. (1970). *Culture and commitment. A study of the generation gap.* New York: Doubleday & Co., Inc.
Menninger, K. (1963). *The vital balance.* New York: Viking Press.
Merikangas, K. (1982). Assortative mating for psychiatric disorders and psychological traits. *Archives of General Psychiatry, 39,* 1173–1180.
Merikangas, K. R., et al. (1985). Marital adjustment in major depression. *Journal of Affective Disorders, 9*(1), 5–11.
Merikangas, K. R., Weissman, M. M., & Prusoff, B. A. (1990). In G. J. Keitner (Ed.), *Depression and families: Impact and treatment.* New York: American Psychiatric Press.
Meyer, A. (1931). Discussion of Dickinson, medical analysis of a thousand marriages. *Journal of the American Medical Association, 97*(8), 534–535.
Millar, J. (1960). The origin of the distinction of the ranks. In W.C. Lehmann, *John Millar of Glasgow, 1735–1801.* Cambridge, MA: Cambridge University Press.
Miller, I. W., Kabacoff, R. I., Epstein, N. B., Bishop, D. S., & Keitner, G. I. (in press). The McMaster Clinical Rating Scale: Reliability and validity.
Miller, J. G. (1978). *General living systems.* New York: McGraw-Hill Book Co.
Miller, J. G., & Miller, J. L. (1980). The family as a system. In C. K. Hofling & J. M. Lewis (Eds.), *The family: Evaluation and treatment.* New York: Brunner/Mazel.
Minuchin, S., Montalvo, B., Guerney, B. G., Jr., Rosman, B. L., & Schumer, F. (1967). *Families of the slums: An exploration of their strucutre and treatment.* New York: Basic Books.
Mitgang, H. (1991, October 19). Separate, still unequal [Review of *Savage inequalities*]. *Louisville Courier Journal,* p. A2.
Moore, R. H., & Moore, B. S. (1976). A typology of family social environments. *Family Process, 15,* 357–372.
Moos, R. H., & Moos, B. S. (1981). *Family environment scale manual.* Palo Alto, CA: Consulting Psychologists Press.
More, L. B. (1913). The cost of living for a wage earner's family in New York City. *Annals of the American Academy of Political and Social Science, 48,* 104–111.
Morgan, L. H. (1908). *Ancient society or researches in the lines of human progress from savagery through barbarism to civilization.* Chicago: Charles H. Kerr.
Morris, J. N. (1964). *Uses of epidemiology* (2nd ed.). Baltimore: Williams & Wilkins.
Morrow, L. (1991, August 12). Busy bodies and crybabies: What's happening to the American character? *Time,* p. 14.

Moynihan, D. P. (1965, March). *The Negro family: The case for national action.* Washington, DC: U.S. Department of Labor.

Murdock, G. P. (1949). *Social structure.* New York: Macmillan.

Myrdal, G. (1944). *An American dilemma.* New York: Harper.

Myers, J. K., Weissman, M. M., Tischler, G. L., Holzer, C. E., III, Leaf, P. I., Orvaschel, H., Anthony, J. C., Boyd, J. H., Burke, J. D., Jr., Kramer, M., & Stoltzman, R. (1984). Six-month prevalence of psychiatric disorders in three communities. *Archives of General Psychiatry, 41*(10), 959–971.

Myerson, A. (1940). Review, mental disorders in urban areas. *American Journal of Psychiatry, 96,* 995–997.

Nasr, S. (1992, March 5). Even among the well-off, the richest get richer. *New York Times,* sec. 1, pp. A1, D24.

NBC News. (1992, August 29). *NBC nightly news* [Television broadcast].

Nimkoff, M. F. (1948). Trends in family research. *American Journal of Sociology, 53,* 477–482.

Norton, A. J., & Moorman, J. E. (1987). Current trends in marriage and divorce among American women. *Journal of Marriage and the Family, 49,* 3–14.

Nuechterlein, K. H., Goldstein, M. J., Ventura, J., Dawson, M. E., & Doane, J. A. (1989). Patient-environment relationships in schizophrenia. Information processing, communication deviance, autonomic arousal, and stressful life events. *British Journal of Psychiatry, 155,* 84–89.

Nye, F. I. (1988). Fifty years of family research: 1937–1987. *Journal of Marriage and the Family, 50,* 305–316.

Ogburn, W. F. (1922). *Social change with respect to culture and original nature.* New York: Viking.

Ogburn, W. F. (1950). *Social change with respect to culture and original nature.* New York: Dell.

Ogburn, W. F., & Nimkoff, M. F. (1955). *Technology and the changing family.* Boston: Houghton Mifflin.

Ogburn, W. F., & Tibbitts, C. (1933). The family and its functions. In W. F. Ogburn (Ed.), *Recent social trends, vol. I.* New York: McGraw-Hill.

Olson, D. H. (1991). Commentary: Three-dimensional circumplex model and revised scoring of FACES III. *Family Process, 30,* 74–79.

Olson, D., McCubbin, H. I., Barnes, H. R., Larsen, A. S., Muxen, M. J., & Wilson, M. A. (1983). *Families: What makes them work.* Beverly Hills, CA: Sage.

Olson, D. H., Portner, J., & Bell, R. (1982). *FACES II: Family adaptability and cohesion evaluation scales.* Department of Family Social Science, University of Minnesota.

Olson, D. H., Portner, J., & Lavee, Y. (1985). *FACES III.* Department of Family Social Science, University of Minnesota.

Olson, D. H., Russell, C. S., & Sprenkle, D. H. (1985). Circumplex model of marital and family systems: VI. Theoretical update. *Family Process, 22,* 68–83.

Owens, S. (1992, August 22). Sex-abusers tag an ugly tool in custody cases. *Louisville Courier Journal,* p. A2.

Park, M. (1800). *Travels in the interior districts of Africa.* New York: F. Tiebout.

Park, R. E. (1950). *Race and culture* (E. C. Hughes, Ed.). Glencoe, IL: Free Press.

Parker, G. (1983). Parental "affectionless control" as an antecedent to adult depression: A risk factor delineated. *Archives General Psychiatry, 40,* 956–960.

Parkes, C. M. (1972). *Bereavement: Studies of grief in adult life.* New York: International Universities Press.

Parsons, E. C. (1906). *The family.* New York: G. P. Putman's Sons, The Knickerbocker Press.

Parsons, T. (1962). Youth in the context of American society. *Daedalus, 91*(1), 97–123.

Parsons, T. (1970). *Social structure and personality.* London: Free Press.

Parsons, T., & Bales, R. F. (1955). *Family, socialization, and interaction process*. Glencoe, IL: Free Press.
Parsons, T., & Skils, E. A. (1951). *Toward a general theory of action*. Cambridge, MA: Harvard University Press.
Parsons, T., & White, W. (1961). The link between character and society. In S. M. Lipset & S. Lowenthal (Eds.), *Culture and Social Character*. New York: Free Press of Glencoe.
Paykel, E. S., et al. (1971). Scaling of life events. *Archives of General Psychiatry, 25*, 340–347.
Paykel, E. S., Myers, J. K., Dienelt, M. N., Klerman, G. L., Lindenthal, J. J., & Pepper, M. P. (1969). Life events and depression: A controlled study. *Archives of General Psychiatry, 21*, 753–760.
Pearson, C. H. (1894). *National life and character: A forecast*. London: Macmillan.
Penrose, L. S. (1944). Mental illness in husband and wife: A contribution to the study of assortative mating in man. *Psychiatric Quarterly Supplement, 18*, 161.
Phillips, K. (1990). *The politics of rich and poor: Wealth and the American electorate in the Reagan aftermath*. New York: Random House.
Phillips, R. (1988). *Putting asunder: A history of divorce in Western society*. New York: Cambridge University Press.
Plato (1952). Republic. In R. M. Hutchins (Ed.), *The great books of the western world*. Chicago: Encyclopaedia Britannica.
Plumb, J. H. (1967, January 1). In Queen Victoria's spacious days. *New York Times Book Review*, p. 1.
Pogrebin, L. C. (1983). *Family politics: Love and power on an intimate frontier*. New York: McGraw-Hill.
Quinton, D., & Rutter, M. (1985). Family pathology and child psychiatric disorder. A four-year prospective study. In A. R. Nicol (Ed.), *Longitudinal studies in child psychology and psychiatry* (pp. 91–134). Chichester, England: John Wiley.
Rabkin, R. (1976). A critique of the clinical use of the double-bind. In C. Sluzki & D. Ransom (Eds.), *Double Bind: The communicational approach to the family* (pp. 287–306). New York: Grune & Stratton.
Radcliffe, D., & Dionne, E. D., Jr. (1992, January 24). The race for president. *Washington Post*, p. A8.
Radloff, L. S. (1975). Sex differences in depression: The effects of occupation and marital status. *Sex Roles, 1*, 249–265.
Radloff, L. S. (1977). The CES-D Scale: A self-report depression scale for research in the general population. *Applied Psychological Measurement, 1*, 385–401.
Rashkis, H. (1968). Depression as a manifestation of the family as an open system. *Archives of General Psychiatry, 19*, 57–63.
Raspberry, W. (1992, May 2). *Violence*. Presentation to Psychiatrists for Better Psychiatry, Washington, DC.
Regier, D. A., Boyd, J. H., Burke, J. D., Jr., Rae, D. S., Myers, J. K., Kramer, M., Robins, L. N., George, L. K., Karno, M., & Locke, B. Z. (1988). One-month prevalence of mental disorders in the United States, based on five Epidemiologic Catchment Area sites. *Archives of General Psychiatry, 45*, 977–985.
Reich, W. (1927). Zur technik der deutung und der widerstandsanalyse. *Internat. Zeitschrift für Psychoanalyse, XIII*.
Reich, W. (1972). *Character analysis* (V. R. Carfagno, Trans.; 3rd ed.). New York: Farrar, Straus and Giroux.
Reiss, D. (1982). The working family: A researcher's view of health in the household. *American Journal of Psychiatry, 139*(11), 1412–1420.
Reiss, D., Gonzalez, S., & Kramer, N. (1986). Family process, chronic illness, and death. *Archives of General Psychiatry, 43*, 795–804.

REFERENCES

Reiss, I. L. (1986). *Journey into sexuality. An exploratory voyage.* Englewood Cliffs, NJ: Prentice-Hall.
Richman, N., Stevenson, J., & Graham, P. (Eds.). (1982). *Preschool to school: A behavioral study.* London: Academic Press.
Reisman, D., Denney, R., & Glazer, N. (1950). *The lonely crowd: A study of the changing American character.* New Haven: Yale University Press.
Robins, L. N., Helzer, J. E., Croughhan, J. L., & Ratcliff, K. S. (1979). *The National Institute of Mental Health diagnostic interview schedule (DIS).* Bethesda, MD: National Institute of Mental Health.
Robins, L. N., Helzer, J. E., Weissman, M. M., Orvaschel, H., Gruenberg, E., Burke, J. D., Jr., & Regier, D. A. (1984). Lifetime prevalence of specific psychiatric disorders in three sites. *Archives of General Psychiatry, 41*(10), 942–948.
Roper, E. (1950). *People's attitudes concerning mental health: A study made in the city of Louisville.* Louisville, KY: Elmo Roper.
Rosenthal, D. (1973). A program of research on heredity in schizophrenia. In S. S. Dean (Ed.), *Schizophrenia: The first ten Dean Award Lectures* (pp. 231–241). New York: MSS Information.
Rosenthal, D., & Kety, S. S. (Eds.). (1968). *Their transmission of schizophrenia.* London: Pergamon.
Rounsaville, B. J., Prusoff, B. A., & Weissman, M. M. (1980). The course of marital disputes in depressed women: A 48-month follow-up study. *Comprehensive Psychiatry, 21*(2), 111–118.
Rowntree, B. S. (1903). *Poverty: A study of town life.* London: Macmillan.
Rüdin, E. (1961). In J. Shields & E. Slater (Eds.), *Handbook of abnormal psychology: An experimental approach.* New York: Basic Books.
Ruestow, P., Dunner, D. L., Bleecker, B., & Fieve, R. R. (1978). Marital adjustment in primary affective disorder. *Comprehensive Psychiatry, 19*(6), 565–571.
Rutter, M. (1966). *Children of sick parents: An environmental and psychiatric study* (Maudsley Monograph 16 of the Institute of Psychiatry). London: Oxford University Press.
Rutter, M., & Madge, N. (1976). *Cycles of disadvantage.* Exeter, NY: Heinemann.
Rutter, M., & Quinton, D. (1977). Psychiatric disorder: Ecological factors and concepts of causation. In H. McGurk (Ed.), *Ecological factors in human development.* Amsterdam: North-Holland.
Salinger, J. D. (1951). *Catcher in the rye.* London: H. Hamilton.
Sandburg, C. (1916). *Chicago Poems.* New York: H. Holt.
Sapir, E. (1930). What is the family still good for? *American Mercury, 19*(74), 145–151.
Schor, J. (1991). *The overworked American: The unexpected decline of leisure.* New York: Basic Books.
Schwab, J. J., Bell, R. A., Warheit, G. J., & Schwab, R. B. (1979). *Social order and mental health: The Florida health study.* New York: Brunner/Mazel.
Schwab, J. J., Stephenson, J. J., & Bell, R. A. (1988). Risk for depression in families over time: a pilot epidemiologic study. *Hospital and Community Psychiatry, 39*(1), 58–62.
Schwab, J. J., Warheit, G. J., & Holzer, C. E., III. (1973). Depressive symptomatology and age. *Psychosomatics, 14,* 135–141.
Seligman, J. (1982). *The transformation of Wall Street: A history of the Securities and Exhcange Commission and modern corporate finance.* Boston: Houghton Mifflin.
Seligman, J. (1990, Winter/Spring). Variations on a theme. *Newsweek,* 38–47.
Selye, H. (1956). *The stress of life.* New York: McGraw-Hill.
Selzer, M. L., Vinokur, A., & van Roijen, L. (1975). A self-administered Short Michigan Alcoholism Screening Test. *Journal of Studies on Alcohol, 36,* 117–126.

Shafii, M., & Shafii, S. L. (1992). *Clinical guide to depression in children and adolescents.* Washington, DC: American Psychiatric Press.
Shaw, G. B. (1913). *The quintessence of Ibsenism.* New York: Hill and Wang.
Sheehy, G. (1976). *Passages: Predictable crises of adult life.* New York: Dutton.
Sherrington, R., Brynjolfsson, J., Petursson, H., Potter, M., et al. (1988). Local susceptibility locus for schizophrenia on chromosome 5. *Nature, 336,* 164–167.
Shields, J., & Slater, E. (1961). Heredity and psychological abnormality. In H. J. Eysenck (Ed.), *Handbook of abnormal psychology: An experimental approach* (p. 313). New York: Basic Books.
Shorter, E. (1975). *The making of the modern family.* New York: Basic Books.
Silver, C. B. (Ed. & Trans.) (1982). *Frederic Le Play: On family, work, and social change.* Chicago: University of Chicago Press.
Singer, M. (1975, February). *The Dean Award lecture.* Paper presented at American College of Psychiatrists, Newport Beach, CA.
Singer, M. T., Wynne, L. C., & Toohey, M. L. (1978). Communication disorders and the families of schizophrenics. In L. C. Wynne, R. L. Cromwell, & S. Matthysse (Eds.), *The nature of schizophrenia.* New York: Wiley.
Singh, B. K. (1980). Trends in attitudes toward premarital sexual relations. *Journal of Marriage and the Family, 42,* 387–393.
Smith, R. M. (1990, Special Edition). A commitment to the family. *Newsweek,* pp. 9–10.
Sorokin, P. (1941). *The crisis of our age.* New York: E. P. Dalton.
Spengler, O. (1929). *The decline of the West.* New York: A. A. Knopf.
Spiegel, J., & Bell, N. (1959). The family of the psychiatric patient. In Silvano Arieti (Ed.), *American handbook of psychiatry, vol. 1* (pp. 114–149). New York: Basic Books.
Spiegel, J. P., & Kluckhohn, F. (1971). *Transactions: The interplay between individual, family and society.* New York: Science House.
Srole, L., & Fischer, A. K. (1986). The Midtown Manhattan longitudinal study: Aging, generations, and genders. In M. M. Weissman, J. K. Meyers, & C. E. Ross (Eds.), *Community surveys of psychiatric disorders.* New Brunswick, NJ: Rutgers University Press.
Srole, L., Langner, T. S., Michael, S. T., Opler, M. K., & Rennie, T. A. G. (1962). *Mental health in the metropolis—The Midtown Manhattan study* (Vol. 1). New York: McGraw-Hill.
Steinbeck, J. (1939). *The grapes of wrath.* New York: Viking.
Stephenson, J. J., Schwab, J. J., & Bell, R. A. (1990). Stressful life events and risk for depression in the family. *Stress Medicine, 6,* 145–155.
Stewart, J. B. (1991). *Den of thieves.* New York: Simon & Schuster.
Stone, L. (1973). *Family and fortune: Studies in aristocratic finance in the sixteenth and seventeenth centuries.* Oxford: Clarendon Press.
Stone, L. (1989). The road to polygamy. *The New York Review of Books, 36*(3), 12–15.
Stonequist, E. V. (1937). *The marginal man.* New York: Charles Scribner.
Strauss, M. A., & Gelles, R. J. (1986). Societal change and change in family violence from 1975 to 1985 as revealed by two national surveys. *Journal of Marriage and the Family, 48,* 465–479.
Strauss, W., & Howe, N. (1991). *Generations: The history of America's future, 1584 to 2069.* New York: William Morrow.
Sullivan, H. S. (1953). The interpersonal theory of psychiatry. New York: W. W. Norton.
Sumner, W. G. (1909). The family and social change. *The American Journal of Sociology, 24*(5), 577–591.
Swift, J. (1965). A modest proposal. In P. Pinkus (Ed.), *A selection of his works* (pp. 477–487). Toronto: McMillan.

Tacitus. (1911). *The works of Tacitus: The history, Germany, and Agricola, & Dialogue on orators, vol. 11* (H. Mattingly, Trans.). London: G. Bell & Sons.
Taylor, C. (1989). *Sources of the self: The making of modern identity.* Cambridge, MA: Harvard University Press.
Terman, L. M. (1938). *Psychological factors in marital happiness.* New York: McGraw-Hill.
Thomas, V. G. (1990a). Determinants of global life happiness and marital happiness in dual-career black couples. *Family Relations, 139,* 174–178.
Thomas, V. G. (1990b). Problems of dual-career black couples: Identification and implications for family interventions. *Journal of Multicultural Counseling and Development, 1*(18), 58–67.
Thomas, W. I. (1923). *The unadjusted girl.* Boston: Little Brown.
Thycydides (1954). *History of the Peloponesian War* (R. Warner, Trans.). Bungay, Suffolk: Chaucer Press.
Toynbee, A. J. (1934). *A study of history.* London: Oxford University Press.
Turner, F. J. (1920). *The frontier in American history.* New York: H. Holt.
Tylor, E. B. (1958). *Primitive culture.* New York: Harper.
Vanfossen, B. E. (1981). Sex differences in the mental health effects of spouse support and equity. *Journal of Health and Social Behavior, 22,* 130–143.
Vaughn, C., & Leff, J. (1976). The influence of family and social factors on the course of psychiatric illness. *British Journal of Psychiatry, 129,* 125–137.
Veroff, J., Douban, E., & Kulka, R. A. (1981). *The inner American: a self-portrait from 1957 to 1976.* New York: Basic Books.
Veyne, P. (1987). The Roman Empire. In P. Veyne (Ed.), *A history of private life: I. From Pagan Rome to Byzantium.* (A. Goldhammer, Trans.). Cambridge, MA: Harvard University Press.
Wallerstein, J. (1989, January 22). Children after divorce: Wounds that don't heal. *New York Times Magazine,* pp. 18–26.
Wallerstein, J. S., Blakeslee, S. (1989). *Second chances: Men, women, and children a decade after divorce.* New York: Ticknor & Fields.
Warheit, G. J. (1979). Life events, coping, stress and depressive symptomatology. *American Journal of Psychiatry, 136,* 502–507.
Warheit, G. J., Holzer, C. E., III, & Schwab, J. J. (1973). An analysis of social class and racial differences in depressive symptomatology: A community study. *Journal of Health and Social Behavior, 14,* 291–299.
Waring, E. M. & Patton, D. (1984). Marital intimacy and depression. *British Journal of Psychiatry, 145,* 641–644.
Watkins, S. C., Menken, J. A., & Bongaarts, J. (1987). Demographic foundations of family change. *American Sociological Review, 52,* 346–358.
Wayward votes. (1991, October 8). *Louisville Courier-Journal,* p. A8.
Weissman, M. M. (1990). Depression and families: A comment. In G. I. Keitner (Ed.), *Depression and families: Impact and treatment* (pp. 187–190). Washington, DC: American Psychiatric Press.
Weissman, M. M. (1991, December). *The epidemiology of depression: Update.* Paper presented at the Paroxetine Investigator's Update, Scottsdale, AZ.
Weissman, M. M., & Paykel, E. S. (1974). *The depressed woman: A study of social relationships.* Chicago: University of Chicago Press.
Weissman, M. M., Paykel, E. S., & Klerman, G. L. (1972). The depressed woman as a mother. *Social Psychiatry, 7,* 98–108.
Weissman, M. M., Tischler, G. L., Holzer, III, C. E., Leaf, P. J., et al., (1984). Six-month prevalence of psychiatric disorders in three communities. *Archives of General Psychiatry, 41*(10), 959–967.

Wells, H. G. (1908). *Socialism and the family* (Vol. 56). Boston: Ball.
Wells, K. B., Stewart, A., Hays, R. D., Burnham, A., Rogers, W., et al. (1989). The functioning and well-being of depressed patients. Results from the medical outcomes study. *Journal of the American Medical Association, 262*(7), 914–919.
Westermarck, E. (1922). *History of human marriage* (5th ed.). New York: Allerton.
Westermarck, E. (1936). *The future of marriage in Western civilization.* New York: Macmillan.
Westley, W. A., & Epstein, N. (1969). *The silent majority: Families of emotionally healthy college students.* San Francisco: Jossey-Bass.
Whyte, W. H. (1956). *The organization man.* New York: Simon & Schuster.
Will, G. F. (1992, January 9). Blaming Japan first. *Washington Post,* p. A21.
Wilson, S. (1955). *Man in the gray flannel suit.* New York: Simon & Schuster.
Wines, M. (1992, May 5). *New York Times,* p. 1.
Winokur, G., Tsuang, M. T., & Crowe, R. (1982). The Iowa 500: Affective disorders in relatives of manic and depressed patients. *American Journal of Psychiatry, 139*(2), 209–212.
World almanac and book of facts 1991. (1990). New York: Pharos.
Wordsworth, W. (1850). *The prelude or growth of a poet's mind: An autobiographical poem.* London: Mofron.
Wrigley, E. A. (1977). Reflections on the history of the family. *Daedalus, 106,* 71–85.
Wynne, L. C. (1984). The epigenesis of relational systems: A model for understanding family development. *Family Process, 23*(3), 297–318.
Wynne, L. C., et al. (1958). Pseudomutuality in the family relationships of schizophrenics. *Psychiatry, 21,* 205–220.
Wynne, L. C., & Singer, M. T. (1963). Thought disorder and family relations in schizophrenics II: A classification of forms of thinking. *Archives of General Psychiatry, 9,* 191–206.
Wynne, L., & Singer, M. (1965). Thought disorder and family relations of schizophrenics, no. 4: Results and implications. *Archives of General Psychiatry, 12,* 201–212.
Wynne, L., Singer, M., Bartko, J., & Toohey, M. (1976). Schizophrenics and their families: Recent research on parental communication. In J. M. Tanner (Ed.), *Psychiatric research: The widening perspective* (pp. 254–286). New York: International University Press.
Yankelovich, D. (1991, February). Presentation at the American College of Psychiatrists, Ft. Lauderdale, FL.
Zimmerman, C. C. (1947). *The family and civilization.* New York: Harper & Brothers.
Zimmerman, C. C. (1959). Frederic Le Play. In *Encyclopaedia Britannica,* vol. 13. Chicago: William Benton.
Zimmerman, C. C. (1972a). 1971 Burgess Award Address: The future of the family in America. *Journal of Marriage and the Family, 323–333.*
Zimmerman, C. C. (1972b). The future of the family in America: II. The rise of the counter-revolution. *International Journal of Sociology of the Family, 2*(2), 1–9.
Zimmerman, C. C., & Frampton, M. E. (1935). *Family and society: A study of the sociology of reconstruction.* Boston: Van Nostrand.

Index

ABC-X Family Crisis Model, 180
Abel, 32
Abortion
 in ancient Rome, 50
 Christianity's view of, 53
Abraham (Old Testament), 52
Abraham, Karl, 165
Academic performance, of children of divorce, 7
Accident rate, 354
Ackerman, Nathan, 167–169, 361–362
Ackerman Institute for Family Therapy, 169
Acquired immune deficiency syndrome (AIDS), 28, 354
Adam, B. N., 78, 184–186
Addams, Jane, 75
Addictive behavior, parental, 350
Adler, Alfred, 165
Adolescents
 depression of, 194, 357
 as family mental health epidemiological study subjects, 299–313
 as family stress cause, 249–250, 376
 of Great Depression, 143–144, 145–146, 180–181
 identity problems of, 133, 134, 138
 mental illness of
  prevalence of, 353
  sex factors in, 271–273, 347–348
 in 1960s, 132–135, 139, 140
 in 1970s, 149
 as psychiatric hospital patients, 26

Adolescents (*Cont.*)
 relationship with parents, 184, 215
 stressors of, 215, 337
 suicide attempts by, 1, 208, 229
Adoptee study, of schizophrenia, 362
Adult children, living at home, 299–313
 mental illness symptomatology, 305–310, 333, 346, 373, 376, 385–386, 389
 parent–child intergenerational boundaries of, 347
Adultery
 in Africa, 74
 in ancient Egypt, 35
 in atomistic families, 119
 as basis for divorce, 34, 48, 52, 53
Advertising, 139
Affective style, in schizophrenic families, 193
African-American families, 3, 70–82
 African origins of, 70–71, 73–74
 characteristics of, 81–82
 children of, with psychiatric disorders, 348
 competence of, 222
 depression in, 207, 208
 dual-career, 210–212
 illegitimacy rate of, 70, 75
 illiteracy rate of, 75
 life cycle study of, 209
 matricentricity of, 78
 northern migration of, 92, 128
 as nuclear family, 79

411

African-American families (*Cont.*)
  racial discrimination toward, 72, 78, 79, 80, 82
  during slavery, 70, 71, 72–73, 74–75, 76, 78
  socioeconomic status of, 79–80
  types of, 81
  urbanization of, 76–77, 92, 128
  violence and, 82
African families, 70–71, 73–74
"Agent blue," 328
Age of consent, 149
Aggression
  of children, 320, 321, 327, 348–349, 387, 389–390
  Freud's theory of, 96
Agriculture, development of, 43, 51–52
Aid for Families with Dependent Children, 14, 17, 248, 307, 308
Airs, Waters, and Places (Hippocrates), 134
Alceste, 62–63
Alcestis (Euripedes), 32, 59
Alcohol abuse
  as family mental illness symptom, 241, 242, 243, 247, 253, 258, 279, 282
  clinical implications of, 333–334
  in families with older children, 267–268, 271, 272, 279, 282, 305, 308, 309–310
  in families with young children, 293, 295
  in Industrial Revolution, 65
  in 1950s, 131
  sex factors in, 243
Amenhotep III, 36, 359
American character
  antifamilism and, 21–26
  in 1950s, 131–132
American Indians
  anthropological studies of, 38, 39, 163
  slaughter of, 87
  Yurok tribe, 134
American Psychiatric Association, 225
American Sociological Association, 91
Amish, 162
Anglo-Saxons
  family life of, 53–56, 58, 63
  individualism of, 116
  wife purchase by, 40
Animals, monogamy of, 34, 41

Anthropology, family research applications of, 162–163, 361
Antifamilism, 6
  the American character and, 21–26
  economic factors in, 20–26
  governmental, 14, 20, 21, 23, 351, 356–357
  indicators of, 354
  in 1960s, 21
  in Russia, 148
Anxiety
  consumerism and, 139
  in interpersonal relationships, 139
  nuclear war–related, 130, 138
  other-directed character and, 136
  sexuality-related, 140
  triangling and, 175–176
  uncertainty-related, 149
Apartments, 93, 95
Aristotle, 48, 120
Arson, 322
Assertiveness training, 152
Assortative mating hypothesis, of depression, 194, 198–199
Astell, Mary, 90
Athena, 48
Athens, 47, 48–49, 69, 120, 136
Atomism, of the family, 69, 118–120, 121, 155
  of disengaged family, 182
  in 1970s, 147
Automobile, social impact of, 104, 109, 129
Autonomy, as basic human drive, 350

Baby boom, 144
Bachofen, J.J., 37–38
Balance theory, 178
Barbarism, 38, 56
Bateson, G., 122
Beavers Systems Model, of family functioning, 216–217
Behavioral approach, to family studies, 179
Bell and Schwab Family Systems Assessment Scale, 231, 365–366
Belsky, J., 223–225
Benedict, Ruth, 163
Bennett, William J., 23
Bereavement
  effect on physical health, 263
  in seventeenth-century England, 61, 62

INDEX

Berkeley Guidance Study, 145–146, 180–181
Bertalanffy, L. von, 171
Berry, Wendell, 27, 28
Betrothal ritual, Anglo-Saxon, 54–55
Bingham Child Guidance Clinic, historical-clinic study of, 315–329, 386–388, 389–390
   children's presenting problems, 318–322
   clinic history and background, 315–316
   families' problems, 322–327
   parents' marital status, 318, 319, 325–326, 327
   study protocol, 316–317
   study sample, 316
Biological basis, of the family, 33, 34, 46, 147
Birth control. *See* Contraception
Birth rate
   decline of, 92
   in 1950s, 124, 131
   in 1989, 131
   in polyandrous societies, 43
   post–World War II, 130
   social character development and, 135
   in World War II, 112
Birth ratio, male:female, 34, 46
Boas, Franz, 163
Bohr, Nils, 87, 169
Bomb shelters, 130
Booth, Charles, 160
Borderline personality disorder, 103
Bowen, Murray, 122, 172, 174–178, 350, 351
Brave New World (Huxley), 147
Breton, André, 104
Bridal veil, 56
Bridal wreath, 56
Britons, ancient. *See also* Anglo-Saxons
   standard of living, 50
Budget, as research tool, 158, 159, 240, 343, 361, 374
Burgess, E.F., 98–99
Burglary, 26
Burgundians, 54, 63
Bush, Barbara, 18, 356
Bush, George
   as education president, 24
   Family and Medical Leave Act veto by, 21

Bush, George (*Cont.*)
   family values and, 18
   1992 Asian trip of, 22
   as vice president, 385
Bush administration, 13–14, 21, 26, 82, 111, 356
Business, wage structure of, 19

Caesar, 50, 53
Cain, 32
Canute, Law of, 58, 56
Capitalism
   of British settlers, 65–66
   holiday celebrations and, 153
   individualism and, 103
   in nineteenth century, 87–88
   nuclear family development and, 57, 58, 59
   romantic marriage and, 58
Career choices, 142–143
   in 1950s, 144
   in 1960s, 145
Catcher in the Rye (Salinger), 132
Catholic Church, marriage ceremony of, 64
Cecrops, 48
Celibacy
   in ancient Rome, 50
   in Anglo-Saxon society, 58
   Christianity's view of, 53
Center for Epidemiologic Studies Depression Scale. *See under* Epidemiological study, of family mental health
Champollion, Jean François, 37
Character
   American
      antifamilism and, 21–26
      in 1950s, 131–132
   definition of, 134
   inner-directed, 135, 136
   other-directed, 135–137, 140
   social, 134, 135–137
   society and, 134–135
   tradition-directed, 135, 136
Character formation, 111, 122. *See also* Personality development
   Freud's theory of, 134
   in 1950s, 131–132
Charles, V., 63
Chicago, University of, 92, 98–99

Chief executive officers (CEOs), divorce of, 4–5, 6
Child abuse, decline of, 185
Childbearing, as social duty, 70, 121–122
Child Behavior Checklist. *See under* Epidemiological study, of family mental health
Childcare
  in dual-career families, 210, 211
  mental illness correlation, 260
  by servants, 50
  women's responsibility for, 13
  for working mothers, 17–18
Childhood, duration of, 43
Child labor, 16–17, 67, 92
Child labor laws, 94
Child neglect, during World War II, 112–113
Childrearing
  in other-directed societies, 136, 136–137
  permissive, 153–154
  skip-generation, 12
  therapists' involvement in, 103
Children
  aggression of, 320, 321, 327, 348–349, 387, 389–390
  average number per household, 9
  as basis of the family, 34
  character formation of, 111, 122, 131–132, 134
  of depressed mothers, 196, 248, 349, 362
  depression in, 154, 322, 328, 348–349, 387, 389–390
  of divorce, 6–9, 129, 137, 140–141, 333
    anxiety of, 2–3
    increasing number of, 6–7
    problems of, 7–8
    support groups for, 3
  as family mental health epidemiological study subjects, 285–299
  family's responsibility for, 111
  federal spending for, 19
  homeless, 15
  institutionalized, 318, 324
  marital relationship and, 221–222, 223–225
  mental illness prevalence among, 27, 353

Children (*Cont.*)
  in nineteenth century, 89
  in 1920s, 100
  in 1950s, 126
  in 1960s, 132
  out-of-wedlock, 3
  parents' love for, 62–63
  poor, 14–18, 19
  as property, 43
  raised by grandparents, 12
  remarriage and, 5
  socialization of, 86, 122, 123–124
    career choices and, 142–143
    Flügel's theory of, 166
    Freud's theory of, 163
    by society, 155
    sociopolitical factors in, 146
    in tradition-directed society, 135
  suicide by, 154, 322, 348–349, 387–390
  therapeutic issues regarding
    parent–child coalition, 345–346
    subclinical cases, 344–345
    trends in problems of, 347–350
Chivalry, 57
Christianity
  slavery and, 70, 71–72
  teachings on the family and marriage, 52–53, 54, 93–94
Christmas, 153
Church attendance, 100
Church Fathers, 53, 69, 120
Cicero, 34, 50
Circumplex Model, of family functioning, 213–216
Citizenship, 38
Civil defense drills, 130, 133
Civilization
  cyclic concept of, 108–109, 118, 355, 356
  decay of, 69
  evolutionary concept of, 108–109
  Morgan's theory of, 38–39
Civil Rights Act of 1964, 23
Civil rights movement, 138
Civil War, 67, 90
Cleopatra, 35
Clinton, Bill, 21
Clowes, William, 72–73
Collins, R., 79, 80, 81
Coats, Dan, 24, 25
Cooley, Charles H., 152

INDEX   **415**

Colonial America, family life in, 65–68
Communication
  by depressed persons, 196, 200–201, 339, 362
  in schizophrenic families, 189, 191, 193, 362
Communication theory, 169, 171
Communism, 134
Community
  decreased importance of, 68
  family's relationship to, 98
  individual's relationship to, 23, 27–28, 150
Competence, family, 219–222
Competition, sexual, 140
Comte, Auguste, 159
Concubinage
  in ancient Greece, 48, 120
  in ancient Israel, 52
  in ancient Rome, 49
Conflict
  marital, depression and, 337, 349–350
  parental
    following divorce, 7
    Freudian theory of, 164
  role-related. *See* Role conflict
  in schizophrenic families, 188
Conflict theory, 179
Consumerism, 138–139, 140
Consumption, family attitudes toward, 143
Contraception
  in ancient Rome, 50
  in 1950s, 127
  post–World War I use of, 98
Contraceptive pill, 138
Contractualism, 110–111
Coronary artery disease, of industrialized populations, 160
Corporations, acceptance of divorce by, 4–5, 6
Corruption, governmental, 24–25
  as social control, 154–155
Cottrell, L.S. Jr, 98–99
Counterculture, 137, 138, 154
Couples interview, 122
Courtesans, in ancient Greece, 48, 120
Courtship, promiscuity as related to, 41–42
Credit card, 138

Crime
  in nineteenth century, 89
  single-parent households and, 26
Criminals, as early American settlers, 67
Cuban missile crisis, 130
Cults, 136
Cultural changes, in 1920s, 104
Cultural norms, internalization of, 124
Culture, definition of, 97
Culture lag, 96–97, 109, 141
Cyclic view, of history, 108–109, 118, 355, 356

Daphnis and Chloe, 59
Darwinian theory, 92, 96.
  applications to family research, 161–162. *See also* Evolutionary theories
David (Old Testament), 52
Decline of the West (Spengler), 130
Defoe, Daniel, 64
Deinstitutionalization, 192
Democracy, of nuclear family, 123
Democracy in America (de Tocqueville), 71–72
Dependency, excessive, 153–154
Depression
  assessment of, 213
  in children, 154, 322, 328, 348–349, 387, 389–390
  in children of divorce, 7
  in divorced/separated persons, 9
  family factors in, 362
  as family mental illness symptom, 237, 238, 241, 242, 243, 248, 252, 253–254, 256, 258, 259
    changes over time, 271, 272, 279, 280–281, 282
  in families with adult children, 305, 306, 307–308, 309
  in families with young children, 291, 293, 294, 295, 299
  family studies of, 194–208
    of assortative mating, 194, 198–199
    of marital interactions, 200–206
    of stressful life events, 206–208
    theories of, 194–195
  intergenerational transmission of, 248
  marital conflict and, 337, 349–350

Depression (*Cont.*)
  peak onset age of, 357
  sex factors in, 243
  theories of, 194–195
De Principia (Newton), 87
De Re Naturem (Lucretius), 33
Desegregation, 133
Detriangling, 176
Developmental approach, in family studies, 178, 179
Diagnostic and Statistical Manual-III-Revised, 227
  Axis IV Severity of Psychosocial Stressors Scale, 245
  Global Assessment of Functioning Scale, 225–226
Diagnostic and Statistical Manual-IV, relational problems classification system, 225, 226
Diagnostic Interview Schedule for Children. *See under* Epidemiological study, of family mental health
Dickens, Charles, 18, 65
Differentiation, 175, 176
  in Great Depression, 143
  mental illness correlation, 259–260
Divorce, 3–6
  in Africa, 74
  among African-Americans, 73, 81
  in ancient Greece, 48
  in ancient Israel, 52
  in ancient Rome, 50, 51
  in Anglo-Saxon society, 54
  by childless couples, 91
  Christianity's prohibition of, 53, 54
  in colonial America, 67–68
  contributing factors in, 129
  in early twentieth century, 92
  economic effects of, 4, 5, 7, 8
  effect on children, 2–3, 7–9, 140
  family research topic, 185
  history of, 34
  Jesus Christ's teaching on, 53
  as marital breakdown indicator, 3–4
  no-fault, 119
  social acceptability of, 4–5
  as social epidemic, 6
  in twentieth century, 68
Divorce laws, 91, 92–93
Divorce: marriage ratio, 129

Divorce rate, 3, 26, 354, 356
  of African-Americans, 81
  death rate correlation, 4
  effect on family structure, 9
  following remarriage, 27
  in nineteenth century, 85, 129
  in 1920s, 100, 101–102
  in 1950s, 124, 129–130, 131
  in 1960s, 114, 131, 138, 155, 166
  in 1970s, 114, 150, 155
  post–World War I, 95, 113, 361
  post–World War II, 112, 113–114, 122, 123, 137, 361
  as stepfamily formation factor, 11
  in United Kingdom, 140
  in World War II, 112
Domestic family, 69, 119, 355
Domestic partners, 10, 116, 354
Dora (Freud's case), 164
Double bind, in communication, 189, 362
Downward social mobility
  of middle class, 19
  of young adults, 306
Dowry, 40, 50, 55
Drug abuse
  as family mental illness symptom, 241, 242, 243, 245, 257
  in families with adult children, 253–254, 267–268, 271, 272, 279, 303, 305, 306, 307, 308, 309–310
  in families with young children, 258–259, 293
  in 1950s, 131
  sex factors in, 243
Dual-career family. *See* Two-income family
DuBois, W.E.B., 73–75, 87–88
Durkheim, Emile, 87, 159
Dysfunctional families, subtypes, 220–221

Eadmund of Aethelstan, 54, 55
Ecological approach, to family studies, 179
Economic factors. *See also* Great Depression; Income; Poverty; Socioeconomic factors
  in antifamilism, 20–26
  effect on family life, 187
  effect on middle class, 18–19
  as stress cause, 245, 246
Economy, definition of, 43

INDEX

Education
  of African-Americans, 72, 73
  in colonial America, 66
  increasing duration of, 147
  in Middle Ages, 56–57
  of women, 67, 90
Ego, in marriage, 141
Ego-ideal, 134
Ego psychology, 102–103, 151–152
Egypt, ancient
  divorce in, 34, 35
  families in, 34–37, 46, 358–359
  mythological depiction of, 31–32
Einstein, Albert, 87, 168
Eisenhower, Dwight D., 128
Ellis, Havelock, 97
Emotional basis
  of the family, 33–34, 99, 100
  of marriage, 60–63
Emotional disorders, in sixteenth-century England, 61–62
Employment, uncertainty about, 149
Empty nest stage, 209, 214, 215
Engaged family system, 224
Engels, Friedrich, 39–40
England. *See also* Anglo-Saxons
  emotional disorders in, 61–62
  poverty in, 18, 88, 89, 160, 361
Enmeshed family, 182
Epidemics, social, 6
Epidemiological study, of family mental health, 363–386
  adolescent and young adult subjects, 299–313
    Center for Epidemiologic Studies Depression Scale scores, 305, 308
    from completing families, 309–310
    from dropout families, 306–309
    education, 301–303
    employment status and occupation, 303
    Family Environment Scale scores, 310–312
    marital status, 304
    physical health status, 303
    sociodemographic characteristics, 301–302
    symptomatic status, 305–310, 333, 346, 385–386, 389
  attrition of subjects, 232–233, 366, 370

Epidemiological study, of family mental health (*Cont.*)
  Center for Epidemiologic Studies Depression Scale data, 241, 242, 248, 370, 372, 377
    from apathetic families, 252, 253
    changes over time, 271, 272–273
    from chronic symptomatic families, 278–279
    from completing families, 295
    from dropout families, 268, 293, 294
    Family Environment Scale scores correlation, 258, 259
    from incidence families, 280–281
    from moral-religious-oriented families, 254
    as predictors of symptomatology, 379
    from remission families, 280
    from structure-oriented families, 253–254
  Child Behavior Checklist Scale data, 242, 248, 250–251, 290–291, 293, 383–384
    from completing families, 294, 295, 297–298
    from dropout families, 268, 293
    from interpersonally effective families, 250–251
  clinical implications of, 331–352
    at-risk family members identification, 333
    for children, 344–350
    comorbidity, 331–332, 334
    depression and social supports, 339–340
    extent of symptomatic distress, 331–332
    Family Environment Scale use, 338–339
    family risk factors, 335–336
    family stress, 336–338
    home visits, 342–343
    individualism versus familism, 350–351
    intergenerational continuity of symptomatology, 333–334, 351
    for poor families, 343–344
    research measures in clinical practice, 340–341
    supportive family therapy, 351–352

Epidemiological study, of family mental health (*Cont.*)
  clinical implications of (*Cont.*)
    symptomatology changes and variability, 332
    treatment-resistant families, 334–335
    videotaping of clients, 342
  concepts and methods of, 364–366
  data management and analysis, 368–369
  Diagnostic Interview Schedules for Children data, 248, 252, 266, 291–293, 295, 368, 383–384 384
    from completing families, 294, 295, 297–298
    from dropout families, 267–268, 293, 308
    from structure-oriented families, 253
  dropout families, 265, 266–269, 370
    Center for Epidemiologic Studies Depression Scale data, 268, 293, 294
    comparison with completing families, 275–276
    sociodemographic characteristics, 266–267
    young children's symptomatology in, 293–294
  Family Environment Scale data, 250–265, 338, 339, 377–378, 388–389
    from apathetic families, 252–253, 254–255
    changes over time, 273–274, 282–283
    from depressed families, 256
    as depression predictor, 259
    dropout/completing families comparison, 269, 270
    from drug-abusing families, 257, 259
    from families with symptomatic children, 255
    family incongruence scores, 250, 256, 257
    from interpersonally effective families, 250–252
    from moral-religious-oriented families, 254
    from panic disorder families, 257
    from phobic families, 257
    as predictors of symptomatology, 257–259, 379–380

Epidemiological study, of family mental health (*Cont.*)
  Family Environment Scale data (*Cont.*)
    from structure-oriented families, 253–254
    subscales and dimensions of, 250, 251
  family life cycle and stress data, 247–250, 376–377
  family structure changes, 372–373
  field procedures and interviews, 367–368
  marital satisfaction data, 261–265, 380–381
  methods, 230–234, 367–368
  recruitment of subjects, 366
  results, 369–386
    adult children's symptomatology, 305–310, 333, 346, 385–386, 389
    extent of symptomatology, 369–371, 388
    family division of labor, 382
    Family Environment Scale scores, 377–378, 388–389
    family goals, 381–383
    family life cycle and stress, 376–377
    family risk factors, 373–376, 388
    genograms, 380
    marital satisfaction, 380–381
    predictors of symptomatic status, 378–380
    symptomatology changes over time, 371–373
    young children's symptomatology, 290–298, 333, 382–385, 389
  sampling, 366–367
  social support system assessment, 246–247
  sociodemographic characteristics, 234–240
    of children, 285–286
    of completing families, 269–273
    of dropout families, 266–267
  stress effects, 244–246, 281, 282, 283, 336–337, 368, 373, 375
    clinical implications of, 336–338
    depression and, 272–273
    life cycle correlation, 247–250, 376–377
    socioeconomic factors in, 275–276

INDEX

Epidemiological study, of family mental health(*Cont.*)
  symptomatology
    chronic, 278–279, 372
    intergenerational continuity of, 333–334, 351
    prevalence rate, 241, 243
  symptomatology changes over time, 274–283
    of chronic symptomatic families, 278–279
    clinical implications of, 332
    of incidence symptomatic families, 280–281
    of remission symptomatic families, 279–280
  treatment-resistant families, 370
  videotaping of subjects, 231–232, 365–366, 367
  young children as subjects, 285–299. *See also* Child Behavior Checklist data; Diagnostic Interview Schedule for Children data
    from completing families, 294–298
    developmental histories, 286
    discipline of, 288–289, 298, 382, 383
    from dropout families, 293–294
    parents' activities with, 290, 299, 382–383
    parents' expectations and values for, 287–288, 298, 299, 382
    parents' time spent with, 289–290, 382–383
    social histories, 286–287
    sociodemographic characteristics, 285–286
    symptomatology, 290–298, 333, 383–385, 389
Epidemiologic Catchment Area studies, 16, 227, 241, 353, 363–364
Epstein, N., 212, 213, 218
Esau (Old Testament), 51
EST, 152
Eugenics, 92
Euripides, 32, 49, 59, 112
Evolutionary theories
  of the origin of the family, 37, 41, 44–45, 86
  of Western civilization, 108–109
Exchange theory, 178

Executives, wives of, 4–5
Existentialism, 130
Exogamy, 40, 43
Expressed emotion
  depressives' reactions to, 200–201
  in schizophrenic families, 192–193, 201
Extramarital sexual activity, in 1920s, 106

Fads, 136
Families of the Slums (Minuchin), 181–183
Familism
  individualism versus, 27, 85, 91, 94, 103–104, 108–112
    clinical implications of, 350–351
  as social duty, 70, 121–122
Family. *See also* History, of the family
  in ancient times, 31–37
  anomic, 356
  atomistic, 69, 118–120, 121, 147, 155, 182
  basic elements of, 99
  biological basis of, 33, 34, 46, 147
  characteristics of, 45
  children as basis of, 34
  in colonial America, 65–68
  companionate, 111
    division of labor in, 260
    Great Depression and, 145
    instability of, 115
    institutional functions of, 129
    in 1950s, 128–129
    post–World War II, 115–116
  crisis of, 1–29
  definition of, 231, 365
  domestic, 69, 119, 355
  emotional basis of, 33–34, 99, 100
  functions of, 21, 86, 123–124
  as haven of refuge, 153
  homosexual, 10
  individual's separation from, 135
  interaction with society, 85–86, 91, 354, 355
  isolated, 32–33
  legal structure of, 147–148
  Le Play's typology of, 158–159
  nontraditional, 10
  poverty of, 14–20
  psychological, 108
  reinstitutionalized, 115
  reorganization of, 115

Family (*Cont.*)
  sociocultural basis of, 46
  stem, 158–159, 361
  traditional, post–World War II, 115
  triple field theory of, 147
  trustee, 68–69, 118, 119, 355
  types of, 10, 118
  unstable, 159, 361
Family Adaptibility and Cohesion Evaluation Scales, 214, 215–216
Family and Medical Leave Act, 21
Family Assessment Device, 196–197
Family dynamics theory, 168
Family Environment Scale. *See under* Epidemiological study, of family mental health
Family functioning models, 212–225, 231, 361–362
  Beavers Systems, 216–217
  Bell and Schwab Family Assessment Scale, 231, 365–366
  of family competence, 219–222
  Family Environment Scale, 219. *See also under* Epidemiological study, of family mental health
  Lewis, 219–222
  McMaster, 212–213
  Olson Circumplex, 213–216
  Pennsylvania State University Infant and Family Development Project, 223–225
  Reiss's Problem-Solving, 217–219
Family research, 157–226
  African-American family studies, 210–212
  anthropological, 162–163, 361
  depression studies, 194–208
  early theories of, 360–361
  family functioning studies, 212–225, 231
  family life cycle studies, 208–210
  family studies, 167–169
  genetic factors studies, 362
  longitudinal studies, 362. *See also* Epidemiological study, of family mental health
  in nineteenth century, 157–162
  obstacles to, 166
  pedigree studies, 161, 162, 191–192, 195, 361, 363

Family research (*Cont.*)
  predictions of
    in 1940s, 121
    in 1950s, 127–128
  psychoanalytic contributions to, 163–167
  schizophrenia studies, 187–194
  social research and, 157–162
  sociological studies, 178–187
  systems theory, 169–171, 174–178
  transactional approach in, 173–174
  trends in, 183–187
Family services, in 1950s, 129–130
Family size
  of atomistic families, 119
  decrease of, 9, 325
  in eighteenth century, 126
  in 1890, 209
  life cycle and, 209
  longitudinal changes of, 318
  in 1940, 209
  in 1950s, 126, 127, 131
  in 1967, 131
  in 1970, 131
Family sociology, 178–187
Family structural changes, 9–12
  grandmother-mother-daughter axis, 28, 365
  as poverty cause, 17
  projected, 28–29
  Quayle on, 23–24
Family studies
  feminist criticism of, 186
  obstacles to, 186
  research approaches to, 178–179
Family system, of employment, 65
Family Systems Assessment Scale, 231, 365–366
Family systems theory, 98, 174–178
Family therapy
  for juvenile delinquency, 181–182
  polarization of, 172–173
  supportive, 351–352
Family therapy movement, 122
Family tree, 341
Family values, 1, 18, 25–26, 356
Father
  abandonment of children by, 148
  authority of, 44
    in African-American families, 76, 77

INDEX

Father (Cont.)
  authority of (Cont.)
    in African families, 74
    in ancient Hebrew families, 47
    in Anglo-Saxon families, 54
    children's psychological health and, 222
    in Great Depression, 106, 143
    loss of, 154
    in 1950s, 126, 129
    in patriarchal families, 158
    in stem families, 158–159
    in unstable families, 159
  personality development role of, 327
  son's relationship with, 125–126, 145
  work-related absence of, 125–126
Federal government, child-oriented spending of, 19
Female-headed families
  African-American, 80, 81
  number of, 155
  poverty rate of, 17
Feminism, 93, 94
Fertility
  in medieval society, 60
  during Industrial Revolution, 65
Feudalism, 135
Field theory, 169
Fleck, S., 122
Flügel, J.C., 165–166
Food stamp program, 15
Franklin, Benjamin, 67
Franks, 54
Free love, 94
French Revolution, mental illness prevalence following, 328
Freud, Sigmund
  aggression theory of, 96
  cases of, 164
  The Interpretation of Dreams, 104
  Oedipus complex theory of, 164–165
  personality development theory of, 134
  psychosexual development theories of, 163–165, 184
  sexuality theories of, 97
  Totem and Taboo, 38, 44
Fricka, 31
Friends, as confidants, 151
Functionalism, 123, 167, 180

Gallic Wars (Caesar), 53
Game theory, 178, 179
Gangs, in Russia, 148
Gang warfare, 130, 131, 132
Gay rights movement, 9
Generalized Contentment Scale, 216
General living systems, 169–171, 228–229, 365
General Living Systems (Miller), 227
Generational differences, in families, 143
Generational research, 142–146, 180–181
Genetics, 162
Genogram, 235–238, 341, 380
George III, 6
Germania (Tacitus), 50, 55
Germanic tribes, 50, 53–54, 58, 86, 120, 169
Gestalt psychology, 169
Ghettoization, 76–77, 128, 131
Gilman, Charlotte Perkins, 93
Global Assessment of Relational Functioning Scale, 225–226
Goals, familial, 340, 381–382
"God is dead" thesis, 87, 130
God's Little Acre (Caldwell), 67
Goodsell, Willystine, 389
Grandmother-mother-daughter axis, 28, 365
Grandparenting, 12
Grapes of Wrath, The (Steinbeck), 109
Great Depression
  adolescents of, 143–144, 145–146, 180–181
  familial effects of, 65, 105–108, 109, 143–146
  intergenerational research about, 143–144, 145–146, 180–181
Great Society, 23–24
Greece, ancient
  decline of, 25, 117, 120
  Egyptian contributions to, 37
  families in, 31, 47–49
    anomic families, 356
    atomistic families, 69, 118
    domestic families, 118
    mythological depiction of, 31
    trustee families, 118, 119
Greed, 21, 26, 156
Greek culture, effect on Roman culture, 50

Greek tragedies, 32
Group for the Advancement of Psychiatry, Committee on the Family, 172–173
Group therapy, 103, 151–152
Guilds, 57
Guilt
  inner-directed character and, 136
  pleasure-related, 144

Happiness, as right, 142
Hapsburgs, 63
Haracleitus, 134
Harrington, Michael, 18
Harris, Marvin, 38, 40, 44
Hatshepsut, 35
Head Start, 14, 23, 322
Hebrews, ancient
  divorce among, 34
  families of, 34–35, 51–52
  father's authority among, 47
Hera, 31
Herd instinct, 136
Hetaerae, 48, 120
High school enrollment, 128
Hill, Reuben, 122, 184
Hippocrates, 134
Hispanic families, 3
History, cyclic view of, 108–109
History, of the family, 31–83, 358–360
  African-American families, 70–82
  in ancient Greece, 31, 47–49, 69, 118, 119, 356
  in ancient Rome, 40, 49–51, 69, 118, 120–121, 356
  in Anglo-Saxon society, 40, 53–56, 58, 63, 116
  current theories of, 44–45
  early theories of, 37–42
  following Industrial Revolution, 64–65
  following the Reformation, 63–64
  in Great Depression, 65, 105–108, 109, 143–144, 145–146
  incest taboo and, 43–44
  Judeo-Christian roots, 51–53
  in nineteenth century, 67, 68, 85–90
  in 1900s, 90–96
  in 1920s, 96–105
  in 1950s, 123–132
  in 1960s, 132–142, 154, 156
  in 1970s, 142–156

History, of the family, *Cont.*
  of nuclear family, 56–60
  post–World War II, 114–123
  in World War II, 112–114
History of Human Marriage (Westermarck), 40–42
Holidays, 153
Homelessness, 15, 18, 109
Homer, 47
Home visits
  by family epidemiological study researchers, 231–232
  by therapists, 342–343
Homicide rate, 354
Homogamy, 141
Homosexual family, 10
Homosexuality, 154
Hoover, Herbert, 99
Hospitalization, as stress cause, 245, 246
Housewife, changing role of, 99
Housework
  in dual-career families, 210, 211
  mental illness correlation, 259–260
  women's responsibility for, 13
Housing, 101
  single-family, 95
Howards End (Forster), 91–92
Human Sexual Response (Masters and Johnson), 184–185
Hume, David, 108
Husband, authority of, 47
  in ancient Hebrew families, 51–52
  in ancient Rome, 49, 120

Identity problems, of adolescents, 133, 134, 138
Ikhnaton, 36
Illegitimacy
  among African-Americans, 70, 75
  among European-Americans, 81
  post–World War II, 114
Illness, parental separation and, 26
Immigrants, child labor among, 16
Incest, 11, 88, 89
Incest taboo, 43–44, 46
Income
  decrease of, 17, 19, 374–375
  during Great Depression, 143, 144
  mental illness correlation, 239, 335–336, 365, 373

INDEX

Income, (*Cont.*)
　upward distribution of, 374
India, patriarchal society in, 40
Individual, separation from family, 135
Individualism
　Anglo-Saxon, 116
　of atomistic families, 69
　of British settlers, 65–66
　of contemporary families, 68
　contractualism and, 110
　decadent, 25
　as divorce cause, 129
　epidemiologic data, 381–382
　excessive, 20–21, 22, 27
　familism versus, 27, 85, 91, 94, 103–104, 108–112
　　clinical implications of, 350–351
　family structure and, 9–10
　Maine's concept of, 40
Individuality, biological basis of, 175
Industrialization, 89–90, 116, 160
Industrial Revolution, 59–60, 64–65, 127
Industry, decentralized, 109–110
Infanticide, 14, 35, 40, 42–43, 48, 50
Infant mortality, 322, 353, 354
Infant–mother bond, 224
Inner-directed character, 135, 136
Institutional approach, in family studies, 178
Interactional approach, in family studies, 178
Intergenerational boundaries
　in child therapy, 345–346
　parent–adult child, 347
Intergenerational continuity, of family mental illness, 189, 333–334, 351
International Classification of Disease, relational problems codes of, 225
International Workers of the World, 88
Interpersonal relations theory, 152
Interpretation of Dreams, The (Freud), 104
Intimacy, 150
　depression and, 204, 205–206, 208
Iran–Contra scandal, 155
Isis, 32
Isolation, 32–33

Jacob (Old Testament), 51, 52
Jason (husband of Medea), 63
Jealousy, male, 41, 42

Jesus, 32, 53
Jobs, lack of meaning of, 139
Johnson, Lyndon, 23
Josephus, 52
Journal of Marriage and the Family, 183, 184, 185, 186
Journey Into Sexuality (Reiss), 184, 185
Joyce, James, 104, 169
Juana la Loca, 63
Jukes family, 161
Juno, 31
Jupiter, 31
Justinian, 53
Justin Martyr, 52
Juvenile delinquency
　in atomistic families, 119
　culture lag and, 97
　in early twentieth century, 89, 91
　Minuchin's study of, 181–183
　in 1920s, 102
　in 1950s, 130, 131
　post–World War II, 114, 122
　in World War II, 113

Kallikak family, 161–162
Kansas Marital Satisfaction Scale, 216
Kapital, Das (Marx), 18
Kaplan, Helen Singer, 5
Kinsey reports, 130, 184–185
Kinship systems
　of ancient Greeks, 47
　of ancient Hebrews, 51
　Anglo-Saxon, 54
　as social organization basis, 38, 40
Kissing, 56
Kluckhohn, Florence, 173–174
Korean War, 130

Labor unions, 88
Landrigan, Philip, 16
Law of the Twelve Tables, 49
Laws, The (Plato), 120
Leah (Old Testament), 51, 52
Leo the Philosopher, 53
Le Play, Frederic, 109, 157–160, 343, 361, 374
Les années folles, 104
Levi-Strauss, C., 44, 45
Lewin, Kurt, 171
Lidz, R., 122

Lidz, T., 122
Life course, family, 210
Life cycle
  of civilization, 108–109
  of family, 166, 179, 208–210
    stress and, 214–216, 247–250, 376–377
Life expectancy
  life cycle and, 209
  in nineteenth century, 86
  rates, 14
Life-style
  Adler's concept of, 165
  diversity of, 187
Lindberg, Charles, 101
Little Hans (Freud's case), 164
Locke, H. J., 98–99
London, poverty in, 18, 89, 160, 361
London, Jack, 18, 39, 361
Lonely Crowd, The (Riesman et al.), 102
Longus, 59
Los Angeles, riots of 1992, 23, 82
Louisville, Kentucky. See Epidemiological study, of family mental health
Love, romantic, 58–59, 61, 63
Lovenson, Harry, 5
Lower-class, value orientations of, 172
Luther, Martin, 63–64
Lycurgus, 134
Lysistrata (Aristophanes), 48–49

MacDonald, M., 61, 62
Mafia families, 118
Maine, Henry, 40
Malachi, 52
Manic-depression, 165, 195
Man in the Grey Flannel Suit (Wilson), 130
Marital adjustment
  of African-Americans, 210–212
  children's effect on, 221–222, 223–225
  depression and, 200–206, 361
  evolutionary trend of, 141–142
  factors in, 106–108
  as family research topic, 185
  longitudinal changes in, 141–142, 323–324
  mental illness correlation, 361, 380–381
  in 1976, 150
  post–World War II, 97–98, 140–141
  public attitudes toward, 141
  in schizophrenic families, 188
  in sixteenth century, 61–62
  of women, 13
Marital breakdown, consequences of, 8
Marital conflict
  depression and, 337, 349–350
  in 1960s, 141
Marriage
  African-American, 76
  ancient Greek, 47, 48, 120
  ancient Hebrew, 52
  ancient Roman, 49, 50–51, 120–121
  Anglo-Saxon, 53–56, 58
  arranged, 47, 63
  brother–sister, 35
  "by use," 34
  childless, 91. See also Marriage, companionate
  civil, 66, 67
  clandestine, 64
  in colonial America, 66, 67
  companionate, 60–61, 108
    definition, 99
    as domestic partnership, 116
    legalization of, 115–116
    in 1950s, 130
    in sixteenth century, 62, 63
    transition from institutional marriage, 210
  in early Christian society, 53
  emotional basis of, 60–63
  exogamous, 40, 43
  as family research topic, 185
  free, 93
  group, 10, 39, 53
  in Middle Ages, 57–59
  monogamous. See Monogamy
  of nobility, 63
  origin of, 37–42, 45
  political, 63
  polyandrous, 10, 40, 42–43, 46
  polygamous, serial, 93
  polygynous, 10, 42, 46, 52
  proxy, 63
  "psychological," 101
  purchase, 49, 55, 73
  Quayle on, 24
  in the Reformation, 63–64
  religious basis of, 33
  romantic, 58–59, 63

INDEX

Marriage, (Cont.)
  social attitudes toward, 6
  subsystem interaction in, 141
  trial, 91
  among Yoruba, 73–74
Marriage age
  of African-Americans, 81
  of ancient Hebrews, 52
  of children of the Great Depression, 144
  in 1890, 209
  family violence and, 185
  increase of, 3
  in medieval society, 60
  in 1940, 209
  in 1950s, 131, 140
  post–World War II, 130
Marriage ceremony
  in ancient Greece, 47
  in ancient Rome, 49
  in Anglo-Saxon society, 55
  Catholic, 64
  of early Christians, 53
Marriage rate, 3
  in 1950, 131
  in 1960, 131
  post–World War II, 113
  in World War II, 112
Marriage vow, 64
Married couple, life expectancy of, 209
Marx, Karl, 39, 130–131
Masters and Johnson, 184–185
Material culture, 97
Materialism, 25
Maternal instinct, 42
Maternity leave, 94
Matriarchive society, 327
Matriarchoid society, 131
Matriarchy, 37–38, 39, 42
  matrilineal descent and, 38, 41
Matricentricity
  of African-American families, 78
  in Great Depression, 143–144
Matrilocal family system, 41, 42
  of Trobriand Islanders, 162–163
McCarthy, Joseph, 134
McCarthyism, 130
McLennan, John, 38, 40, 43
McMaster Clinical Rating Scale, 213
McMaster Family Assessment Device, 213

McMaster Model, of family functioning, 212–213, 218
Mead, George Herbert, 152
Mead, Margaret, 163
Measles, 15
Medea, 59, 63
Media, family crisis coverage by, 2
Menninger, William C., 172
Mental health services, in 1960s, 140
Mental illness
  Ackerman's theories of, 167–169
  age factors in, 333
  of children of divorce, 7
  of divorced/separated persons, 9
  epidemiological study of. See Epidemiological study, of family mental health
  family research in, 171–173
  genetic factors in, 161–162
  increase of, 322–323, 328–329
  in Industrial Revolution, 64–65
  of industrialized populations, 64–65, 160, 161
  intergenerational continuity of, 189, 333–334, 351
  pedigree studies of, 161, 162, 191–192, 195, 361, 363
  physical health correlation, 243
  poverty-related, 15–16
  prevalence of, 241, 328, 353, 357
  sex factors in, 333
  in sixteenth-century England, 61–62
  social attitudes toward, 6
  socioeconomic factors in, 15–16, 239–240, 335–336, 365, 373–375
Mentally ill, deinstitutionalization of, 192
Mexican-American families, 81
Middle Ages
  emotionality of family life in, 61
  family development in, 56–59, 69
  romantic love in, 58–59, 61
  trustee families in, 118
Middle class
  African-American, 77, 79–80, 210–212
  British, 91–92
  child socialization strategies of, 155
  declining economic status of, 18–19
  in nineteenth century, 87
  in 1960s, 138
  suburbanization of, 68, 131
  value orientations of, 172

Mid-life crisis, 249–250
Military-industrial complex, 128
Millar, John, 33–34, 41
Miller, James Grier, 227, 365
Minnesota Multiphasic Personality Inventory, 219
Mobility, geographic, 109, 115, 129, 209–210
Model Cities Act, 23
Model T, 104
Modest Proposal, A (Swift), 24
Monogamy, 38–39
  in ancient Rome, 49
  of animals, 34, 41
  definition of, 10
  evolution of, 39
  of Germanic tribes, 50
  in Middle Ages, 58
  religious basis of, 93–94
  serial, 4–5, 27, 137
  theories of, 39, 40–42
Monotheism, in ancient Egypt, 36
Morgan, Lewis Henry, 38–39, 43
Mortality rate
  divorce rate correlation, 4
  in Industrial Revolution, 65
Mosaic law, 52
Mosbacher, Georgette, 5
Mosbacher, Robert, 5, 23
Moses (Old Testament), 36
Mother
  depressed, 196, 248, 349, 362
  of disorganized family, 182
  employed, 13–14
    child care for, 17–18
  homeless, 15
  schizophrenogenic, 187–188, 189, 190
  status of, in Great Depression, 143–144, 145–146
Mother Courage and Her Children (Brecht), 112
Mother–daughter relationship, 145–146
Motherhood
  African-American women's attitudes toward, 76
  as women's primary role, 94
Mothers, The (Briffault), 42
Motion pictures, sexual behavior and, 129
Moynihan, Patrick, 14–15
Multigenerational emotional process, 177
Mutterrecht, Das (Bachofen), 37

Mystical Bedlam (MacDonald), 61
Mythology, families in, 31–32

Napier, Richard, 61
Napoleon Bonaparte, 37
Narcissism, 150, 152, 153, 154
  of adult children, 304
  of parents, 189
"Narcissistic," 156
National Divorce Reform League, 85
National League for the Protection of the Family, 85
Naturem, De Re (Lucretius), 33
Nefertiti, 36
Neurosis
  Adler's theory of, 165
  Freud's theory of, 164–165
Nimkoff, M. F., 126–128
1984 (Orwell), 147
Nineteenth Amendment, 96
Nuclear family
  African-American, 79
  characteristics of, 123
  democratic structure of, 123
  in Egyptian mythology, 31–32
  isolation of, 123, 124, 152–153
  origin of, 56–60
  parental role differentiation in, 124, 125
  as reflection of society, 141
  in sixteenth century, 62
  as societal subsystem, 123, 125
  universality of, 46
Nuclear war, anxiety about, 130, 138

Oakland Growth Study, 143, 180–181
Object relations theory, 122, 123, 130–131, 152
Obsessive-compulsive disorder, 344
Oedipus complex, 164–165
  resolution of, 125
  among Trobriand Islanders, 162–163
Ogburn, W. F., 96–97, 98–99, 126–128
Old Testament, 51–52
Olson Circumplex Model, of family functioning, 213–216
Oresteia, The (Euripides), 32
Organization Man (Whyte), 130
Organizations, participation in, 150, 151
Origin of Species (Darwin), 37, 86
Osiris, 32

INDEX

Other America, The (Harrington), 18
Other-directed character, 135–137, 140
Ozarks, Highlander families of, 109

Panic disorder
    as family mental illness symptom, 241, 242, 243, 253–254, 257, 258, 271, 279, 291–293, 305, 306
    sex factors in, 243
Parental factors, in schizophrenia, 187–194
Parent–child relationship
    in Africa, 74
    in atomistic families, 119
    Flügel's theory of, 165–166
    in Great Depression, 142–146
    historical-clinical study of, 319, 320, 321, 327–328, 387
Parents
    attitudes toward divorce, 8–9
    of depressives, 195
    juvenile, 182
    in 1950s, 129
    nonevolved, 182
    personality stabilization of, 123–124, 220
    role differentiation of, 124, 125
Park, Mungo, 70–71
Park, R. E., 77
Park, Thomas, 71
Parsonian theory, 125, 138, 167, 180
Parsons, Elsie Clewes, 90–91, 115–116
Parsons, Talcott, 123–126
Paternity, 38
Patriarchy
    in ancient Greece, 47
    in ancient Rome, 49
    development of, 37, 40, 41, 51–52
    Le Play's theory of, 158
    of the Puritans, 62
Paul (apostle), 53
Paul, Jean, 87
Pedigree studies, of mental illness, 161, 162, 361, 363
    of depression, 195
    of schizophrenia, 191–192
Peloponnesian War, 48–49, 356
Pennsylvania State University Infant and Family Development Project, 223–225
Pensions, for widows, 94

People of the Abyss (London), 18, 89, 361
Pericles, 48, 49, 120
Peripheral males, 182
Personality
    culture/social structure relationship of, 123, 125, 162–163
    definition, 98
Personality development
    as family function, 98, 100, 124
    father's role in, 327
    in 1960s, 133
Personality development theory, 125, 142
Personality disorders, 102
Personality functions, of the family, 100, 123–124
Personality stabilization, 123–124, 220
Phenomenological approach, to family studies, 179
Philip the Handsome, 63
Phobias, as family mental illness symptoms, 241, 242, 253–254, 257, 258, 268, 279, 294, 297, 305, 306
Physical abuse
    of children, 185
    of homeless mothers, 15
Physical health
    marital adjustment correlation, 262–263
    mental illness correlation, 243
    social support and, 375–376
Pilgrims, 63
Plantations, 66
Plato, 23
    The Laws, 120
    The Republic, 48, 134
Plutarch, 120
Polyandry
    definition of, 10
    in early societies, 40
    economic basis of, 42–43, 46
Polygamy, serial, 93
Polygyny
    of ancient Hebrews, 52
    definition of, 10
    economic basis of, 42, 46
Pompeii, 50
Poor Laws, 60
Population decline, in other-directed societies, 135
Population growth, social character development and, 135

Populist movement, 88
Pornography, in nineteenth century, 88–89
Poseidon, 48
Poverty, 14–20
  of African-American families, 77, 79, 80
  children living in, 353, 354
  clinical implications of, 343–344
  depression and, 207–208
  in early twentieth century, 89, 92
  in England, 18, 88, 89, 160, 361
  illness and, 353
  as life-cycle stage, 208
  as mental illness risk factor, 239, 335–336, 365, 373–375
  Minuchin's research regarding, 181–183
  in nineteenth century, 88
  primary, 160
  secondary, 160
Poverty rate, 3
  increase of, 374
  of two-parent households, 24
Prayer, 100
Premarital sexual behavior
  generationally related attitudes toward, 185
  of women, public attitudes toward, 126
Prenuptial agreements, 40
Principia, De (Newton), 87
Prisoners of war, 22
Private property, 39
  common ownership of, 40
  patriarchy and, 51–52
Problem-Solving Model, of family functioning, 217–219
Professions, women in, 90, 93
Promiscuity
  as courtship, 41–42
  in prehistoric societies, 37–38, 41–42
Prostitution
  in nineteenth century, 89
  in World War I, 95–96
Protestant Reformation, 63–64, 135
Pseudomutuality, 191, 194, 362
Psychoanalytic theory
  family research applications of, 163–166, 167–169
  in 1920s, 102–103
  in 1970s, 152

Psychoanalytic theory (*Cont.*)
  object relations and, 130–131
  post–World War II, 122–123
Psychosexual development, Freudian theory of, 163–165, 184
Ptahhotep, maxims of, 36
Public education. *See also* Schools
  of poor children, 14
Public health, 86
Punic Wars, 49, 90
Puritans, 61–62, 66, 67, 86

Quayle, Dan, 18, 23
Quayle, Marilyn, 18
Quintessence of Ibsenism, The (Shaw), 93

Rachel (Old Testament), 51, 52
Racial discrimination, 72, 78, 79, 80, 82
Reactives generation, 28–29
Reagan, Ronald, 4, 6, 23, 154
Reagan administration, 14, 21, 23, 26, 111, 322, 356
Recreational activities
  in 1920s, 100
  in 1950s, 128
Reformation, 63–64, 135
Reich, Wilhelm, 102
Reiss, D., 217–219
  Problem-Solving Model, of family functioning, 217–219
Reiss, I., 184, 185
Relationships, types of, 110
Relativity theory, 87, 104, 169
Religion
  as basis of the family, 33, 47, 49
  decreasing importance of, 10, 128
  as monogamy basis, 93–94
Remarriage
  children and, 5
  divorce rate following, 349, 356
  social acceptability of, 4–5
Remarriage rate, 26–27
Renaissance, 69, 135
  Carolingian, 119
  women's status in, 57
Reproduction, socialization of, 152
Republic, The (Plato), 48, 134
Republican National Convention of 1992, 1, 18
Robinson Crusoe (Defoe), 32–33

INDEX

Role changes, familial, 13–14
  in 1950s, 129
Role conflict
  in depression, 204
  marital, 151
  in transactional therapy, 174
Role differentiation, parental, 124, 125
Role theory, 125, 167
Rome, ancient
  Christianity in, 69
  decline of, 25, 86, 117, 120–121
  families in, 49–51, 69
    anomic, 356
    atomistic, 118
    domestic, 118
    mythological depiction of, 31
    trustee, 118
  other-directed individuals in, 136
  patriarchal society of, 40
  wife capture in, 40
Roosevelt, Franklin D., 183
Rorschach test, for schizophrenic family members, 190, 191
Rosetta stone, 37
Rosita, Pennsylvania, 160
Rowntree, B. S., 160, 161
Rudin School, 162
Russia, antifamilism in, 148

Sade, Comte Donatien de, 27
Sarah (Old Testament), 52
Sartre, Jean-Paul, 130
Savagery, 38
Savings and loan disaster, 24–25
Schizophrenia
  family studies of, 187–194
  pedigree studies of, 162, 361
Schoenberg, Arnold, 104, 169
Schools
  funding reductions for, 24
  lunch programs, 14
  moral instruction by, 24
Scientific Retrieval System, 233
Scotch-Irish, 66–67
Secularism, 10, 87, 109, 127, 129
Segregation
  of African-Americans, 72, 128
  age-related, 144–145
Self-esteem, peer-dependency of, 153–154

Self-interest, 152
Self-sufficiency, 150
Self-theory, 152
Seneca, 51
Servants
  as childcare givers, 50
  indentured, 67
  sexual exploitation of, 88
Sex education, 94, 107
Sex roles, 382
  following American Civil war, 90
  in Great Depression, 143–144
Sexual abuse, within stepfamilies, 11
Sexual basis, of the family, 46
Sexual harassment, 28
Sexuality
  Christianity's view of, 52–53
  contemporary, 154
  in 1960s, 140
  post–World War I research in, 97–98
  research landmarks in, 184
Sexual satisfaction, of married couples, 264–265, 381
Shame, tradition-directed character and, 136
Shaw, George Bernard, 93
Short Michigan Alcohol Screening Test, 232
Single-parent families
  crime and, 26
  increase of, 348, 354
  as mental illness risk factor, 335, 373
  parent–child coalition in, 346
  poverty rates of, 17, 24
Situational approach, in family studies, 178
Skip-generation rearing, 12
Slavery, African-American families in, 70, 71, 72–73, 74–75, 76, 78
Slaves, in colonial America, 66
Smith, Adam, 108
Social basis, of the family, 33–34
Social change
  evolutionary concepts of, 96
  mental illness and, 328
  rate of, 96–97
  as stress cause, 355
Social character, 134, 135–137
Social control, governmental corruption as, 154–155

Socialization
  of children, 86, 122, 123–124
    career choice and, 142–143
    Flügel's theory of, 166
    Freud's theory of, 163
    by society, 155
    sociopolitical factors in, 146
    in tradition-directed societies, 135
  of reproduction, 152
Social relations, 180
Social self, 167–168
Social support
  depression and, 207, 339–340
  mental health correlation, 246–247, 339–340
  as stress mediator, 375–376
Society
  character and, 134–135
  family's relationship to, 85–86, 354, 355
Sociocultural basis, of the family, 46
Socioeconomic factors, in mental illness, 15–16, 207–208, 239–240, 335–336, 365, 373–375
Solomon, 52
Solon's laws, 69
Sorokin, Pitrim, 108–109, 389
Spanish-American War, 88
Sparta, 48–49, 134
Specialization, 109, 139
Spencer, Herbert, 43, 159
Spengler, Oswald, 108–109
Spiegel, John, 172, 173–174
Spouse abuse, decline of, 185
Stalking, 28
Standard of living, 139
Statistical Package for the Social Sciences, 368, 368
Stealing, by children, 320, 321, 322
Stem family, 158–159, 361
Stepchildren, 10–11
Stepfamilies, 3, 10–12
Stravinsky, Fedorovich, 104, 169
Stress, familial, as mental illness risk factor, 206–208, 231, 244–246, 272–273, 281, 282, 283, 363, 373
  clinical implications of, 336–338
  life cycle correlation, 247–250, 376–377
  schizophrenia and, 193
Structure-function approach, in family studies, 178, 179

Studies on Hysteria (Breuer and Freud), 165–166
Study of History (Toynbee), 130
Substance abuse. *See also* Alcohol abuse; Drug abuse
  sex ratio of, 243
Suburbia, middle-class relocation to, 68, 131
Suffrage, women's, 96
Suffragettes, 93
Suicide
  by adolescents, 1, 208, 229
  anomie/alienation-related, 87
  by children, 154, 322, 348–349, 387–390
  in early twentieth century, 89
Superego, 134, 163, 327
  father's role in development of, 125–126
Support groups. *See also* Social support
  for children of divorce, 3
Surrealism, 104, 169
Sweden, mental illness prevalence in, 328–329
Symbolic interaction theory, 179
Systems theory, 125, 168, 169–171, 179, 187

Tacitus, 50, 53, 86
Taxation, 19
Technoculture, effect on family structure, 9
Ten Commandments, Egyptian prototype of, 36, 359
Terentia, 50
Teutonic mythology, families in, 31
Teutonic tribes. *See* Germanic tribes
Thematic Apperceptive Test, 191
Therapy
  increasing reliance on, 125
  post–World War II growth of, 123
  predictors of family response to, 218–219
Thomas, V. G., 210, 211
Thomas, W. F., 98–99
Tobacco Road (Caldwell), 67
Tocqueville, Alexis de, 21–22, 27, 103
Togetherness, as basic human drive, 175, 350
Totem and Taboo (Freud), 38, 44

Totemism, 40
Tradition-directed society, 135, 136
Transactional approach, to family studies, 173–174
Transference, 164
Transient nature, of American family, 129
Trial of Euripides, The (Aristophanes), 49
Triangling, 175–176, 362
Triple field theory, 147
Trobriand Islanders, 162–163
Trojan Women, The (Euripides), 112
Trustee family, 68–69, 118, 119, 355
Tuberculosis, 15, 65, 354
Turner, Frederick Jackson, 88
Tutankhamen, 36
Two-income family
  African-American, 210–212
  decline of, 324
  household work division in, 13
Tylor, Edward, 43

Uncertainty, as anxiety cause, 149
Uncertainty principle, 87, 169
Union of Soviet Socialist Republics, antifamilism in, 148
Unmarried parents, 318, 325–326, 327, 354
Unmarried persons, 3
  African-American, 81
  in ancient Rome, 51
  in colonial America, 66
  European-American, 81
  as families, 10
Unstable family, 159, 361
Upward Bound, 14
Urban areas, problems of, 354
Urbanization
  of African-Americans, 76–77, 92, 128
  after Civil War, 116
  as divorce cause, 129
  in early twentieth century, 92
  effect on family functions, 127
  in 1950s, 129
Urban life, deterioration of, 68

Value orientations, 172
Values, family, 1, 18, 25–26, 356
  effect of Great Depression on, 144
Veterans, of World War II, 114

Videotaping
  of family epidemiologic study subjects, 231–232, 365–366, 367
  of therapy sessions, 342
Vietnam War, 128, 138, 151, 152, 156
Violence
  in African-American community, 82
  familial, 183, 184, 185–186
Virgin Mary, the, 32
Voltaire, François, 105

Wages, sexual equality of, 93
Wage structure, of business, 19
War. *See also* specific wars
  divorce rate following, 4
  effect on family, 360
  effect on women's status, 114
War on Poverty, 23
Watergate, 151, 154, 155, 156
Wealth, upward distribution of, 20–21
Wedding cake, 47
Wedding ring, 56
Welfare, 14–15, 17, 148, 293–294, 307
  Quayle on, 23
Well-being, personal growth and, 149–150
Wells, H. G., 93
Westermarck, Edward, 40–42, 43–44, 45
West Side Story (Bernstein, L.), 131
White House Conference on Children, 144–145
Whooping cough, 15
Widowers, physical health of, 263
Widows
  pensions for, 94
  physical health of, 263
Wife capture, 40
Wilson, Pete, 14
Wives
  role of, 5
  of second marriage, 5, 6
Women. *See also* Mother
  African, 71
  African-American, 74–75, 76, 78, 80–82
  in colonial America, 66
  divorced
    in ancient societies, 34
    economic status of, 4, 5, 8
  education of, 67, 90

Women (*Cont.*)
  employment of
    in early twentieth century, 92
    in Great Depression, 146
    impact on family, 187
    in Industrial Revolution, 65
    in nineteenth century, 67
    in 1920s, 100
    in 1950s, 126, 128, 129
    legislation regarding, 94
    post–World War II, 130
    in World War II, 113
  professional, 90, 93
  stalking of, 28
  status and rights of, 142
    African-American women, 75
    in ancient Egypt, 35
    in ancient Greece, 48–49
    in ancient Israel, 52
    in ancient Rome, 49, 50–51
    in ancient societies, 34
    in Anglo-Saxon society, 54, 56
    in colonial America, 66
    in early Christian society, 53
    industrialization and, 116
    in Middle Ages, 57
    in nineteenth century, 67
    in 1950s, 126, 127, 129

Women (*Cont.*)
  status and rights of (*Cont.*)
    in pioneer society, 116
    in Renaissance, 57
    war and, 114
    working-class, 159
Women's rights movement, 9, 90, 93, 138
Work, lack of meaning of, 139
Workers, Le Play's classification of, 159
World Health Organization, child psychiatric disorders classification of, 225
World war(s), divorce rate following, 4
World War I, 95–96
World War II, 112–114
Wotan, 31
Wright, Carroll D., 85
Wynne, L.C., 172

Yeats, William Butler, 104
Yoruba, 73–74
Youth culture
  of 1950s, 132
  of 1960s, 137–138
  of 1970s, 149
Yurok Indians, 134

Zeus, 31
Zimmerman, Carle, 108–110, 389